CONCEPTS IN
Dental Public Health

Jill Mason, MPH, RDH

Associate Professor
OHSU School of Dentistry
Portland, Oregon

LIPPINCOTT WILLIAMS & WILKINS
A **Wolters Kluwer** Company

Philadelphia • Baltimore • New York • London
Buenos Aires • Hong Kong • Sydney • Tokyo

Acquisitions Editor: John Goucher
Managing Editor: Kevin Dietz
Marketing Manager: Hilary Henderson
Production Editor: Jennifer Ajello
Designer: Doug Smock
Compositor: Nesbitt Graphics
Printer: RR Donnelly & Sons—Crawfordsville

351 West Camden Street
Baltimore, MD 21201

530 Walnut Street
Philadelphia, PA 19106

Printed in the United States of America

Library of Congress Cataloging-in-Publication Data

Mason, Jill (Jill Dee)
  Concepts in dental public health / Jill Mason.
    p. ; cm.
  Includes index.
  ISBN 13: 978-0-7817-4488-1
  ISBN 10: 0-7817-4488-1
    1. Dental public health. 2. Health promotion. I. Title.
  [DNLM: 1. Oral Health. 2. Community Health Planning. 3. Health Promotion. 4. Public Health. WU 113 M399c 2004]
  RK52.M287 2004
  362.19'76—dc22   2004048685

The publishers have made every effort to trace the copyright holders for borrowed material. If they have inadvertently overlooked any, they will be pleased to make the necessary arrangements at the first opportunity.

To purchase additional copies of this book, call our customer service department at **(800) 638-3030** or fax orders to **(301) 824-7390**. International customers should call **(301) 714-2324**.

Visit Lippincott Williams & Wilkins on the Internet: http://www.LWW.com. Lippincott Williams & Wilkins customer service representatives are available from 8:30 am to 6:00 pm, EST.

07 08 09
3 4 5 6 7 8 9 10

Preface

You are about to venture into an aspect of the dental profession that may be a new realm to you—one not considered as a career possibility. Enter with an open mind, and you can find rewards also not previously considered. Did you enter the profession because you "want to work with people" or "want to help people"? Now is the chance to explore new avenues for that personal goal.

This textbook provides an overview of dental public health in greater depth than the traditional view of community dental hygiene. It includes the basic community education and health promotion focus and expands to provide a broader view of the core principles and competencies expected at all levels of involvement in public health practice, from part-time volunteer work to career professions in public health practice.

As depicted on the cover of the text, dental public health involves many entities coming together around a central focus—improving the public's oral health. When each piece of the puzzle is in place, the infrastructure is strong and the benefit to the public is enhanced.

Each chapter in this text is written by a leader in the dental public health community. All have advanced education and expertise in public health. Although primarily written for the dental hygiene student, it is also useful for other health care providers working in public health settings.

The modular format of the text is specifically designed to allow for flexibility in depth of content or order of presentation for different curricula and teaching styles. Each module centers on a core content area of public health. To accommodate different curricula, the modules can be used in a different sequence than presented. The text also can be used for multiple courses, in the event that public health content is presented in various courses (e.g., statistics, ethics, research, health education, and community dental hygiene). Additionally, the chapter layout allows flexibility.

Key terms and competencies are listed at the beginning of each chapter to guide the learner's study of core concepts. The key terms are often used in public health practice and appear on National Board Examinations. The competencies are from the American Dental Education Association Competencies for Entry into the Profession of Dental Hygiene. These competencies are not used verbatim in all dental hygiene programs for purposes of accreditation; however, they are the guiding principles for assuring that students are competent for practice and, therefore, a useful tool to guide the learner's study and aid the instructor's efforts toward that end. Various learning activities are provided for groups or individuals to use inside or outside the classroom. In addition, review questions and answers are provided to reinforce main ideas. Resources, including Web sites and search terms, are listed for use with the learning activities or for more in-depth study and reference.

Module 1: Introduction to Dental Public Health. This module is an introduction to the core principles of public health, with a brief, historical overview of dental public health. This module also highlights more recent trends and the many career opportunities in public health, together with a global perspective of public health from various countries.

Module 2: Program Planning and Evaluation. This module is a primer of public health program planning and evaluation. The module takes the familiar framework of assessment, diagnosis, planning, implementation, and evaluation and expands it from the patient care setting to its application in public health settings.

Module 3: Health Promotion and Oral Health Education. This module describes the necessary elements of health promotion and health education programs and model programs and provides resources and instruction for creating culturally appropriate materials for use in these programs.

Module 4: Epidemiology and Research. This module provides an overview of epidemiologic and research principles, both for evaluating public programs and for critically reviewing literature. It also describes the various forms of scientific communication and includes instruction on how to prepare a written article, an oral presentation, and a poster session or table clinic. The chapter on biostatistics uses specific dental examples and builds from the simple concepts of statistical terminology and central tendency to more advanced concepts, such as logistic regression. Sections of the chapter can be selected for study to meet the needs of the individual program curriculum.

Module 5: Ethics and the Law in Public Health Practice. Most ethics texts focus on individual ethics and private practice implications. This module includes basic ethical concepts and terminology and the process of how laws are developed. In addition, it expands the principles to the public health arena, to assist advocacy and social justice efforts for populations.

Module 6: National Board Preparation. This module presents a personalized system and checklist to prepare for the Community Dental Hygiene section of the National Board Dental Hygiene Examination (NBDHE). The module includes sample questions in the testlet format of the NBDHE.

Acknowledgments

So many people—So little space

To the contributors and reviewers whose perseverance, dedication, and suggestions enhanced the outcome—thank you.

To Ellen Grabarek, whose vision was the impetus for the whole endeavor.

To Mom, Dad, and Marc, who always knew me better than I knew myself—I miss you.

To Erin and Lauren: Your patience and understanding are phenomenal beyond your years!

Contributors

Editor:

Jill Mason, MPH, RDH
Associate Professor
Oregon Health & Science University
School of Dentistry
Portland, OR

List of Contributors:

Gail Aamodt, MEd, RDH
Assistant Professor
Department of Dental Hygiene
Northern Arizona University
Flagstaff, AZ

Rachel L. Badovinac, DMD, MS
Department of Oral Health Policy and
    Epidemiology
Harvard School of Dental Medicine
Boston, MA

Ann Overton Dickinson, MS, RDH
Professor, Dental Hygiene
St. Louis Community College—Forest Park
St. Louis, MO

Chester W. Douglass, DMD, PhD
Professor, Harvard School of Dental Medicine
Professor, Harvard School of Public Health
Boston, MA

LCDR Travis L. Fisher, BS, MPA, RDH
United States Public Health Service

Ellen S. Grabarek, MPH, CHES, RDH
Assistant Professor
Department of Dental Hygiene
Northern Arizona University
Flagstaff, AZ

Denise Muesch Helm, MA, RDH
Director and Associate Professor
Department of Dental Hygiene
Northern Arizona University
Flagstaff, AZ

Beverly A. Isman, MPH, ELS, RDH
Dental Public Health Consultant
Davis, CA

Robert Isman, DDS, MPH
California Department of Health Services
Sacramento, CA

Kathy Phipps, DrPH, RDH
Associate Professor
Oregon Health & Science University
Portland, OR

LCDR Karen J. Sicard, MPH, RDH
United States Public Health Service

Kneka P. Smith, MPH, RDH
Arizona Department of Health Services
Office of Oral Health
Phoenix, AZ

Pamela Zarkowski, MPH, JD, RDH
Professor and Executive Associate Dean
University of Detroit Mercy
    School of Dentistry
Detroit, MI

Table of Contents

INTRODUCTION TO
DENTAL PUBLIC HEALTH

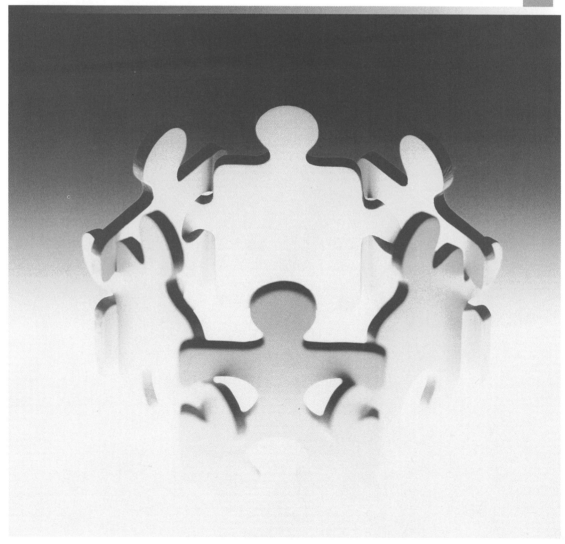

History and Principles of Dental Public Health

1

Objectives

After studying this chapter and completing the study questions and activities, the learner will be able to:
- Define dental public health.
- Define common public health terms.
- List three core functions of public health.
- Describe what constitutes a public health problem.
- Describe the four phases in the history of public health.
- Explain the motivation for the newest phase of public health.
- Identify key organizations and events that have shaped dental public health.
- Identify federal agencies involved in public health activities.

KEY TERMS

American Board of Dental Public Health
American Dental Hygienists' Association
American Association of Public Health Dentistry
American Public Health Association
Association of State and Territorial Dental Directors

Canadian Association of Public Health Dentistry
Community
Core functions of public health
Dental public health
Health
Healthy People 2010
Institute of Medicine
Maternal and Child Health

National Center for Health Statistics
National Institute of Dental and Craniofacial Research
Pan American Health Organization
Public health
Social Security Act
Surgeon General's Report on Oral Health
World Health Organization

The American Dental Education Association competencies addressed in this chapter include[1]:

HP.1:   Promote the values of oral and general health and wellness to the public and organizations within and outside the profession.
PGD.3:   Access professional and social networks and resources to assist entrepreneurial initiatives.

Introduction

As you begin to explore the public health aspects of the oral health profession, you will find both differences and similarities to your clinical experiences. This chapter highlights the history and philosophy of dental public health, the structure of the profession, and the goals of public health. You may find many of your clinical skills in treatment planning, problem solving, and critical thinking are valuable in identifying and solving public health issues in the communities in which you choose to practice. It is the aim of this text to provide you with the skills and knowledge necessary to be a valuable contributor in the community in which you practice. It is essential that all dental care providers, regardless of practice location and mode, are aware of the unique problems in ensuring oral health for all members of society and participate in the solutions.

WHAT IS DENTAL PUBLIC HEALTH?

If someone were to ask you about your **health,** how would you respond? Great? Good? Poor? Lousy? Do you think only of your physical status and not your mental mindset? Over time, many people have attempted to define health. Webster defines health as "physical and mental well-being; freedom from disease."[2] This is an abbreviated version of the often-used definition established in 1948 by the **World Health Organization** (WHO)[3]: "health is a state of complete physical, mental, and social well-being and is not merely the absence of disease or infirmity." How does one know when they have complete physical, mental, and social well-being? What about the multitude of people who live with chronic diseases, such as diabetes or hypertension, and consider themselves healthy? Even given the availability of a definition by a preeminent health organization like WHO, can one definition suffice for all of the nuances and individual perceptions that surround health?

Attempting to define health as a dichotomy when it is, in reality, a continuum continues to present difficulties.

A similar difficulty is present when defining **public health.** If health is difficult to define, how does one define public health? A definition presented by Winslow[4] in 1920 is still used today. He defined public health as "the science and art of preventing disease, prolonging life, and promoting physical health and efficiency through organized **community** efforts." The definition does not define what constitutes a healthy public so much as it provides a description of the professional discipline of public health and the method used by that profession to attain or maintain public health. In 1955, J.W. Knutson[5] also defined the discipline, reflecting the community nature of public health as, "Public health is people's health. It is concerned with the aggregate health of a group, a community, a state, or a nation." In 1988, the **Institute of Medicine** (IOM)[6] defined the mission of public health as ". . . fulfilling society's interest in assuring conditions in which people can be healthy." Interestingly, this last definition includes "society's interest" as a component in the attainment of the public's health. As you will encounter throughout this text, the interest, acceptance, and input from recipients of public health interventions are important elements of public health practice.

If we add dental care to our exploration of the definition of health, we next attempt to define dental public health. **Dental public health** is one of nine specialties of dentistry recognized by the American Dental Association. The definition of dental public health adopted by the **American Board of Dental Public Health** (ABDPH), the governing body for the specialty, defines dental public health as:

"The science and art of preventing and controlling dental diseases and promoting dental health through organized community efforts. It is that form of dental practice that serves the community as a patient rather than the individual. It is con-

cerned with dental health education of the public, with applied dental research, and with the administration of group dental care programs, as well as the prevention and control of dental diseases on a community basis."[7]

The **Canadian Association of Public Health Dentistry** similarly defines public health dentistry:

"Dental public health is concerned with the diagnosis, prevention, and control of dental diseases and the promotion of oral health through organized community efforts. Dental public health serves the community as the patient rather than the individual, through research, health promotion, education, and group dental care programs."[8]

These definitions incorporate the concept of the community as the patient, rather than the individual, a key concept of public health that you will encounter throughout this text. The definitions also articulate the importance of public education, research, and program administration to control disease on a community level; however, they may fall short in addressing the impact of societal changes and the role played by various models of health care. In addition, the ABDPH definition was adopted prior to the increased acceptance of the term *oral health* rather than *dental health,* while the Canadian version uses the term oral health. This terminology has changed, replacing the term dental health with oral health to emphasize more than just teeth in the oral cavity. Professionals recognize that oral cavity health extends beyond dental care of the teeth and supporting structures. However, the general public has been slower to make the connection beyond teeth and gums. With oral health now known to be so influential in the general health of the body and vice versa, it is time to update the definitions and incorporate a broader scope for ensuring the public's oral health. The term oral health also encourages other groups to readily join the effort in improving the public's oral health when the effort is not so closely aligned with the term dentistry. Unfortunately, den-

tistry is too often seen as an exclusive profession, keeping a distance from the rest of the health care system. This may be perceived as a barrier for other partners outside the oral health professions who may join in our efforts. Other groups interested in oral health may include other health care provider groups, citizen coalitions, philanthropic organizations, third-party payers, schools, faith organizations, and businesses.

The most distinctive difference between public health practice and private practice is the concept of the community as the patient. In private practice, the patient is the person currently in the dental chair and care is provided based on the individual's needs and desires. In public health, even in a clinical setting, the care decisions for the person in your chair are impacted by the larger community and the setting in which the person is treated. Dental public health positions require skills in assessing and diagnosing community oral health needs; planning, implementing and evaluating community-based oral health programs; providing educational services; applying research; using epidemiology; formulating policy; advocating; and understanding the organization of health care. The specific competencies for community involvement stated in the Competencies for Entry into the Profession of Dental Hygiene (American Dental Education Association [ADEA])[1] and the competencies for dental public health practitioners[7,9] express the specific skills needed for practice or employment in dental public health. These will be explored in more detail in Chapter 4. In addition, all of the dental hygienist roles described by the **American Dental Hygienists' Association**[10] (advocate/change agent, health educator, clinician, consultant, researcher, and administrator) illustrate the close alignment between dental hygiene and public health practice. It should not be overlooked that all dental professionals can and should become involved in community public health efforts. A clear understanding of public health principles is necessary for all oral health practitioners to meet this challenge. It is the ethical responsibility of all health care practitioners to work toward improvement of the health of the community, especially for those who have limited access to care or cannot advocate for themselves.

CORE PUBLIC HEALTH PRINCIPLES

Public health is often an invisible infrastructure until crisis occurs. The public health infrastructure includes all governmental and nongovernmental entities that provide any public health services.[11] From how many public health measures have you personally benefited?

One recent trend in business and government is increased accountability. For example, schools are expected to be accountable to the public for the educational achievement of their students, businesses must be more accountable to clients and investors, and government entities must be more accountable to the taxpayers who fund their programs. In this era of demand for greater accountability, it is incumbent on schools, businesses, and governments to develop methods to evaluate and ensure quality in their respective endeavors. Dental public health practice is not without guidelines, competencies, goals, and expectations at all levels of practice. Several groups, such as the Institute of Medicine, the **American Public Health Association,** and the **Association of State and Territorial Dental Directors** (ASTDD), have developed frameworks to assess progress, quality, and success in public health.[6,12,13] These frameworks work well to elucidate the nature of public health practice.

In 1988, the Institute of Medicine[6] delineated the **core functions of public health** agencies as assessment, policy development, and assurance (Box 1-1). This landmark report prompted the public health community to look closely at services provided and, in 1994, developed a statement of core public health functions that are considered essential public health services (Box 1-2).[12]

All of these important public health functions are interrelated and continuous and based on evidence provided by research to form a strong foundation for public health practice. This interrelationship is illustrated in Figure 1-1 by the diagram

---

BOX 1-1 The Role of the Government in Public Health—Core Functions of Public Health Agencies

Assessment: Each public health agency regularly and systematically collects, assembles, analyzes, and makes available information on the health of the community, including statistics on health status, community health needs, and epidemiologic and other studies of health problems.
Policy Development: Each public health agency exercises its responsibility to serve the public interest in the development of comprehensive pubic health policies by promoting use of the scientific knowledge base in decision making and leading in the development of public health policy.
Assurance: Public health agencies assure their constituents that services necessary to achieve agreed upon goals are provided by encouraging actions by other entities, requiring such action through regulation or providing services directly. Each public health agency involves key policy makers and the general public in determining high-priority personal and communitywide health services, which the government guarantees to every member of the community.

Source: The Future of Public Health. Institute of Medicine. National Academy of Sciences, 2002.[6] Available at: http://www.nap.edu/openbook/0309038308/html.7.html.

BOX 1-2 Essential Public Health Services

What Public Health Does (The Purpose of Public Health):

- Prevents epidemics and the spread of disease
- Protects against environmental hazards
- Prevents injuries
- Promotes and encourages healthy behaviors and mental health
- Responds to disasters and assists communities in recovery
- Assures the quality and accessibility of health services.

How Public Health Serves (The Practice of Public Health)(Essential Services):

- Monitors health status to identify and solve community health problems
- Diagnoses and investigates health problems and hazards in the community
- Informs, educates, and empowers people about health issues
- Mobilizes community partnerships and actions to identify and solve health problems
- Develops policies and plans that support individual and community health efforts
- Enforces laws and regulations that protect health and ensure safety
- Links people to needed personal health services and assures the provision of health care when otherwise unavailable
- Assures a competent public and personal health care workforce
- Evaluates effectiveness, accessibility, and quality of personal and population-based health services
- Researches for new insights and innovative solutions to health problems.

Source: Public Health in America, Fall 1994. Public Health Functions Steering Committee.[12] Available at: www.health.gov/phfunctions.public.htm. Accessed February, 2004.

developed by the Public Health Functions Steering Committee.[12]

Following this report of essential public health functions, the Association of State and Territorial Dental Directors further developed (1997) the list of services as it relates directly to dental public health services provided at the state level (Box 1-3).[13]

These guidelines, used at national, state, and local levels, provide a unified framework for all public health efforts, allowing all public health programs to work toward common goals. The common framework also allows for better collaboration, sharing of information, and documentation of success among public health partners.

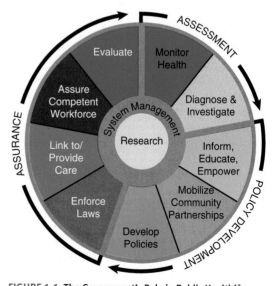

FIGURE 1-1 The Government's Role in Public Health[12]

BOX 1-3 Essential State Dental Public Health Services

Assessment
Assess oral health status and needs
Analyze determinants
Assess fluoridation status water systems
Implement oral health surveillance systems

Policy Development
Develop plans and policies through a collaborative process
Provide leadership
Mobilize community partnerships

Assurance
Inform, educate, and empower the public
Promote and enforce laws
Link people to oral health services; assure availability, access, and acceptability
Support primary and secondary prevention
Assure the capacity and expertise of the public and personal health workforce
Evaluate effectiveness, accessibility, and quality of oral health services
Conduct research and support demonstration projects

Source: Guidelines for state and territorial oral health programs: Essential public health services to promote oral health in the United States (2001 Revision). The Association of State and Territorial Dental Directors. Available at: http://www.astdd .org. Accessed February 2004.[13]

DEFINING A PUBLIC HEALTH PROBLEM

After defining the role of public health and the essential services that should be provided, what constitutes a public health problem that warrants resources applied toward its solution? If the public health workforce responded to all public concerns regarding health, it would result in a reactive, knee-jerk, inefficient, and ineffective response to society's health needs.

The current criteria used to define a public health problem are (1) a condition or situation that is a widespread actual or potential cause of morbidity or mortality, and (2) a perception on the part of the public, the government, or public health authorities that the condition is a public health problem.[14] This definition allows a broad interpretation of a public health problem in that "widespread," "potential," and "perception" can all be interpreted differently in different situations with different threats to the public. Bioterrorism, West Nile Virus, Severe Acute Respiratory Syndrome (SARS), automobile safety, water purification, and oral disease may be seen as more or less a problem depending on whom you ask. Later chapters will describe methods for identifying public health problems and developing solutions.

HISTORY OF PUBLIC HEALTH

Public health has traversed through three phases into a current, fourth phase that is centered on the current societal needs of the times and the progression of industrialization and technology in the world. During the first phase (1849–1900), public health activities were related to the elimination and control of diseases that grew out of rapid industrialization and crowded and poor living conditions. Many activities were aimed at reducing the morbidity and mortality of such diseases as cholera, polio, and plague. Efforts, therefore, were directed at basic sanitation methods.

In the second phase (1880–1930), population-based prevention strategies were possible with advances in bacteriology and immunizations, reducing the effects of infectious diseases. Immunization programs were an outgrowth of this phase.

Continued advancements in technology from 1930–1975 allowed a further shift to the treatment of disease through increasingly complex medical treatments. Interventions in this third phase occurred increasingly in hospitals rather than with community-based public health measures. During this phase, many major infectious diseases, such as smallpox, were eradicated and cures for many acute health problems were developed.

The current, or fourth, phase arises from the realization that technology may be strikingly effective in the treatment or cure of acute health problems but ineffective in managing chronic lifestyle diseases and controlling the spiraling cost of high technology health care. The value of technology is limited because of the lack of availability to all members of the public and the inability to correct the most prevalent diseases we now face, those that occur as a result of longer life expectancy gained from earlier phases of public health and lifestyle choices. This current phase now emphasizes a broader approach to health. It goes beyond prevention of specific diseases to encompass the concept of overall wellness. Health promotion strategies are used to encourage healthy lifestyles, resulting in a reduced risk of multiple problems. For example, choosing not to smoke or choosing to stop smoking can reduce the risk for lung cancer, hypertension, periodontal disease, heart disease, or emphysema.

Will terrorist actions, such as the events of September 11, 2001, and the SARS outbreak, cause us to look again at our public health infrastructure and our ability to respond to new public health threats, such as bioterrorism? Will we enter a new phase of public health? Will we strengthen the protection from and rapid response to unknown or undefined threats to health? The quick responses and measures taken to stop the spread of the SARS epidemic indicate how rapid information transfer and global cooperation can protect the public's health and highlight how important cooperation and information sharing can be in preventing a world disaster.

HISTORIC HIGHLIGHTS IN DENTAL PUBLIC HEALTH

No text would be complete without setting the stage for what is to come by exploring the path by which we have traveled. Knowing where we have been helps us understand where we are and where we are going. Several key events have shaped the profession of dental public health to make it what it is today.

The dental hygiene profession originated in 1906 as Dr. Alfred C. Fones began a course of study for his assistant, Irene Newman.[15] This early profession was centered in public health practice. The dental hygienist was prepared to provide education and treatment in the community setting and to work as an advocate for dental care. The preventive nature of the dental hygiene profession is still a perfect fit in the public health arena as envisioned by Alfred Fones. Even today, the mission of the American Dental Hygienists' Association (ADHA) is "to improve the public's total health."[16]

Public health continues to be an arena in which oral health professionals work together and with other groups to improve the oral health of the communities in which they work and live. It is sad to think that the original purpose of the dental hygiene profession has blurred because of the fear that dental hygienists may be a threat to dental practices and the public. This perception has resulted in the limitations put on dental hygiene licensure and practice through restrictive dental practice acts, which are only now starting to reverse, with more states allowing dental hygienists to practice in other than private settings and under less restrictive supervision requirements. State dental practice acts are also evolving to allow dental hygienists to perform services not permitted in the past. However, it will be some time before Fones' vision is truly fulfilled.

A key public health event occurred in August 1935. The **Social Security Act,**[17] passed by Congress, established unemployment compensation and benefits for the elderly. In addition, it provided aid to the individual states for health and welfare activities, including grants for **Maternal and Child Health** (MCH). Because oral health services were included in maternal and child health block grants, many states established dental public health units within their health department structure. The number of dental public health units grew so rapidly that, in 1937, a group of state dental administrators founded the American Association of Public Health Dentists (AAPHD), which was changed in 1983 to the **American Association of Public Health Dentistry,** reflecting the expanded membership that included dental hygienists, health educators, and others. In 1977, the AAPHD voted to allow dental hygienists to be voting members of the organization, becoming the first and only sponsoring organization of a dental specialty to allow full membership to dental hygienists.[18]

The 1940s saw many dental public health developments. During World War II (WWII), the dental services of the armed forces expanded considerably. This was a direct result of the poor oral health status of the young recruits being inducted, which shed light on the extensive dental needs of the United States population.[19] Dental services for the armed forces increased during WWII because of selective service rejections, resulting from about 10% of potential recruits failing the military physical examination. The recruits lacked the necessary six opposing teeth in each arch to meet the military

standard.[19] To accommodate the manpower needs for the war, selective service requirements were again lowered twice before the end of the war. The growth in armed forces services and the need to treat large groups of people efficiently and effectively became the seed for the concept of the community as the patient, which has remained a core concept for dental public health practice. The armed forces experience led to the development in 1948 of the National Institute of Dental Research (NIDR) to address the national dental problem.[19] The NIDR was eventually changed to the **National Institute of Dental and Craniofacial Research** (NIDCR), reflecting a broader perspective about oral growth and development.

In 1945, controlled clinical trials of water fluoridation began in Grand Rapids, Michigan, and Newburgh, New York. These trials forever changed the smiles of America and led to the establishment of water fluoridation as a safe, effective means of preventing dental caries. Indeed, water fluoridation, considered one of ten great public health achievements of the 20th Century,[20] is supported by all major health professional organizations (Box 1-4).

In 1951, public health dentistry was recognized as the seventh of what are currently nine specialties in dentistry. The ADHA is currently considering developing special emphases in dental hygiene practice, one of which would be public health.

In January 2000, the Department of Health and Human Services launched **Healthy People 2010,** a comprehensive, nationwide health promotion and disease prevention plan.[21] It builds on similar documents of 1990 and 2000 and contains 467 objectives designed to be a framework for improving the health of the nation during the first decade of the 21st century. There are 28 focus areas, each representing a public health area, including oral health. The objectives serve as targets for the health of the nation for the year 2010 and provide a basis for comparison and a focus for health agencies at all levels to participate in the goals of the nation. Tracking of progress is the responsibility of the **National Center for Health Statistics,** which provides a centralized location for informa-

BOX 1-4 Ten Great Public Health Achievements of the 20th Century

Vaccination
Motor vehicle safety
Workplace safety
Infectious disease control
Reduction in death from coronary heart
  disease and stroke
Safer and healthier food
Healthier mothers and babies
Family planning
Fluoridated drinking water
Recognition of tobacco use as a health
  hazard

Source: Ten Great Public Health Achievements—
United States, 1900–1999. Centers for Disease Control
and Prevention. MMWR 1999;48(12):241–243.[20]

tion and data related to the objectives. More about this effort will be discussed in Chapter 2.

The **Surgeon General's Report on Oral Health** was released in May 2000.[22] This was the first Surgeon General's Report on Oral Health in the more than 50-year history of Surgeon General Reports. The report highlights the fact that oral health is better now than ever before in history. The report's primary message is that oral health is essential to the general health and well-being of all Americans and that it can be achieved by all Americans. However, the report also illustrates the profound disparities that exist in oral health in America—children, the elderly, members of racial and ethnic groups, and those with disabilities and complex health conditions are at greater risk for oral disease. The report calls for a national partnership to provide opportunities for individuals, communities, and the health professionals to work together to maintain and improve the nation's oral health. It is too early to know the full impact of this report on

oral health in America; however, public health dentistry professionals are taking the charge seriously.

PUBLIC HEALTH INFRASTRUCTURE

The fabric of the public health infrastructure in the United States is an example of a broad, sweeping network of many entities, working at all levels of government and society to protect the health of Americans. A constant challenge in public health is that efforts are occurring on so many fronts that coordination and collaboration are often difficult. However, the Internet and common goals and frameworks allow for better communication and easier access to information. This network is often invisible to the beneficiaries of the efforts; however, all of these protections and core functions of a public health infrastructure are part of our everyday lives. The dental public health network also appears at all levels of society. Many local, national, and international governmental agencies include a dental public health component and opportunities for dental public health careers. Chapter 4 highlights many of these career opportunities in greater detail.

The United States Government will be used here to illustrate a public health and dental public health infrastructure. In the United States, the President's Cabinet includes leading officials of the fifteen departments of the government. Within these departments are many agencies responsible for essential services in public health. Figure 1-2 highlights the departments and agencies with significant dental public health functions. Many of these agencies work together and in tandem with schools, community organizations, philanthropic organizations, and others to accomplish their goals. Similar infrastructures also occur at local, state, provincial, and international levels.

Global health also affects the health of the local population. With the increased ability to travel throughout the world, health concerns can quickly transfer from one country or area of the world to another and become a global public health problem. Infectious and life-threatening diseases, such as

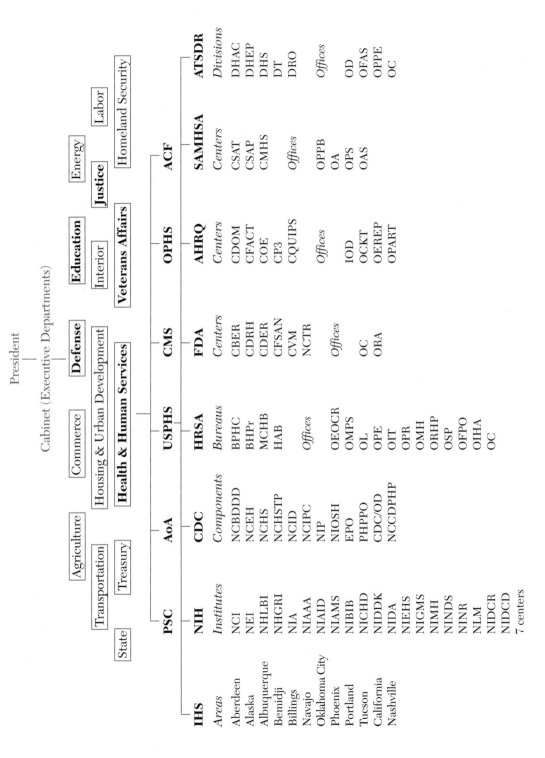

FIGURE 1-2 United States—Federal Infrastructure of Public Health Services (see Appendix II for a listing of the acronyms and their meanings)

SARS and HIV/AIDS, are a leading concern. The effect of global movement of people from one country to another also affects the need for a strong oral health infrastructure. Therefore, it behooves public health professionals and agencies from various countries to work together to solve problems, eradicate disease, and protect people from newly developing threats. Certain, more notable, global entities involved in public health endeavors are the World Health Organization (WHO) and the **Pan American Health Organization** (PAHO).

The WHO headquarters is located in Geneva, Switzerland. Their objective is attainment of the highest possible level of health by all peoples.[23] WHO acts as the directing and coordinating authority on international health work and proposes regulations and makes recommendations about global public health practices. The World Oral Health Report 2003 states that oral diseases are a major public health problem and that increased emphasis should be on developing global policies in oral health promotion and oral disease prevention.[24] One priority is more effective coordination with other WHO programs and external partners.

The PAHO headquarters is located in Washington, DC. It is an international public health agency that includes all 35 countries in the Americas.[25] Its mission is to strengthen national and local health systems and to improve the health of the peoples of the Americas. PAHO collaborates with such entities as Ministries of Health, governmental agencies, nongovernmental organizations (NGO), universities, social security agencies, and community groups.

SUMMARY

Much of public health, which has evolved with time, is an invisible infrastructure that has been developed to protect the health of the public. Public health activities occur at all levels of government and society and include efforts to improve the

 Learning Activities

1. List public health services from which you have personally benefited.
2. Develop your own definition of dental public health.
3. Choose a governmental agency with oral health responsibilities and write a description of its mission, activities, budget, and role in the dental public health infrastructure.
4. Write a reflection paper discussing what constitutes good oral health.
5. Choose a particular oral health problem in your community and create a list of organizations or community groups in your community that would be important partners in an oral health coalition formed to address the problem (e.g., early childhood caries, fluoridation of the com-

munity's water supply, school fluoride rinse program).
6. Write a reflection paper on the pros and cons of the public health infrastructure being "invisible."
7. Identify a public health problem and describe why it constitutes a public health problem.
8. Compare and contrast the three sets of competencies for public health practitioners (i.e., Council on Linkages, American Board of Dental Public Health, and the American Dental Education Association).
9. Choose a state, province, or a country other than the United States and investigate the dental public health infrastructure of the chosen area.

public's oral health. Core functions of public health entities and competencies for public health professionals guide public health practice. The dental public health profession has a rich history of working to improve the oral health of the public. In addition, the mission of the dental hygiene profession and the professional roles of dental hygienists are a reflection of the natural fit between dental hygiene and public health, which was envisioned by Dr. Alfred Fones as he prepared the first dental hygienist.

RESOURCES

American Association of Public Health Dentistry. Available at: http://www.aaphd.org. listserves available on site

American Public Health Association. Available at: http://www.apha.org

Association of State and Territorial Dental Directors. Available at: http://www.astdd.org

World Health Organization. Available at: http://www.who.int

Pan American Health Organization. Available at: http//:www.paho.org

U.S. Government official Web portal. Available at: http:// www.firstgov.gov

---

Review Questions

1. The third phase of public health included all of the following EXCEPT the:
   a. treatment of disease with complex medical treatment.
   b. eradication of smallpox.
   c. intervention through hospitalization rather than the community.
   d. cure for acute health problems.
   e. effective management of chronic, lifestyle-related diseases.

2. State dental public health units originally developed as a result of the:
   a. establishment of the American Association of Public Health Dentistry.
   b. need for recruits during World War II.
   c. Surgeon General's Report.
   d. Maternal and Child Health grants to states.
   e. creation of the National Institute of Dental Research.

3. The controlled clinical trials of water fluoridation began in:
   a. 1937.
   b. 1942.
   c. 1945.
   d. 1948.
   e. 1953.

4. The primary reason for developing the National Institute of Dental Research was to:
   a. provide a central agency to monitor state fluoridation efforts.
   b. address the national dental problems discovered through selective service rejections.
   c. create educational opportunities for dental public health professionals.
   d. make dentistry more visible at the National Institutes of Health.
   e. study the cost-effectiveness of community water fluoridation.

5. Core functions of public health include:
   a. assessment.
   b. policy development.
   c. assurance.
   d. funding of oral health programs.
   e. a, b, and c.

REFERENCES

1. American Dental Education Association. Competencies for entry into the profession of dental hygiene, exhibit 7. J Dent Educ 2003;67(7):1–5. Available at: http://www.adea.org/cepr. Accessed January 2004.
2. Webster's New World Dictionary. Simon and Schuster, 1995.
3. World Health Organization. Preamble to the Constitution Adopted by the International Health Conference, New York, June 19–22, 1946.
4. Winslow CEA. The untilled fields of public health. Modern Med 1920;2:183–191.
5. Knutson JW. What is public health? In: Pelton WJ, Wisan JM, eds. Dentistry in Public Health, 2nd Ed. Philadelphia, PA: WB Saunders, 1955.

6. The Future of Public Health. Institute of Medicine, Committee for the Study of the Future of Public Health. Washington, DC: National Academy Press, October 1988.

7. American Association of Public Health Dentistry/American Board of Dental Public Health. Competency statements for dental public health. J Public Health Dent 1998; 58(Suppl. 1):119–122.

8. Canadian Association of Public Health Dentistry. Available at: http://www.caphd-acsdp.org/about.html. Accessed February 2004.

9. Core competencies for public health professionals. Council on Linkages Between Academia and Public Health Practice. Washington, DC: Public Health Foundation, 2001. Available at: http://phf.org/Link.htm.

10. Types of dental hygiene careers. American Dental Hygienists' Association Online. Available at: http://www.adha.org/careerinfo/types.htm. Accessed September 2002.

11. Chapter 23: Public Health Infrastructure. In: Healthy People 2010 (Conference Edition; two volumes). Washington, DC: Department of Health and Human Services, January 2000.

12. Public Health in America. Fall 1994. Public Health Functions Steering Committee. Available at: http://www.health.gov/phfunctions.public.htm. Accessed February 2004.

13. Guidelines for state and territorial oral health programs: Essential public health services to promote oral health in the United States (2001 Revision). The Association of State and Territorial Dental Directors. Available at: http://www.astdd.org. Accessed February 2004.

14. The practice of dental public health. In: Burt BA, Eklund SA, eds. Dentistry, Dental Practice, and the Community. 5th Ed. Philadelphia, PA: WB Saunders,1999, p 36.

15. Motley WE. History of the American Dental Hygienists' Association, 1923–1982. Chicago, IL: American Dental Hygienists' Association, 1983, p 21.

16. Profile of ADHA—Mission Statement. Available at: http://www.adha.org/aboutadha/profile.htm. Accessed February 2004.

17. Social Security Act of 1935. Available at: http://www.usconstitution.com/SocialSecurityActof1935.htm. Accessed February 2004.

18. Application for Continued Recognition of the Specialty of Dental Public Health. Submitted by the American Association of Public Health Dentistry to the American Dental Association, 1986. Available at: http://www.aaphd.org/docs/history.htm. Accessed January 2003.

19. Harris RR. Dental Science in a New Age: A History of the National Institute of Dental Research. Rockville, MD: Montrose Press, 1989, p 78–91.

20. Ten Greatest Public Health Achievements—United States, 1900–1999. Centers for Disease Control and Prevention. MMWR 1999;48(12):241–243.

21. Healthy People 2010 (Conference Edition; two volumes). Washington, DC: Department of Health and Human Services, January 2000.

22. Oral Health in America: A Report of the Surgeon General—Executive Summary. Rockville, MD: DHHS, National Institute of Dental and Craniofacial Research, National Institutes of Health, 2000.

23. World Health Organization (WHO). About WHO. Available at: http://www.who.int/about/en/. Accessed February 2004.

24. WHO Oral Health Report for 2003. Comm Dent Oral Epid 2003;31(Suppl. 1):3–23. Available at: http://www.who.int/oral_health/media/en/orh_report03_en.pdf. Accessed January 2004.

25. Pan American Health Organization (PAHO). About PAHO. Available at: http://www.paho.org/english/paho/about_paho.htm. Accessed February 2004.

Trends in Dental Public Health

2

Objectives

After studying this chapter and completing the study questions and activities, the learner will be able to:
- Discuss the reasons for oral health disparities and the lack of access to care.
- Describe at least five public health strategies for reducing oral health disparities and access problems.
- Discuss trends in oral health care financing and community-based public health programs.
- Describe potential reasons for a fragile dental public health infrastructure.
- Give examples of multidisciplinary collaborations to address oral health problems.
- Discuss how advances in science and information technology influence the field of dental public health.
- Locate resources for creating culturally relevant health communication strategies.
- Discuss the goal of evidence-based practice and obstacles to implementing this approach in public health settings.

KEY TERMS

Anticipatory guidance
Capitation
Community coalitions
Cultural relevance
Dental health professional
   shortage areas
Dental home
Evidence-based practice
Gatekeeper
Health communication

Healthy People 2010
Integration of oral health and
   general health
Interdisciplinary
Leadership development
Literacy
Loan forgiveness program
Media advocacy
Mobile and portable services
Oral health disparities

Oral health infrastructure
Plain language movement
Public health care financing
   programs
Risk assessment
Safety net dental clinics
Social marketing
Teledentistry
Volunteerism

The American Dental Education Association competencies addressed in this chapter include[1]:

HP.1:   Promote the values of oral and general health and wellness to the public and organizations within and outside the profession.

HP.4:   Identify individual and population risk factors and develop strategies that promote health-related quality of life.

CM.1:   Assess the oral health needs of the community and the quality and availability of resources and services.

CM.4:   Facilitate client access to oral health services by influencing individuals and/or organizations for the provision of oral health care.

CM.5:   Evaluate reimbursement mechanisms and their impact on the patient's/client's access to oral health care.

Introduction

"It was the best of times, it was the worst of times; it was the age of wisdom, it was the age of foolishness; it was the epoch of belief, it was the epoch of incredulity; it was the season of Light, it was the season of Darkness; it was the spring of hope, it was the winter of despair; we had everything before us, we had nothing before us. . ."

Charles Dickens (1812–1870)

This quotation from *A Tale of Two Cities* by Charles Dickens captures the seemingly opposing perspectives that have characterized the field of dental public health for the last few decades. It reflects the vicissitudes of public health, as well as the importance of considering different perspectives on an issue. Students who learn ideal public health practices while in school often do not realize how much the fields of public health and dental public health fluctuate in response to overall societal, medical, economic, and political changes. Traditional approaches that have been previously successful may no longer be relevant. Dental hygienists must be aware of trends that affect the public's oral health and the way that professional care is delivered and financed.

Public health professionals who stay energized by new challenges that arise on a daily basis may also be frustrated by ongoing budget fluctuations and bureaucratic processes that appear to be inflexible and outdated. One day may be highlighted by a successful fluoridation campaign and the next by a request to cut 20% from the oral health program budget to redirect funds to homeland security and bioterrorism. Dental public health professionals face an environment, therefore, in which they need to be flexible, proactive, up-to-date, creative, and compassionate. Those who succeed have learned the importance of maintaining a sense of balance—between a career and personal/family interests, idealism and reality, personal integrity and compromise, and innovation and patience. This chapter addresses certain trends in the United States that challenge dental public health practice and certain ways that organizations, communities, and professionals are meeting these challenges.

ORAL HEALTH DISPARITIES AND ACCESS TO CARE

Oral Health Disparities

Although oral health problems affect everyone, certain population subgroups, defined by demographic factors such as age, sex, race or ethnicity, socioeconomic status, primary language, geography, medical or disability status, and behavioral lifestyles, experience higher levels of oral disease. They are said to have **oral health disparities** in comparison with other groups. Non-Hispanic Blacks, Hispanics, American Indians, and Alaska Natives generally have the poorest oral health of the racial and ethnic groups in the United States.[2]

BOX 2-1 Oral Health Needs and Disparities

- Dental caries is the most common chronic childhood disease—five times more common than asthma and seven times more common than hayfever.
- Poor children suffer twice as much dental decay as their more affluent peers and the disease is more likely to be untreated; this trend continues into adolescence.
- Recent national survey data suggest that a higher proportion of Mexican American children aged 12 to 23 months experience dental caries than other racial/ethnic groups.
- American Indian/Alaska Native children aged 2 to 4 have five times the rate of dental decay of all U.S. children.
- In 1996, only 30% of Mexican Americans, 32% of non-Hispanic Whites, and 41% of non-Hispanic Blacks aged 12 to 17 were free of caries in their permanent teeth.
- Uninsured children are 2.5 times less likely than insured children to receive dental care. For each child without medical insurance, there are at least 2.6 children without dental insurance.
- Fewer than 20% of Medicaid-covered children received a single preventive dental service in a recent yearlong study.
- More than 51 million school hours are lost each year to dental-related illness; poor children suffer nearly 12 times more restricted activity days than higher-income children.
- A greater percentage of non-Hispanic Blacks aged 18 and older have missing teeth compared with non-Hispanic Whites.
- Male African Americans have the highest incidence of oral and pharyngeal cancers in the United States; their 5-year survival rates are also lower.
- Nasopharyngeal cancer incidence and mortality rates among Chinese and Vietnamese populations are many times higher than other groups.
- American Indian/Alaska Native populations have much greater rates of dental caries and periodontal disease in all age groups than the general U.S. population. The high prevalence of diabetes is a contributing factor.
- Small-scale studies show that populations with mental retardation or other developmental disabilities have higher rates of poor oral hygiene and periodontal treatment needs than the general population.
- Almost two thirds of community residential facilities for persons with disabilities report inadequate access to dental care for their residents.
- Sixty-five percent of child abuse cases involve head and oral-facial trauma.
- Oral clefts are more common among North American Indians (3.7 per 1,000 live births) and more common among Whites than Blacks (1.7 versus 0.5 per 1,000 live births).

Source: Oral Health in America: A Report of the Surgeon General. Rockville, MD: DHHS, NIDCR, NIH, 2000.[3]

Limited knowledge of and access to preventive oral health measures and professional care have contributed to these disparities. Box 2-1 summarizes some statistics to highlight the extent of the problem.

What is being done to address these disparities?

1. **Healthy People 2010** is a national health promotion and disease prevention initiative that includes the goal of eliminating health

disparities among different segments of the population. Oral health, with 17 objectives, is a separate focus area, but it is also woven into many other focus areas, such as maternal and child health, cancer, diabetes, access, and infrastructure.[4] A new Healthy People 2010 Oral Health Toolkit has been developed to help states and communities translate the Healthy People oral health objectives into action.[5] Healthy People 2010 is discussed in relationship with program planning in Chapter 5.

2. In April 2003, the Surgeon General issued A National Call to Action, a framework for oral health action and strategies for collaboration to reduce disparities and improve oral health.[6] The report calls for action on the part of individuals and groups in five areas: (1) change perceptions of oral health; (2) overcome barriers by replicating effective programs and proven efforts; (3) build the science base and accelerate science transfer; (4) increase oral health workforce diversity, capacity, and flexibility; and (5) increase collaboration. National organizations, such as the Association of State and Territorial Dental Directors (ASTDD), the American Association of Public Health Dentistry (AAPHD), and local oral health coalitions, are using this framework to develop strategic plans and implement activities.

3. Lack of comparable data at state and local levels hinders attempts to document improvements in oral health, despite continuing efforts to refine data collection and analysis for oral health indicators. The National Oral Health Surveillance System (NOHSS), developed jointly by the ASTDD and the Centers for Disease Control and Prevention (CDC), is one attempt to collect and analyze comparable data. On the NOHSS Web site, data for the following eight oral health indicators can be displayed in tables, graphs, and maps for the nation and each state that submitted data: (1) dental visits, (2) teeth cleaning, (3) complete tooth loss, (4) fluoridation status, (5) dental caries experience, (6) untreated dental caries, (7) dental sealants,

and (8) cancer of the oral cavity and pharynx. These data can be used to advocate for more resources to address oral health disparities and to track improvements in oral health. More information on the NOHSS is included in following chapters.

4. State and local health departments, dental schools, and dental hygiene programs can play a role in reducing oral health disparities by conducting research using measures that yield comparable data. To increase regional resources as part of its Plan to Eliminate Craniofacial, Oral, and Dental Health Disparities, the National Institute of Dental and Craniofacial Research (NIDCR) has funded two initiatives: (1) four Regional Research Centers on Minority Oral Health, and (2) five Centers for Research to Reduce Oral Health Disparities to encourage **interdisciplinary** research across components of academic health centers and with community-based agencies and organizations. Also as part of the Disparities Plan, NIDCR and CDC collaborated on the formation of the Dental, Oral, and Craniofacial Data Resource Center to consolidate health and disease data from multiple sources. CDC also funds a network of Prevention Research Centers across the country, some of which are conducting interdisciplinary oral health research.

Demographic Shifts

The U.S. population is aging, with the fastest growing segment aged 85 years and older. By 2030, persons aged 65 and older will constitute about 20% of the population. In 1999, about one half of the elderly lived in only nine states (CA, FL, IL, MI, NJ, NY, OH, PA, TX).[7] Most older persons remain in the community, with fewer than 5% living in nursing homes and 3% residing in assisted living facilities.[7] The number of persons with disabilities living in the community, regardless of age, continues to increase. About 20% of Americans have a disability, with 10% having a severe disability that limits daily functions. With improved oral care, these groups retain their teeth longer, increasing the demand for comprehensive services that can be provided in different settings. This presents a challenge to planners, academic faculty, and clinicians. In a 2002 American Dental Education Association (ADEA) survey of graduating dental students, most students felt they were well prepared for providing oral health care for a diverse society; however, students noted the following areas in which they did not feel as well prepared: practice management, care for disabled and geriatric patients and those with HIV/AIDS, and interacting with medical colleagues.[8]

More than one of four Americans is Black, Hispanic, or Asian/other non-Hispanic; this proportion will increase to one of three Americans by 2020.[2] Nearly one of 10 U.S. residents is foreign-born, the majority of Hispanic or Asian/Pacific Islander origin. Many arrive in the United States with significant unmet oral health needs, inadequate finances, and a limited knowledge of the English language. When seeking care, they find themselves in a cultural and communication disconnect with a predominantly Caucasian and predominantly English-speaking dental and dental hygiene workforce and with limited resources to pay for care. They may not receive timely care or any care and are more likely to have negative health encounters.

The number of oral health professionals representing minority groups in the United States is disproportionate to the distribution of these groups in the population. Although the percentage of minority dental students has increased from 13 to 34% since 1980, most of the increase has been among Asian/Pacific Islander students. There actually has been a 15% decline in the number of underrepresented minority first-year dental students, particularly Black/African American and Hispanic/Latino students.[9] The field of dental hygiene is even less ethnically diverse. Relatively few faculty members in dental or dental hygiene schools are ethnic minorities.

These ethnic and cultural discrepancies between the oral health workforce and the general population create a number of challenges. Appropriate role models and mentors are lacking for students and graduates from ethnic minority groups who wish to work in dental public health settings. Designing effective community-based oral health promotion and disease prevention programs that are **culturally relevant** to different groups (incorporating health beliefs, dietary considerations, and communication styles from each group) is difficult. Dental hygienists who provide services in large metropolitan school districts often find themselves working with children and families that represent more than 240 different language groups. Although language assistance for limited English proficient (LEP) persons (including use of bilingual staff, interpreters, and translation of written materials) has been required for years for programs and health care providers who receive federal funding (including Medicaid and Medicare), resources and monitoring are inadequate. Groups, such as Volunteers in Health Care, have created manuals and training programs to help providers overcome language and literacy barriers.[10]

Access to Care

There are pronounced geographic shifts in the U.S. population, with southern and western states increasing in population, and in the number of oral health personnel. The oral health workforce, like the general population, however, is aging, and many professionals choose to work part-time. Some states project they will lose 30 to 50% of their oral health workforce to retirement in the next decade. This situation is mirrored in public health and academic settings.

More than 90% of active dentists and dental hygienists work in private practice.[3] Many general dentists and specialists do not participate in publicly financed programs such as Medicaid or the State Children's Health Insurance Program (SCHIP), placing a burden on community clinics that treat underserved populations. Recent efforts through the American Dental Association, Oral

Health America, The National Foundation of Dentistry for the Handicapped, and Special Olympics promote private sector **volunteerism** to provide free or reduced-fee preventive services and oral health care to individuals who can't afford private sector care, especially children, disabled individuals, and frail elders. This does not begin to solve the dental access problem, however.

An estimated 25 million people reside in areas lacking adequate oral health services. In 2001, the Department of Health and Human Services Bureau of Primary Health Care (BPHC) reported 1,480 designated **Dental Health Professional Shortage Areas** (DHPSAs).[7] DHPSAs are geographic areas, special population groups (e.g., low-income or Medicaid populations), or facilities (e.g., correctional institutions) designated by the federal government as having a shortage of oral health personnel. This designation qualifies these entities for various federal programs (e.g., community health centers and sites where health professionals may be able to practice and have all or a portion of their government-subsidized student loans forgiven). A database of dental and other health professional shortage areas can be found on the BPHC Shortage Designation Branch home page (Box 2-2).

Numerous community nonprofit and for-profit clinics have emerged to serve as **safety net dental clinics.** The oral health care safety net is where people go because (1) they do not have a regular source of care or they choose it as their regular source of care, (2) they know there is a sliding fee scale or that their Medicaid card will be accepted, (3) they will not be turned away when they are in pain and cannot afford care, and (4) the clinic is close to home, or for various other reasons. It helps people who otherwise fall through the cracks in oral health care. Unfortunately, there are not enough clinics to meet the growing need and demand for care. The Safety Net Dental Clinic Manual is available online to help communities make decisions about building or expanding safety net clinics (Box 2-2).

The federal government supports Federally Qualified Health Centers (FQHCs), community/ migrant/homeless health center programs located in medically or dentally underserved communities. In 2001, 530 of these centers included on-site oral health programs, employing more than 1,200 oral health professionals to provide services including primary and preventive oral health care and outreach to more than 1.4 million people. This represents only 14% of the total health center users, however. To increase the proportion of centers that provide on-site oral health care, the Bureau of Primary Health Care issued an initiative in 2002 that required new clinics or expansion of existing clinics to include oral health care to receive funding.

Another solution to the access problem is to take the services to where populations live, work, or spend a significant amount of time, such as to the schools. Many community-based programs that use self-propelled mobile vans, mobile trailers that are parked at sites, and portable dental equipment that will fit into an automobile or truck, are providing services to underserved populations. These **mobile and portable services** are particularly efficient for conducting dental sealant programs. A manual to help communities implement high-quality mobile and portable dental care systems is available online (Box 2-2).

To address the lack of or maldistribution of dental specialty services in rural or isolated areas, **teledentistry** is helping general practitioners seek needed consultation from specialists for certain patients and reducing travel time and expenses for families. Teledentistry uses electronic information and communications technology to provide and support health care provided in distant locations. Digital radiography and other computer and video applications, as well as Integrated Services Digital Network (ISDN) lines, make this type of service possible. Teledentistry may eventually enable more dental hygienists to practice in areas where a dentist is not always available for diagnosis and consultation. It also has applications for continuing education and dentist–laboratory communication.

One potential solution to certain access problems is to change restrictive state dental practice

BOX 2-2 Helpful Web Sites

Web Site	Address
Healthy People 2010 Resources	http://www.healthypeople.gov
Office of the Surgeon General	http://www.surgeongeneral.gov/library
Centers for Disease Control and Prevention (CDC), Oral Health Resources	http://www.cdc.gov/OralHealth
CDC Prevention Research Centers	http://www.cdc.gov/prc
National Oral Health Surveillance System	http://www.cdc.gov/nohss
National Institute of Dental and Craniofacial Research Dental, Oral and Craniofacial Data Resource Center	http://drc.nidcr.nih.gov/
Health Resources & Services Administration (HRSA) Bureau of Primary Health Care	http://bphc.hrsa.gov/
Bureau of Primary Health Care Dental Health Professional Shortage Areas	http://belize.hrsa.gov/newhpsa/newhpsa.cfm.
HRSA Maternal and Child Health Bureau	http://mchb.hrsa.gov/
HRSA Bureau of Health Professions	http://bhpr.hrsa.gov/
National Maternal and Child Oral Health Resource Center	http://mchoralhealth.org
Administration for Children & Families (ACF) Head Start Bureau	http://www2.acf.dhhs.gov/programs/hsb/
Indian Health Service	http://ihs.gov
Association of State & Territorial Dental Directors (ASTDD)	http://www.astdd.org
American Association of Public Health Dentistry (AAPHD)	http://www.aaphd.org
American Public Health Association	http://www.apha.org
Oral Health America	http://www.oralhealthamerica.org
Special Olympics Special Smiles	http://www.specialolympics.org
National Foundation of Dentistry for the Handicapped	http://www.nfdh.org/Services.html
Northeast Wisconsin Technical College Community Dental Health Certificate Prog.	http://www.nwtconline.com
Safety Net Dental Clinic Manual	http://www.dentalclinicmanual.com
Mobile and Portable Dental Manual	http://www.mobile-portabledental manual.com
The National Literacy and Health Program (Canada)	http://www.nlhp.cpha.ca/
Harvard School of Public Health. Health Literacy Studies	http://www.hsph.harvard.edu/healthliteracy.
Synopses of State and Territorial Dental Public Health Programs	http://www2a.cdc.gov/nccdphp/doh/ synopses/index.asp
ASTDD Best Practices	http://www.astdd.org click on Best Practices
Cochrane Oral Health Group	http://www.cochrane-oral.man.ac.uk/
National Governors Association	http://www.nga.org
National Conference of State Legislatures	http://www.ncsl.org

acts that prevent dental hygienists from practicing without the supervision of a dentist, that limit state licensure to practitioners who have successfully passed a state clinical board, and that prevent dental hygienists from receiving direct reimbursement from third-party payers, such as Medicaid or private dental insurers. Recent legislation has expanded the role of dental hygienists in several states to promote better access to preventive services, although it is too soon to document the impact on preventive oral health services delivery.[11] As of September 2003, 17 states allowed dental hygienists to provide services in certain settings under various forms of unsupervised practice and less restrictive supervision. This is addressed in more detail in Chapters 16 and 17.

Financing of Public Health and Oral Health Care

Unlike medical care, a large portion of oral health care is financed privately, either as out-of-pocket payments made directly to a dentist or through employment-based dental insurance benefits. Since 1960, these two sources have financed more than 93% of all dental expenditures.[3] Nationally, the public paid out-of-pocket for 43% of dental expenditures, but for only 15% of total health care expenditures (including dental) in 2001.[12]

The two largest **public health care financing programs** are Medicare and Medicaid. In 2001, the Medicare program provided health insurance coverage for more than 40 million people who were aged 65 and older, certain people with disabilities, and persons with kidney failure. Since its inception in 1965, with a few minor exceptions, Medicare has never provided coverage for oral health services.

Medicaid is a jointly funded, federal–state health insurance program for certain low-income and needy people. It covers approximately 36 million individuals, including children, seniors, people who are blind or have other disabilities, and people who are eligible to receive federally assisted income maintenance payments. Oral health services under Medicaid are mandatory for children, but are one of about 34 health and health-related services that are considered optional for adults. In difficult economic times, cash-strapped states may cut these optional benefits to save money and preserve other programs. In 2000, 31 state Medicaid programs offered full or limited oral health coverage for adults and seven states offered no coverage. By 2003, when only three states were not facing budget deficits, only 15 states were continuing or proposing to offer full or limited adult oral health benefits, and the number of states offering no coverage had increased to 16.

These program descriptions illustrate the traditionally limited or fragmented coverage afforded to oral health care by public programs. In 2001, state and federal public programs covered less than 6% of oral health expenditures nationally, but 43% of all personal health care expenditures.[12] State and federal governments convey an unfortunate message to the public about the importance of oral health by covering virtually no oral health services in Medicare and deeming the coverage of adult oral health services optional for state Medicaid programs. In contrast to medicine, the relative scarcity of dental insurance and the absence of managed care in existing dental plans means that those people who seek care always have to assume at least some responsibility for their oral health costs.

The State Children's Health Insurance Program is a relatively new, jointly funded federal–state program that provides health insurance coverage for children up to age 19 whose families do not qualify for Medicaid and whose incomes are generally less than twice the federal poverty level ($34,100 for a family of four in 2003). During 2002, 5.3 million children were enrolled in SCHIP for at least part of the year.[12] Although oral health coverage is not a mandatory component of SCHIP (unless the program is an extension of the state's Medicaid program), all states have elected to offer at least some oral health coverage to eligible children. However, the extent of coverage is dependent on funding and, in difficult economic times, states often tend to view oral health coverage as one of the more expendable benefits.

In addition to the major publicly financed oral health care programs noted above, the wide range of community-based programs—community clinics, school-based sealant programs, preschool fluoride supplement programs, nursing home oral health programs—are funded through various sources, such as federal, state, and local governments; corporate sponsors; foundations and other philanthropic organizations; sliding fee schedules; and private donations. The one thing common to most of these programs is that they are typically underfunded relative to public need and demand.

Insurance is a major determinant of oral health care utilization. Most full-time employees in medium-sized and large businesses are covered for at least some oral health care benefits, but fewer small businesses offer such benefits. Although more than 14% of children younger than 18 have no form of public or private medical insurance, more than twice as many—23 million children—have no dental insurance.[13] Although more than 15% of persons aged 18 and older have no form of medical insurance, three times as many—more than 85 million persons—have no form of dental insurance.[14]

Health insurance plans can be broadly divided into two large categories: (1) indemnity plans (also referred to as reimbursement plans), and (2) managed care plans. With indemnity plans, the insurer pays a specific amount for a specific service or set of services; therefore, these plans are often referred to as fee-for-service plans.

There are three basic types of managed care plans: (1) health maintenance organizations (HMOs), (2) preferred provider organizations (PPOs), and (3) point-of-service (POS) plans. See Box 2-3 for definitions of these managed care plans. All managed care plans involve an arrangement between the insurer and a selected network of health care providers. All offer policyholders financial incentives to use the providers in that network. There are usually specific standards for selecting providers and formal steps to ensure that quality care is delivered.

When managed care programs first began in the 1940s, an underlying principle was that pro-

BOX 2-3 Basic Types of Managed Care Plans

Health Maintenance Organizations (HMOs)
HMOs, or their dental equivalents (dental maintenance organizations [DMOs] or dental health maintenance organizations [DHMOs]), provide health care services on a prepaid basis, meaning that HMO/DMO members pay a fixed monthly fee, regardless of how much care is needed in a given month. In most cases, HMO/DMO members must receive their care from providers and facilities within the HMO/DMO network.

Preferred Provider Organizations (PPOs)
PPOs are plans under which patients select a provider from a network or list of providers who have agreed, by contract, to discount their fees. In PPOs that allow patients to receive treatment from a nonparticipating provider, patients will be penalized with higher deductibles and copayments. PPOs are usually less expensive than comparable indemnity plans.

Point-of-Service (POS) Plans
POS plans are arrangements in which patients with a managed care plan have the option of seeking treatment from an "out-of-network" provider. The reimbursement for the patient is usually based on a low table of allowances, with significantly reduced benefits than if the patient had selected an "in-network" provider.

viding and paying for preventive services would ultimately reduce the costs of health care. Even today, many managed care plans are in the forefront of prevention and offer wellness and other preventive programs that traditional indemnity insurance plans may not cover.

Managed care plans are typically paid a fixed amount per enrollee per month, regardless of whether that individual actually uses the services the plan offers. This arrangement is referred to as **capitation.** Although the plans themselves are capitated, providers participating in the plans may be reimbursed in several different ways (e.g., they may also receive a capitation fee, but they may also be paid fee-for-service or be salaried by the plan).

In many managed care plans, a primary care provider (e.g., pediatrician, family practitioner, general dentist, and, sometimes, pediatric dentist) controls referral to specialists (i.e., the patient cannot independently see a specialist). This is referred to as the **gatekeeper** function.

ORAL HEALTH INFRASTRUCTURE AND INTEGRATION WITH PUBLIC HEALTH

Infrastructure at the National, State, and Local Levels

As noted in the Surgeon General's Report on Oral Health and A National Call to Action, the lack of personnel with oral health expertise at all levels in public health programs remains a serious problem and, ultimately, may result in a decline in the public's health. Oral Health America, a national nonprofit organization, has issued an Oral Health Report Card for states since 2000, using the categories of Prevention, Access to Care, Oral Health Infrastructure, Health Status, and State Policies.[15] During that period, the national average has remained a C, reflecting that much work still needs to be done to reduce oral health disparities and to improve the **oral health infrastructure**—those programs and people who assure the public's oral health. State and local oral health programs vary in funding sources, staffing patterns, and range of activities. Differences in state oral health programs

are reflected in the ASTDD annual Synopses of State and Territorial Dental Public Health Programs. Reports about dental public health "best practice" approaches to improve the infrastructure can be accessed through the ASTDD Best Practices Web site.

Workforce

Recruiting members of underrepresented ethnic groups into oral health and allied health professions and, therefore, into dental public health positions has been difficult. For example, recruitment continues to be a problem for the Indian Health Service and for tribal clinics that want to hire members of their own communities.

Student indebtedness plays a major role in decisions to enter dental school and then to work in private practice or in public health. In 2002, the mean graduating debt of dental students was $107,503.[8] About 29% of the graduating seniors in 2002 reported use of Health Professions Student Loans and 6.5% received scholarships from one of the uniformed services, the Indian Health Service, or the National Health Service Corps. Only 5.7% reported they would be participating in a federal or state **loan forgiveness program.** Unfortunately, graduates who practice in the National Health Service Corps or the Indian Health Service to pay off student loans or scholarship obligations often leave after their obligations are finished.

Lower salaries for university faculty and public health positions have deterred some dental and dental hygiene graduates from pursuing these options, despite other benefits that they gain. Only about 9% of students planned on entering government service immediately on graduation; declines were noted in the percentage of ethnic minorities who planned on doing so.[8] When asked about long-term plans for practice, 1.6% indicated they would practice in government service and 1.5% indicated teaching/administration or research. Only 0.1% of the seniors had applied for further education in the specialty of dental public health.

Only about 145 dentists are board certified in dental public health.

Options for dental hygiene and dental assisting graduates to pursue advanced education in dental public health are limited, although some possess MPH or DrPH degrees. Many do not wish to enroll in a formal degree program but would rather work part-time or full-time and pursue a specialty certificate or participate in a fellowship or residency program. Northeast Wisconsin Technical College has initiated an online community dental health certificate program to help fill this gap. ADHA's public health council may partner with other organizations to create additional options and career tracks.

Public health agencies are experiencing a void in the number of experienced dental public health professionals who can fill management or policy positions. Numerous national organizations and government agencies are trying to alleviate this situation by promoting **leadership development** through already existing leadership institutes, public policy fellowships, or by creating new opportunities for skill development in public health, management, and information technology.

Integration of Oral Health into General Health and Public Health

The Surgeon General's Report, Oral Health in America, called for the **integration of oral health and general health**—thinking of the mouth as an integral part of the whole body rather than as "separate territory" that only dental professionals can enter.[3] This concept is important for assuring the sustainability of community-based oral health programs. Oral health concepts can be integrated into and funded by programs on nutrition, cancer, HIV/AIDS, osteoporosis, birth defects, diabetes and cardiovascular disease prevention, tobacco cessation, prenatal counseling, school-readiness initiatives, efforts to maintain the functional status of the elderly, and military readiness for action.

Integrating primary medical care and oral health care to prevent oral disease in young children is the focus of numerous collaborative projects and publications. In 1994, the National Center for Education in Maternal and Child Health published *Bright Futures: Guidelines for Health Supervision of Infants, Children, and Adolescents,* a framework for health professionals to provide developmentally appropriate health promotion and disease prevention services to children and their families.[16] *Bright Futures in Practice: Oral Health* followed in 1996 to help oral health and other health care professionals address the oral health needs of children within this framework.[17] New editions will be introduced periodically to reflect advances in science and new models of education. The basis for these guidelines is (1) **risk assessment**—assessment of risk factors and protective factors for dental caries, periodontal disease, malocclusion, and oral injury, and (2) **anticipatory guidance**—counseling families about their children's current oral health status and what to expect at upcoming developmental stages. This approach now has been adopted by many groups and is becoming the cornerstone of clinical and community-based infant and child oral care programs.

Other models for integration include: (1) teaching general dentists the skills to treat young children and recognize other childhood health problems, (2) promoting a child's first oral health assessment/dental visit by age one, (3) assuring that each child has a "medical home" and a "**dental home**"—a continuous, accessible source of care, (4) incorporating oral health screening/referral, education, and fluoride varnishes into primary care and well child visits, and (5) increasing interprofessional education and communication via the Internet. Head Start is an example of a national program that promotes such integration.

Mobilizing Assets Through Coalition Building

The role of government in health care has always been a contentious issue and continues to be a focus of arguments on covering the uninsured, prescription drug benefits, cutbacks in Medicaid services, and laws/regulations governing the health care industry. Many public health professionals and members of advocacy groups have turned to community-based solutions to solve health issues and have applied practices from other cultures and countries to arrive at new approaches. The concepts "Think globally; act locally" and "It takes a village to raise a child" are readily applicable to today's crises in health care and oral health care.

Communities are recognizing the need for broad and diverse input into promotion of oral health and provision of oral health services, where anyone, not just oral health professionals or government employees, can have a role. They realize that coordination of health, education, social and other services is needed to ensure healthy individuals and healthy communities. Public/private partnerships, **community coalitions,** and volunteerism are now the primary focus of many funding streams from foundations and government agencies. Staff of state oral health programs who are frustrated with the slowness of bureaucracy and an inability to advocate directly with lawmakers are experiencing new successes when community groups advocate for improvements in oral health and leverage various resources to fund and implement programs. Oral health coalitions have helped initiate significant changes in legislation, regulations that impact dental hygiene practice and public financing of care, and promotion of community-based preventive programs. Recent communication efforts have focused on increasing the general public's knowledge of oral health, including strategies to advocate with policymakers and legislators for public policy changes and increased resources. To show their commitment to oral health, the National Governors' Association funded a series of Oral Health Policy Academies from 2000-2001 that enabled 21 states to follow a structured approach to the development of state oral health action plans. The National Council of State Legislatures has also held conferences on various issues related to access to oral health care and oral health workforce needs.

APPLICATION OF TECHNOLOGY AND SCIENTIFIC RESEARCH

Influence of Information Technology

Health professionals today are inundated with information that affects the way they practice. Many older professionals are challenged by computers and find it difficult to learn new communication systems, putting them at a disadvantage for keeping professionally current. Rapid dissemination of information in various formats through electronic media, particularly the Internet, is enabling people to learn about innovations in a timely manner and to share them with others. Health professionals often are in the difficult position of trying to keep ahead of consumer knowledge levels, answer questions based on reliable information, and correct misperceptions. Unfortunately, increased consumer expectation of practitioner knowledge and skills has contributed to a litigious society, with clinicians paying high malpractice premiums and adopting a defensive mind-set. On a more positive note, people are more aware of their rights and responsibilities as health care consumers. People with difficulty understanding and navigating the health care system and communicating with their providers now have more opportunities to find helpful resources. All of these factors are changing the way health professionals and consumers communicate.

Health Communication Strategies

New health communication strategies are slowly being incorporated into public health approaches to improving oral health. **Health communication** is the "study and use of communication strategies to inform and influence individual and community decisions that enhance health." Its emerging importance is reflected in its inclusion as a separate focus area in Healthy People 2010.[4] Two health communication strategies that are used in public health are (1) **social marketing,** a technique used to increase public awareness of the relationship of behaviors to diseases and to influence people to take action,[18] and (2) **media advocacy,** the strategic use of various media outlets and formats to increase awareness and knowledge of issues.[19] These concepts are discussed in more depth in Chapter 9.

FrameWorks Institute has used these techniques in research on oral health for more than 5 years, examining public understanding of children's oral health to help engage and mobilize advocates and the general public to address this issue. Using this research, funded by the Washington Dental Service and others, FrameWorks designed and managed a public campaign on oral health for children in the state of Washington. The "Watch Your Mouth" campaign has now become a model for replication in other states and communities.[20]

Other strategies in the United States attempt to address the health needs of people with limited English language skills. The National Literacy Act of 1991 defined **literacy** as ". . . ability to read, write, and speak in English and compute and solve problems at levels of proficiency necessary to function on the job and in society, to achieve one's goals, and develop one's knowledge and potential."[21] In 2000, 45% of the adult U.S. population read at an eighth grade level or lower. About 45% of English-speaking adults are estimated to have limited literacy skills that interfere with their ability to handle basic skills involved in seeking and receiving health care.[22] Health literacy is important for learning oral health knowledge, completing health applications and forms, following health recommendations, purchasing oral health care products, promoting oral health to others, communicating with oral health care providers, and navigating various aspects of an oral health care system. One model for improving health literacy is to integrate health concepts and skills into adult education, General Educational Degree (GED) programs, and English as a Second Language (ESL) classes. A recent trend, particularly in government and in public health, is the **plain language movement.**[23] Although there is no standard definition, it means that people who use

documents written in plain language can quickly and easily (1) find what they need, (2) understand what they find, and (3) act on that understanding.

All of these strategies emphasize the importance of identifying appropriate communication and health promotion approaches for each audience. Because the "one size fits all" approach does not work, programs must learn how to customize their messages and approaches to different groups to be culturally relevant. There continues to be a lack of evidence for the effectiveness of oral health education and health promotion to improve oral health.[24] Evaluating effectiveness and efficiency of interventions, therefore, has assumed more importance so that oral health promotion efforts can be more evidence-based. Resources that programs can use to plan and manage health communication programs are included in Box 2-4. Additional information on creating appropriate communication tools will be presented in Chapter 10.

Evidence-Based Practice

In the last decade, evidence-based health care has served as a catalyst for new avenues for health services research and a focus on health outcomes. The goal of **evidence-based practice** is to facilitate timely translation of research findings into clinical and community practices that result in improved oral health. This requires a decision-making process based on integration of new evidence for effectiveness with expert opinion, clinical and community experience, and professional judgment. Various barriers exist, however, to prevent widespread use of this approach in clinical or certain public health settings (Box 2-5).

Research on diffusion of innovations demonstrates that it takes at least 10 years for practitioners to adopt new materials or techniques.[26] Research on many new clinical and preventive techniques has not yet been translated to their use with various population groups in private practice or public health settings. Before evidence-based practice can be fully implemented in clinical and

BOX 2-4   Helpful Publications

Berkowitz B, Wolff T. The spirit of the coalition. Washington, DC: American Public Health Association, 2000.

CDCynergy 2001. Your guide to effective health communication. Available at: http://www.cdc.gov/communication/cdcynergy.htm.

Centers for Disease Control and Prevention. Scientific and Technical Information. Simply Put. 2nd Ed. Atlanta, GA: CDC, 1999. Available at: http://www.cdc.gov/od/oc/simpput.pdf.

The interface between medicine and dentistry in meeting the oral health needs of young children. Washington, DC: Children's Dental Health Project, 2003. Available at: http://www.cdhp.org.

Crall JJ, Edelstein BL. Examples of state efforts to improve oral health and access. Available at: http://www.cthealth.org.

Institute of Medicine. Speaking of Health: Assessing Health Communication Strategies for Diverse Populations. Washington, DC: The National Academies Press, 2002. Available at: http://www.nap.edu/catalog/10018.html.

Isman B. Get into the race to get people healthy. Contemp Oral Hyg 2003;3(1)26–27.

Making health communication programs work. NIH Publication No. 02-5145.2002. Available at: http://cissecure.nci.nih.gov/ncipubs/details.asp?pid=209.

Community roots for oral health. Guidelines for successful coalitions. Olympia, WA: Washington State Department of Health, 2000. Available at: http://www.cdc.gov/oralhealth/library.

Writing and designing print materials for beneficiaries: A guide for state medicaid agencies. Health Care Financing Administration (CMS) Pub. #10145, October 1999.

BOX 2-5   Barriers to Implementing Evidence-Based Dentistry

- Insufficient research or inconclusive evidence
- Poor quality research
- Inadequate or ineffective dissemination of evidence
- Faculty not basing their teaching on evidence-based approaches
- Clinicians not reading or hearing about new research or not wanting to learn the new skills
- Expecting clinicians to document and evaluate clinical oral health outcomes for their patients
- Convincing third-party payers to reimburse based on new practice guidelines
- Implementing standard diagnostic codes.

Adapted from Mertz B, Manuel-Barkin C, Isman B, O'Neil E. Improving oral health care systems in California. San Francisco, CA: UCSF Center for the Health Professions, 2000.[25]

public health settings, however, additional research is needed, especially to develop reliable and valid measures of oral health outcomes. The ADHA has recognized the importance of this type of practice, sponsoring the Fourth National Research Conference in 2000, devoted entirely to evidence-based approaches.[27] The Cochrane Oral Health Group, one of several groups that perform evidence-based reviews, has completed a number of oral health reviews. Additional information about evidence-based oral health promotion programs is found in Chapter 8.

SUMMARY

Many trends in the field of dentistry, dental hygiene, and public health create challenges for students and professionals who wish to work in the field of dental public health. Major challenges include reducing oral health disparities, increasing access to preventive services and oral health care, integrating oral health into general health and public health efforts, mobilizing assets through new collaborations and community partnerships, and using new technologies and evidence-based practices.

New skills that are needed to meet future dental public health challenges include

- Interdisciplinary teams: working with new partners such as social scientists, epidemiologists, evaluation specialists, and multimedia specialists.
- Community coalition building: increasing support and ownership for oral health programs,

 Learning Activities

1. Use one chapter or a section of a chapter in the Healthy People 2010 Oral Health Toolkit and design a lesson plan for teaching a General Educational Development (GED) class about the Healthy People initiative and the oral health objectives.

2. Choose one of five actions cited in the National Call to Action to Promote Oral Health, and discuss ways that you or your class can "answer the call."

3. Find oral health statistics for your community or state. Compare statistics from 10 to 20 years ago to more recent statistics. How have they changed? What do you think contributed to these changes?

4. Check to see if your state has held a dental summit or Head Start oral health forum. If so, review the proceedings, action plan, and recommendations. Present to your class what barriers to care were identified and what the recommended actions were to address the problems. Discuss roles that dental hygiene students and practicing dental hygienists can play in implementing the recommendations.

5. Interview someone in the state Medicaid program about how enrollment of families, enrollment of dental providers, and coverage and reimbursement rates for various oral health services have changed in the last 5 years.

6. View the ASTDD Synopses of State and Territorial Dental Public Health Programs and compare four states on such characteristics as population, infrastructure, dental director's time, funding sources, and range of programmatic activities.

7. Develop recruitment tools to interest underrepresented ethnic groups in public health professions, especially dental public health.

8. Interview the state oral health program director, a member of the state staff, or a city or county dental director to learn ways that oral health is integrated into other health programs and activities.

9. Interview a dental researcher or a member of the dental hygiene faculty. Ask how advances in science and technology have changed the way they do research, access information, and teach in the past 5 to 10 years.

10. Use one or more of the health communication resources listed in this chapter and critique some of the health promotion approaches or materials that are used in community-based programs.

creating solutions to local issues, and assuring sustainability of programs.

- New communication channels: learning to design and disseminate key messages to different target audiences using new technologies.
- Outcome-based evaluation: looking at the impact of programs on oral health rather than just program logistics and numbers of people served.
- Management of young professionals: relating to a group that expects participatory decision making and has different communication skills and styles.
- Methods for imparting dental public health history and experience: making the lessons of the past relevant to the present and the future.

RESOURCES

Box 2-2 lists Web sites and Box 2-4 lists publications mentioned in the text, as well as additional resources that provide valuable information.

Review Questions

1. Which of the following persons is least likely to have difficulty accessing dental care?
   a. A frail, elderly woman who is homebound
   b. A 20-year-old, male, Hispanic, migrant agricultural worker
   c. A 40-year-old female American Indian in an isolated Alaskan village
   d. A 59-year-old state government worker
   e. A 2-year-old who lives in a single-parent family with his five brothers and is eligible for but not enrolled in Medicaid

2. Which of the following is NOT a true statement?
   a. Dental caries is the single most common chronic children's disease.
   b. Over 50% of child abuse cases involve head and oral facial trauma.
   c. Uninsured children are 2.5 times less likely than insured children to receive dental care.

   d. Less than 200 school hours are lost to dental-related illness each year.
   e. African American males have the highest incidence of oral and pharyngeal cancers in the United States and their 5-year survival rates are lower than the rest of the population.

3. The Surgeon General's Report, A National Call to Action to Promote Oral Health, covers five actions. Which of the following is NOT one of the actions?
   a. Change public perceptions of oral health
   b. Increase oral health workforce diversity, capacity, and flexibility
   c. Build the science base and accelerate science transfer
   d. Overcome barriers by replicating effective programs and proven efforts
   e. Promote more disciplinary rather than interdisciplinary collaborations

4. Which of the following is NOT an example of a national effort that involved collaboration of various partners?
   a. National Call to Action to Promote Oral Health
   b. The Surgeon General's Report, Oral Health in America
   c. National Oral Health Surveillance System
   d. Centers for Research to Reduce Oral Health Disparities
   e. Cincinnati Community Health Center

5. All of the following trends may increase access to care EXCEPT:
   a. teledentistry.
   b. mobile and portable dentistry.
   c. making Medicaid an entitlement program for children.
   d. less restrictive dental and dental hygiene state practice acts.
   e. volunteerism.

6. Which of the following is an accurate representation of a current dental public health workforce issue?

a. Ethnic representation in the dental public health workforce does not mirror representation in the population served by public health programs.

b. Too many graduates are applying for dental public health advanced education programs.

c. Salaries for dental public health positions are not much different than salaries in private dental or dental hygiene practice.

d. Currently, there are many options for dental hygienists to pursue advanced education or credentialing in dental public health.

e. The number of dental professionals applying for government jobs has increased in the past few years.

7. All of the following are considered barriers to implementing evidence-based dental public health practice EXCEPT:

a. the time it takes for practitioners to adopt new research.

b. the translation of techniques used successfully in private practice with individual patients to a community-based population approach.

c. not having enough scientists to review previous studies.

d. the lack of funded oral health research in community-based settings.

e. convincing third-party payers to reimburse based on new practice guidelines.

REFERENCES

1. American Dental Education Association. Competencies for entry into the profession of dental hygiene, exhibit 7. J Dent Educ 2003;67(7)1–5. Available at: http//www.adea.org/cepr. Accessed January 2004.

2. A plan to eliminate craniofacial, oral, and dental health disparities. National Institute of Dental and Craniofacial Research, 2002. Rockville, MD: DHHS, NIH, NIDCR. Available at: http://www.nidcr.nih.gov/research/healthdisp/hdplan.pdf. Accessed February 2004.

3. Oral Health in America: A Report of the Surgeon General. Rockville, MD: Department of Health & Human Services (DHHS), National Institute of Dental and Craniofacial Research. (NIDCR), National Institutes of Health (NIH), 2000. Available at: http://www.surgeongeneral. gov/

library/oralhealth/default.htm. Accessed February 2004.

4. Healthy People 2010: Objectives for Improving Health. Washington, DC: U.S. Government Printing Office, 2001. Available at: http://www. healthypeople.gov. Accessed February 2004.

5. Healthy People 2010 Oral Health Toolkit. Bethesda, MD: NIDCR, NIH, 2004. Available at: http://www.nidcr.nih.gov.

6. A national call to action to promote oral health. Rockville, MD: DHHS, Public Health Service (PHS), NIH, NIDCR, Spring 2003.

7. Dental care considerations of disadvantaged and special care populations. Rockville, MD: Health Resources & Services Administration (HRSA), Bureau of Health Professions, 2001.

8. Weaver RG, Haden NK, Valechovic RW. Annual ADEA survey of dental school seniors: 2002 graduating class. J Dent Educ 2002;66(12): 1388–1404.

9. Valachovic RW, Weaver RG, Sinkford JC, Haden NK. Trends in dentistry and dental education. J Dent Educ 2001;65(6):539–561.

10. Jacobs EA, Goldin GI. A Volunteers in Health Care Guide to Overcoming Language Barriers. Part I: For clinicians. Pawtucket, RI: Volunteers in Health Care, 2002. Available at: http://www.volunteersinhealthcare.org/manuals/VIH.Lang.Barriers.Manual.pdf. Accessed February 2004.

11. The future of oral health. Trends and issues. 2003. American Dental Hygienists' Association. Available at: http://www.adha.org/downloads/future_of_oral_health.pdf. Accessed February 2004.

12. National health care expenditures projections: 2002–2012. Centers for Medicare and Medicaid Services. Available at: http://cms.hhs.gov/statistics/nhe/projections-2002/proj2002.pdf. Accessed February 2004.

13. Vargas CM, Isman RE, Crall JJ. Comparison of children's medical and dental insurance coverage by socioeconomic characteristics, United States, 1995. J Public Health Dent 2002;62(1): 38–44.

14. National Health Interview Survey (NHIS) 1995. Data tabulated by the Office of Analysis, Epidemiology, and Health Promotion. Atlanta, GA: National Center for Health Statistics (NCHS), Centers for Disease Control and Prevention, 2000.

15. Keep America Smiling. Oral Health in America. Chicago, IL: Oral Health America, 2003.

16. Green M, ed. Bright Futures: Guidelines for Health Supervision of Infants, Children, and Adolescents. Arlington, VA: National Center for Education in Maternal and Child Health, 1994.

17. Casamassimo P. Bright Futures in Practice: Oral Health. Arlington, VA: National Center for Education in Maternal and Child Health, 1996.

18. Bolig R. Social marketing and health communications. Am J Health Commun 1997; Spring: 12–16.

19. Wallach L, Dorfman L. Media advocacy: A strategy for advancing policy and promoting health. Health Educ Q 1996;23(3):293–317.

20. Children's Oral Health. Kids Count E-Zine. FrameWorks Institute, 2003, No. 2. Available at: http://www.frameworksinstitute.org/clients/oralhealth.shtml. Accessed February 2004.

21. PL 1-2-73. The National Literacy Act of 1991. July 25, 1991.

22. Scott BS. Low literacy: A health care quality issue. Closing the Gap 2003;Jan/Feb:14–15.

23. Locke J. The plain language movement. Am Med Writers Assoc J 2003;18(1):5–8.

24. Kay E, Locker D. Effectiveness of oral health promotion: A review. London, England: Health Education Authority, 1999.

25. Mertz B, Manuel-Barkin C, Isman B, O'Neil E. Improving oral health care systems in California. San Francisco, CA: UCSF Center for the Health Professions, 2000.

26. Rogers EM. Diffusion of Innovations, 3rd Ed. New York: The Free Press, 1983.

27. Fourth National Research Conference: An Evidence-Based Approach in Dental Hygiene Practice, Education, and Research. J Dent Hyg (online Suppl.), Spring 2001. Available at: http://www. adha.org/publications/nrc. Accessed February 2004.

Global Perspectives of Oral Health

3

Objectives

After studying this chapter and completing the study questions and activities, the learner will be able to:

- Identify three major barriers to health care.
- Understand the development and education of nondentist providers around the world.
- Describe different models for the use of nondentist providers in public health.
- Discuss the relationship between socioeconomic position and oral health disparities.

KEY TERMS

Aboriginal health worker
Atraumatic restorative technique
    (ART)
Dental nurse

Dental therapist
Financial barrier
Health disparities
Indian Health Service

Midlevel provider
Personal/cultural barrier
Socioeconomic position
Structural barrier

The American Dental Education Association competencies addressed in this chapter include[1]:

C.2:   Adhere to state and federal laws, recommendations, and regulations in the provision of dental hygiene care.

C.3:   Provide dental hygiene care to promote patient/client health and wellness using critical thinking and problem solving in the provision of evidence-based practice.

CM.1:   Assess the oral health needs of the community and the quality and availability of resources and services.

CM.4:   Facilitate client access to oral health services by influencing individuals and/or organizations for the provision of oral health care.

PGD.1:   Identify alternative career options within health care, industry, education, and research and evaluate the feasibility of pursuing dental hygiene opportunities.

Introduction

Chapter 1 introduced the concept of public health; Chapter 2 identified trends and disparities in public health. Oral health care is an evolutionary process influenced by oral health needs, financial resources, and manpower supplies. Like most **health disparities,** oral health is directly related to **socioeconomic position.**

This chapter outlines global oral health problems and prevention efforts. It is important to expose the learner to health care models beyond the borders of their own delivery systems. Various countries have developed alternative methods of delivering oral health care to meet the oral health needs of that country. Provider shortages and high rates of dental disease have led to educating nondental providers to perform basic restorative and emergency care procedures, easing the burden on the dentist provider. Some countries have developed alternate methods of fluoride delivery to address oral health. In the United States, some states have revised state practice acts to allow dental hygienists to perform specific procedures under general supervision or unsupervised in settings where people have limited access to care. These settings include community clinics, nursing homes, and other programs and facilities serving high risk or disadvantaged populations (e.g., children, people of lower socioeconomic position, older adults, and people with disabilities).

The World Health Organization's (WHO) World Oral Health Report 2003 indicated that because of the high prevalence and incidence in all regions of the world, oral disease is a major public health problem.[2] Many changing disease patterns are linked to changing lifestyles that include diets rich in sugar, widespread use of tobacco, and increased consumption of alcohol. The report also stated that traditional treatment of oral disease is costly in several industrialized countries and not feasible or possible in most low- and middle-income countries.

BARRIERS TO CARE

Barriers to oral health care can take many forms. The barriers may be **structural, financial,** and/or **personal/cultural.** Structural barriers are related to the number, type, concentration, location, or organizational configuration of health care providers. Providers face barriers and economic challenges to developing practices in low-income areas. Many providers have large loan debts, and the cost of establishing a practice in low-income areas can be tremendous. Public programs and community health care facilities are seeing rapidly increasing caseloads as the result of the high cost of oral health care in the private practice sector, decreasing numbers of providers accepting Medicaid, and a broader definition of dental indigence.

Financial barriers limit access because of a patient's inability to pay for a service or providers who choose not to provide care for those with limited finances. Currently, in the United States, millions of Americans do not have dental insurance coverage, making access to care more difficult.

Personal/cultural barriers inhibit patients from seeking care or following provider recommendations based on personal or cultural beliefs. These beliefs include fear of providers of different cultural backgrounds and races, fear of the system, belief in their own healers, and culturally accepted attitudes and beliefs. For example, children on many reservations receiving care from the **Indian Health Service** want "silver teeth" or stainless steel crowns on their front teeth, while children from another cultural background may prefer a different treatment.

ORAL HEALTH THROUGHOUT THE WORLD

Oral disease is one of the most prevalent problems throughout the world. Dental caries and periodontal disease represent most of the problem, but edentulism, oral cancer, orodental trauma, maloc-

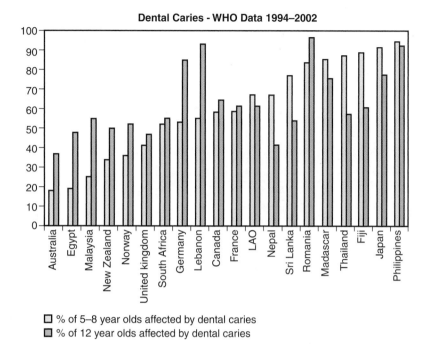

FIGURE 3-1 The Percentage of Children With Dental Caries in the World Population. Source: World Health Organization. Global Oral Health Data Bank. Geneva, Switzerland: World Health Organization, 2002. Available at: http://www.whocollab.od.mah.se/index.html.)[3]

clusion, and craniofacial anomalies also contribute. Dental caries affect 60 to 90% of schoolchildren and the majority of adults (Fig. 3-1).[3,4] Severe periodontitis, which may lead to tooth loss, affects 5 to 15% of most populations.[4] Edentulousness ranges from 6 to 78% among countries around the world (Fig. 3-2).[3,4] Oral and pharyngeal cancers are related to tobacco and alcohol use and vary dramatically by country.

This high prevalence of oral disease has the greatest effect on disadvantaged populations that have limited access to care. However, common, modifiable risk factors provide opportunities for reducing this burden. Health promotion programs for other diseases in which lifestyle choices are emphasized may also directly or indirectly promote oral health. In addition, the development of nondentist providers and various models of care delivery have developed in response to oral disease problems.

DEVELOPMENT OF NONDENTIST PROVIDERS

Currently, across the world, nondentist providers are being educated and used to perform many procedures that are restricted to the dentist in many health care systems. More than 30 countries worldwide have developed dental therapists or dental nurses to provide basic restorative care; extraction of primary and, in some instances, permanent teeth; pulpotomies and stainless steel crowns; and, in some countries, basic orthodontics. Educational programs range from 6 months to a little longer than 2 years—at a fraction of the cost of educating a dentist. These countries, realizing that there were problems with access to care and limited financial resources, have found successful methods of meeting the needs of the people.

One might question the quality of these programs and whether or not care from these

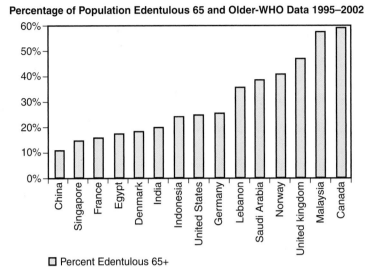

FIGURE 3-2 The Percentage of the World Population Edentulous at Age 65.
Source: World Health Organization. Global Oral Health Data Bank. Geneva, Switzerland: World
Health Organization, 2002. Available at: http://www.whocollab.od.mah.se/index.html.)[3]

providers is of the quality expected by the public. Studies reviewing the quality of care have been supportive, and access to oral health care has increased in countries such as New Zealand, where up to 95% of school-aged children receive care.

The type of dental services delivered by nondentist providers in many countries is varied. Table 3-1 illustrates the diversity of treatment provided by **dental nurses/dental therapists** in 13 countries. In reviewing studies that described the type of treatment provided by dental nurses in other countries, seven countries include diagnosis and treatment planning. Dental nurses in all 13 countries are permitted to extract deciduous teeth, and dental nurses in 7 of 13 countries are allowed to extract permanent teeth. Dental nurses in 11 of the countries are able to prepare teeth for restorations and place composite or amalgam restorations. Only Cambodia limits dental nurses to placing temporary restorations. Furthermore, eight countries allow emergency care to people of all ages to be rendered by a dental nurse. New Zealand limits emergency care by dental nurses to patients who are aged 14 years or younger, while dental nurses in Singapore are able to provide emergency care to patients who are be-

tween the ages of 4–12 years. Dental nurses in 12 countries are able to provide local anesthetic, and dental cleaning and oral hygiene instruction are provided in all countries.

In addition to the 13 countries listed in Table 3-1, 17 other countries are using dental nurses. These countries include Brunei, Burma, Ceylon, Costa Rica, Ghana, Haiti, Hong Kong, Italy, Paraguay, Senegal, Sierra Leone, Sudan, South Vietnam, Taiwan, Uganda, Sri Lanka, and Zambia.

United States

Although the oral health of the United States' population has improved significantly during the last 30 years as a result of community water fluoridation and sealants, a large population of people exists whose needs are not being met. Low-income minority children continue to have high rates of oral disease and poorer oral health. These disparities exist because of limited access to services by low-income populations. This access is generally affected by low dentist participation in Medicaid programs, an overall shortage of dentists to meet the needs of the population, restrictive state laws prohibiting the use of

TABLE 3-1 DENTAL PROCEDURES PERFORMED BY NONDENTIST PROVIDERS

COUNTRY	X-DECID	X-PERM	PREP TEETH	PL COMPO	PL AMAL	EMERG TX	L ANES	SCALE	OHI	DIAGNOSE	PULPOT	SSC
New Zealand	yes	no	yes	yes	yes	yes, up to age 14	yes	yes	yes	yes	no	no
Canada	yes	yes	yes	yes	yes	yes	yes	yes	yes	no	yes	yes
Papua New Guinea	yes	yes	?	?	?	yes	?	yes	yes	?	?	?
Malaysia	yes	no	yes	yes	yes	yes	yes	yes	yes	no	no	no
United Kingdom	yes	no	yes	yes	yes	no	yes	yes	yes	no	no	no
Australia	yes	no	yes	yes	yes	yes	yes	yes	yes	yes	yes	yes
Colombia	yes	yes	yes	yes	yes	?	yes	yes	yes	no	?	?
Singapore	yes	no	yes	yes	yes	yes, age 4–12	yes	yes	yes	yes	no	no
Thailand	yes	no	yes	yes	yes	yes	yes	yes	yes	yes	no	no
Jamaica	yes	yes	yes	yes	yes	yes	yes	yes	yes	yes	?	?
Cuba	yes	yes	yes	yes	yes	?	yes	yes	yes	no	?	?
Africa	yes	yes	yes	yes	yes	yes	yes	yes	yes	yes	?	?
Cambodia	yes	yes	no	ART	no	yes	yes	yes	yes	yes	no	no

Key:

X-Decid = extract deciduous
X-Perm = extract permanent
Prep Teeth = prepare teeth
Pl Compo = place composites
Emerg Tx = emergency treatment
L Anes = local anesthetic

Scale = scale teeth
OHI = oral hygiene instruction
Diagnose = diagnose oral disease
Pulpot = pulpotomy
SSC = place stainless steel crown
ART = atraumatic restorative technique

nondentist providers, lack of oral health insurance for patients, and lack of patient awareness and understanding.[5]

The dental nurse concept was experimented with in the United States in the early 1970s. Four expanded-function dental hygiene programs were developed in conjunction with dental hygiene educational programs. This research demonstrated no significant difference in performance between the expanded functions of dental hygiene students and dental students. Since the 1970s, additional research has not been pursued.

More recently, certain states have changed their dental practice acts and initiated alternative models of care using dental hygienists. Connecticut developed an alternative model allowing dental hygienists with at least 2 years experience to provide care in public health facilities without a dentist's supervision. In New Mexico, an alternative model was developed as a "collaborative" practice; a dental hygienist may develop a collaborative agreement with one or more consulting dentists. South Carolina allows licensed dental hygienists to provide selected services in public health settings without prior authorization from a dentist, including screenings, oral prophylaxis, and sealants. Dental hygienists may provide additional treatment after receiving authorization from a consulting dentist.[5] Other states that have expanded dental hygiene practice include Minnesota,

Montana, Oregon, and Washington. In addition, certain government public health service agencies, such as the Indian Health Service, are developing alternative models of oral health care delivery. Community health care workers from remote villages in Alaska have been sent to New Zealand to attend the dental nurse educational program.

Canada

The Canadian dental therapist program was established in 1972 following a 3-year pilot program in 1968. This 3-year educational program is unique because dental therapists are provided education in interceptive orthodontics, child development, children's emotional response, and public speaking, as well as preparing teeth and placement of restorative materials, extracting permanent and deciduous teeth, providing local anesthetic, and providing preventive and periodontal treatment.[6]

New Zealand

New Zealand was the first country to use nondentist personnel, specifically dental nurses, to help with the acute shortage of dentists and high oral disease rates. After an intense 2-year educational program, dental nurses can extract deciduous teeth, prepare and place composite and amalgam restorations, administer local anesthetic, diagnose oral disease, provide oral health instruction, and provide oral cleanings to children aged 4 to 12. In addition, they can provide emergency care for children up to 14 years of age. This care is provided under the general supervision of the supervisory dentist. Programs are visited monthly by supervisory dental nurses to assess the quality of oral health care being rendered, record keeping, and grooming.

The introduction of the dental nurse by the New Zealand Dental Association brought strong opposition and was described "a menace to the public" and an "injustice to prospective dental students."[7] Consideration and development of the dental nurse began in 1914 during World War I. A significant percentage of military recruits were rejected because of dental problems, and 90% of the children suffered from dental disorders. This prompted the government to take action and, in 1921, the first dental nurse educational program began. By 1941, the Manpower Regulation Act declared dental nurses an "essential" occupation.[7] It is interesting to note that these programs were set up as individual schools and not part of a university. Dental nurses are not taught to use x-rays and are not permitted to use medical and dental libraries in an attempt to prevent students from learning and trying techniques that are not taught or prescribed by the program. The employment of dental nurses is restricted to the government.[8]

The New Zealand government believes that health care is the right of every citizen rather than a luxury.[9] Currently, the program is completely voluntary, and 60% of preschool and 95% of school children use the services of the school dental nurse. In 1925, 78.6 teeth were extracted per 100 teeth filled compared with 2.5 teeth extracted per 100 filled in1974.[9] This program has become so successful at saving children's teeth that the extraction of permanent teeth is no longer taught.[9] This program has been so successful that more than 30 countries throughout the world have developed programs using the dental nurse concept.

Currently, New Zealand does not have any dental hygienists and dental nurses are only trained to provide preventive care to children up to the age of 12. Because of the aging population and periodontal conditions, the need for a provider similar to the dental hygienist in the United States is currently being considered.

Australia

The Australian dental therapist can be employed through the government or private practice under the direction of a dentist. The dentist is solely responsible for the dental welfare of the patient. After 2 years of education, a dental therapist can prepare teeth and place amalgam or composite materials, scale teeth, administer local anesthetic, provide oral health instruction, and take radiographs. In addition to dental therapists, the

Australian government has developed **Aboriginal health workers.**[10] Access to health care in rural and remote areas is greatly limited. Although approximately 2% of the total Australian population is aboriginal, they comprise a high percentage of the rural population. Because of limited access, aboriginal health workers were developed. Responsibilities of an aboriginal health worker include screening and assessing, managing health care equipment and facilities, and interpreting information to the patient. An oral health care component was added to the aboriginal health worker in 1979 that focuses on preventive dental education and noninvasive emergency procedures to effect pain relief.[11]

Cambodia

More than 80% of the Cambodian population lives in rural areas and does not have access to oral health care. A national survey in 1991 demonstrated high rates of dental caries and periodontal disease. Dentists were reluctant to work in these rural areas due to the lack of facilities and equipment. Working with the Ministry of Health and instituted by World Concern (an American, nongovernmental organization), the dental therapist program was developed in 1992. The program is approximately 4 to 5 months long, in addition to 1 year of basic nursing education.[12] On completion of the educational program, the dental nurses are given a set of instruments and the materials needed to provide basic preventive and curative needs, which include oral health education, local anesthetic, scaling, the **atraumatic restorative technique** (ART), and extraction of teeth.[12] This provides the population with basic care at a cost the country can afford.

Africa

The dental therapist was initiated in 1955 in Tanzania. After 3 years of education, a dental therapist can extract diseased teeth, place simple restorations, perform limited prosthetic procedures, and scale teeth. In 1979, the program was reevaluated and oral health education and treatment for school children was added.[13] Dental therapists primarily work in district hospitals and spend approximately 40% of their time providing school services, 40% providing clinical care, and 20% providing oral health education and miscellaneous administrative procedures.

Singapore

A dental nurse in Singapore provides care to children aged 4–14. The dental nurse program is a 2-year educational course; to attain certification, this is followed by 1 year of field experience under the direct supervision of a dental officer. Dental nurses perform standard cavity preparations and the placement of fillings in deciduous teeth, extractions of deciduous teeth, relief of pain, pulp capping, oral hygiene instructions, and simple scaling. They work in schools, hospitals, mobile dental clinics, and dental health education units under the professional control and supervision of a dental officer who routinely visits the clinics. A dental officer performs all initial examinations; however, the dental nurse performs subsequent routine examinations at 6-month intervals.[14]

EFFICIENCY OF ALTERNATE MODELS OF ORAL HEALTH CARE DELIVERY

Overall, studies report the cost for providing dental services by a nondentist provider as lower than that provided by a dentist. The studies also indicate that more quality services could be provided at lower cost. This cost-benefit trend has been noted in the medical profession with the introduction of **midlevel providers.** Nielson-Thompson reported that physician assistants and nurse practitioners could substitute for 63% of physician services at 38% of the physician's cost. It was also reported that nurse practitioners could effectively provide between 75 to 80% of adult primary care services and up to 90% of pediatric care services. Therefore, these professionals can provide quality care to more people at a lower cost.[15]

If the cost to train a nondentist provider who can provide definitive treatment takes one half of the time and resources necessary to train a dentist, it can be anticipated that the cost to deliver care will be lower. Soricelli reported dental nurses could increase production by 400%, cutting operating costs in half.[16] Lobene et al. concluded that nondentist providers could increase the dentist's capacity to provide quality treatment for more people at the lowest possible cost.[17] Roder investigated studies related to the New Zealand dental nurse and found the annual cost per patient was 50% less than care provided by a general dentist.[8]

Success in other countries and research in the United States clearly demonstrate that nondentist providers can be taught to provide basic restorative and emergency care. The use of nondentist providers to perform services traditionally done by the dentist can, in fact, provide greater quantity of services with higher quality at a lesser cost than has heretofore been provided. The time and cost factor to train and produce this provider amounts to a small fraction of that required to train the traditional dentist. The application of this method can be a primary factor in meeting the needs of the public, satisfying the ideal philosophy of the profession.[16]

GLOBAL PREVENTION EFFORTS

In addition to different models of care delivery, numerous countries have developed prevention and health promotion measures to reduce oral disease rates. These initiatives include community water fluoridation, fluoride supplements, fluoridated milk and salt, fluoride varnish, and xylitol gum. These prevention efforts will be described in more detail in Chapter 8.

The health disparities across regions and countries present a dynamic challenge in addressing oral disease. The WHO has developed worldwide priority action areas for oral health.[2] The first action area is centered on the use of fluorides. Not only should community water fluoridation be promoted worldwide where applicable, but also other modes of fluoride therapy, including toothpaste, milk fluoridation, and salt fluoridation, should be promoted as well.

The second action area is associated with diet, nutrition, and oral health. Many oral diseases are affected by changing lifestyles related to diet and nutrition. This is an opportunity to partner with other programs to address common risk factors for disease.

Preventing tobacco use and tobacco use cessation is a third action area. This also is an opportunity for integrating with other programs.

WHO has also targeted both ends of the age spectrum. It has launched programs in schools and with youth populations to control oral health risks for young people. In addition, the staggering growth in the older population worldwide presents a challenge, both in numbers of people and the impaired mobility to obtain access to care.

Finally, oral health systems have been targeted for improvement. These include examining various models of care delivery, developing new categories of personnel to fit a country's need, payment systems, information and surveillance systems, and building and strengthening research programs.

SUMMARY

Oral disease is one of the most prevalent diseases in the world, causing considerable morbidity, particularly for disadvantaged populations. Oral disease has many risks common to other diseases affected by lifestyles. To address these problems, many countries have developed nondentist providers to help ease the burden of care needed. In addition, the World Health Organization has set priorities for a coordinated effort for addressing oral disease and disparities worldwide.

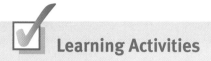
Learning Activities

1. Describe three types of barriers to health care.
2. Discuss the challenges public health dentistry faces in trying to improve access to oral health care.
3. Compare and contrast the different models of oral health care delivery systems used in the world today.
4. Describe the "perfect" model of oral health care delivery and provide reasons why.

Review Questions

1. What barriers are faced when accessing oral health care?
   a. Structural
   b. Cultural
   c. Financial
   d. Personal
   e. All of the above

2. Approximately how many countries worldwide use dental therapists or dental nurse providers to provide oral health care?
   a. 20
   b. 30
   c. 80
   d. 100
   e. 120

3. All of the following groups have limited access to oral health care EXCEPT:
   a. minorities.
   b. poor children.
   c. rural residents.
   d. people of low socioeconomic position.
   e. working professionals.

4. What organization monitors health issues on a global scale?
   a. Centers for Disease Control and Prevention
   b. European Association for Public Health
   c. Pan American Health Organization
   d. World Health Organization
   e. National Institutes of Health

5. Structural barriers to oral health include:
   a. the number, type, and distribution of health care providers.
   b. personal belief systems.
   c. fear of the oral health care system.
   d. lack of dental insurance.
   e. perceived need for care.

6. Alternative models for health care delivery:
   a. have been successful worldwide.
   b. indicate nondentist providers provide quality care.
   c. indicate nondentist providers are less expensive to educate.
   d. indicate that nondentist providers can provide care without supervision.
   e. All of the above.

REFERENCES

1. American Dental Education Association. Competencies for entry into the profession of dental hygiene, exhibit 7. J Dent Educ 2003;67(7)1–5. Available at: http://www.adea.org/cepr. Accessed February 2004.
2. Petersen PE. The World Oral Health Report 2003–Continuous Improvement of Oral Health in the 21st Century. Oral Health Programme, Noncommunicable Disease Prevention, and Health Promotion. Geneva, Switzerland: World Health Organization, 2003, p 1–45. Available at: http://www.who.int.
3. Global Oral Health Data Bank. Geneva, Switzerland: World Health Organization, 2002.

4. World Health Organization. WHO Oral Health Country/Area Profile. Available at: http://www.whocollab.od.mah.se/index.html.

5. Nolan L, Kamoe B, Harvey J, et al. The effects of state dental practice laws allowing alternative models of preventive oral health care delivery to low-income children: January 2003. Report by Center for Health Services Research and Policy.

6. Keenan GW. The Saskatchewan dental nurse: An expanded duty auxiliary. J Can Dent Assoc 1975;6:344–345.

7. West NM. The New Zealand dental nurse: Part I. Virginia Dent J 1980;57(2):40–45.

8. Roder DM. The employment of dental nurses. J Public Dent Health 1978;38(2):159–171.

9. Roberts MW. The New Zealand dental nurse program. Public Health Rev 1975;4(1):69–82.

10. Paeza T, Steele L, Tennant M. Development of oral health training for rural and remote Aboriginal health workers. Aust J Rural Health 2001;9:105–110.

11. Graebner AFH. The Western Australian dental therapist—A new member of the dental team. CAL 1975;38(8):27–28.

12. Mallow PK, Klaipo Ratanakiri M, Penh P, Durward C. Dental nurse training in Cambodia—A new approach. Int Dent J 1997;47(3):148–156.

13. Mosha HJ, Mgalula NE. Tanzania oral health workers' views on the relevance of their training to their duties. East African Med J 1996;73(7):443–447.

14. Howe R. The dental nurse program in Singapore. J Dent Educ 1975;39(8):542–543.

15. Nielsen-Thompson N, Brine P. Expanding the physician-substitute concept to oral health care practitioners. J Public Health Policy 18(1):80–97.

16. Soricelli D. Implementation of the delivery of dental services by auxiliaries —The Philadelphia experience. Am J Public Health 1972;62(8):1077–1087.

17. Lobene RR, Berman K, Chaisson LB, Karelas HA, Nolan LF. The Forsyth experiment in training of advanced skills hygienists. J Dent Educ 1974;38(7):369–379.

Professional Opportunities in Dental Public Health

4

Objectives

After studying this chapter and completing the study questions and activities, the learner will be able to:

- Compare and contrast dental public health practice with private practice.
- Describe skills and abilities necessary for dental public health positions.
- Describe dental public health opportunities in different sectors of the workforce.
- Identify how dental public health positions are funded.

KEY TERMS

Agency for Healthcare Research
   and Quality (AHRQ)
Agency for Toxic Substances and
   Disease Registry (ATSDR)
American Dental Education
   Association (ADEA)
American Dental Hygienists'
   Association's Types of Dental
   Hygiene Careers
Career opportunities
Centers for Disease Control and
   Prevention (CDC)
Commissioned Corps (USPHS)
Council on Linkages between
   Academia and Public Health
   Practice

Department of Defense
Department of Education
Department of Health and Human
   Services (DHHS)
Department of Justice
Department of Veterans Affairs
Food and Drug Administration
   (FDA)
Health Resources and Services
   Administration (HRSA)
Indian Health Service (IHS)
National Institutes of Health (NIH)
National Spit Tobacco Education
   Program (NSTEP)

Prevent Abuse and Neglect
   through Dental Awareness
   (P.A.N.D.A.)
Public health practice
Special Olympics Special Smiles
   (SOSS)
Substance Abuse and Mental
   Health Services Administration
   (SAMHSA)
United States Public Health
   Service (USPHS)
Women, Infant, Children (WIC)
   Program

The American Dental Education Association competencies addressed in this chapter include[1]:

C.5:   Continuously perform self-assessment for lifelong learning and professional growth.

CM.3:   Provide community oral health services in a variety of settings.

PGD.1: Identify alternative career options within health care, industry, education, and research and evaluate the feasibility of pursuing dental hygiene opportunities.

PGD.3: Access professional and social networks and resources to assist entrepreneurial initiatives.

Introduction

What type of person chooses a career in public health? Are you a dreamer, creative, compassionate, people-oriented, innovative, flexible, patient, or organized? Do you enjoy variety, intellectual challenge, bringing people together around an issue, and the reward of helping people attain better health? Public health dentistry may be the career for you!

This chapter explores the many and varied **career opportunities** for dental hygienists to engage in **public health practice** and discusses the necessary knowledge and skills to participate at many different levels. Opportunities in this field are only limited by the imagination. The choice to build a career in public health can lead to a stimulating and rewarding career, as you will discover from the interviews of people who have chosen this field included in this chapter. The multitude of paths that lead from being a learner to a career in dental public health cannot all be depicted in one chapter or even one book. Careers in dental public health encompass a broad scope of activities, including administrative activities, program planning and evaluation, financial management, education, clinical services, legislative activities, personnel management, research, and many other facets of the oral health and business arenas. The job responsibilities of a particular position can vary widely based on the employment setting. The employment settings discussed in this chapter

highlight the many contributions dental hygienists can make in the field of public health.

As you read in Chapter 1 and will discover in greater depth in Chapter 5, many of the skills in assessment, diagnosis, planning, and evaluation developed as a student clinician in preparation for private practice can be valuable and transferable to public health practice. The profession of dental hygiene is focused on prevention of disease, as is public health. This philosophical cornerstone provides a natural entree into a career in public health. That entree may occur when you provide a presentation to a second grade class about the merits of brushing daily. Public health dental hygienist? Not really, but public speaking ability, good communication skills with diverse groups, and developing appropriate educational tools are necessary skills for a public health professional. The entree may occur when you volunteer on a mobile dental van, treating disadvantaged populations. Public health dental hygienist? Not really, but knowledge of epidemiology, oral health disparities, and financing mechanisms for dental care for disadvantaged populations is important knowledge for a public health professional. You may be asked as a parent to coordinate the school fluoride rinse program using volunteer parents at your child's school. Public health dental hygienist? Not really, but skills in personnel management, program planning and evaluation, and public relations are critical skills for the public health professional. Many small or short-term opportunities provide a way to explore the field of public health and are a vital component of the commitment to better oral health for the public.

With these opportunities, you may find a desire to pursue a career in dental public health. This chapter highlights opportunities for careers in public health and discusses the skills and knowledge needed and includes the career paths of people who have chosen to devote their careers to public health.

COMPETENCY IN DENTAL PUBLIC HEALTH

Chapter 1 discussed the most distinctive difference between public health practice and private practice—the concept of the community, rather than an individual, as the client. Dental public health positions frequently require skills in assessing and diagnosing community oral health needs; planning, implementing, and evaluating community-based oral health programs; providing educational services; applying research and epidemiology; formulating policy; advocating; and understanding the organiza-

tion of health care and government. The necessary skills and knowledge base are addressed in the various competency documents that have been developed by experts in the field of dental public health.

Several organizations have developed written sets of skills and knowledge required of public health practitioners in different settings. The **American Dental Education Association** (ADEA) provides "Competencies for Entry Into the Profession of Dental Hygiene,"[1] which includes specific core competencies for the newly graduating dental hygienist's complex role in the community (Box 4-1). Dental hygiene programs use this as a curriculum guide for accreditation and for teaching the role of dental hygienists in the community.

The ADEA also lists competencies for other areas of dental hygiene practice. This document is the one from which all competencies listed at the beginning of each chapter of this text are drawn. It includes the knowledge, psychomotor skills, communication skills, and attitudes needed in this field of study. These are basic skills for working in entry-level positions in public health. In addition, the American Dental Hygienists' Association (ADHA) developed the **Types of Dental Hygiene**

BOX 4-1 ADEA Community Involvement Competencies for Entry Into the Profession of Dental Hygiene

CM.1: Assess the oral health needs of the community and the quality and availability of resources and services.

CM.2: Provide screening, referral, and educational services that allow clients to access resources of the health care system.

CM.3: Provide community oral health services in a variety of settings.

CM.4: Facilitate client access to oral health services by influencing individuals and/or organizations for the provision of oral health care.

CM.5: Evaluate reimbursement mechanisms and their impact on the patient's/client's access to oral health care.

CM.6: Evaluate the outcomes of community-based programs and plan for future activities.

(Source: American Dental Education Association. Competencies for entry into the profession of dental hygiene, Exhibit 7. J Dent Educ 2003;67(7):1–5. Available at: http://www.adea.org/cepr. Accessed February 2004.)[1]

BOX 4-2 Dental Hygiene Careers

- Administrator/Manager
- Change Agent
- Clinician
- Consumer Advocate
- Educator
- Researcher

(Source: Types of dental hygiene careers. American Dental Hygienists' Association Online. Available at: http://www.adha.org/careerinfo/types.htm. Accessed January 2003.)[2]

Careers[2], which includes specific roles for dental hygienists: administrator/manager, change agent, clinician, consumer advocate, educator, and researcher (Box 4-2). Many, if not all, of these roles are encompassed in a public health career.

Two additional organizations have developed competencies for public health professionals. The first is the **Council on Linkages Between Academia and Public Health Practice.**[3] These competencies, developed by the Public Health Functions Steering Committee, relate to the 10 Essential Public Health Services discussed in Chapter 1. Competency in skills and knowledge needed in eight domains or areas for each of the 10 Essential Public Health Services is outlined in the document, including skills in analysis/assessment skills, basic public health sciences skills, communication skills, community dimensions of practice skills, cultural competency skills, financial planning and management skills, leadership and systems thinking skills, and policy development/program planning skills (Box 4-3).

These competencies provide a framework for public health practitioners from front line staff to senior level staff to supervisory/management level staff. More specific and detailed than the ADEA competencies, they are used by federal, state, and local agencies and organizations as a key part of workforce development. The competencies have been used to guide the development of public health courses, curricula, and training priorities.

The second organization that has developed competency statements specifically for dental public health is the American Association of Public Health Dentistry (AAPHD) in conjunction with the American Board of Dental Public Health (ABDPH).[4] These performance indicators set up the knowledge and practice base by which this specialty of dentistry is recognized. The competencies were developed primarily for dentists seeking to become specialists in dental public health and, as such, require advanced training in dental public health. However, they also are an excellent guideline for any professional in dental public health with advanced responsibilities in their job position.

These many perspectives on the knowledge and skills needed for public health practice are useful in understanding the nature of public health practice and the various levels at which a dental hygienist may participate in that profession. One may participate as a community-based dental hygienist by participating in the activities mentioned earlier, such as a school fluoride volunteer or volunteering on a mobile dental van with a dis-

---

BOX 4-3 Eight Domains of Skill and Knowledge for Public Health Professionals

- Analytic/Assessment Skills
- Basic Public Health Sciences Skills
- Communication Skills
- Community Dimensions of Practice Skills
- Cultural Competency Skills
- Financial Planning and Management Skills
- Leadership and Systems Thinking Skills
- Policy Development/Program Planning Skills

(Source: Council on Linkages Between Academia and Public Health Practice. Core Competencies for Public Health Professionals. Washington, DC: Public Health Foundation, 2001.)[3]

advantaged population. Or, one can choose to pursue a career as a public health professional by expanding their scope of knowledge and skills and becoming a researcher, state program administrator, or health policy consultant.

The cameos in this chapter highlight the many pathways to a career in public health and the many possible paths to take when you have entered a public health career. It is possible to combine a private practice career and a public health career, be involved in improving the public's health solely as a community volunteer, or become a dental public health career professional.

CAREER OPPORTUNITIES IN DENTAL PUBLIC HEALTH

Many careers in public health may be new to dental hygiene students. Most dental hygiene students enter school expecting to enter and remain in private practice for their entire careers. This chapter takes the opportunity to expose the student to many other career path options. Career pathways in dental public health may develop in many different ways and be funded from many different sources. A position may be at the federal, provincial, state, or county/local level, funded by public tax dollars. It may be in education, research, or industry, funded by public or corporate entities. It could even be as a self-employed contractor or consultant in health policy, prevention, or education, funded by a philanthropic organization, coalition, or health maintenance organization. Perhaps, it may be a volunteer position or other method of becoming involved in the health of the community in which you practice.

Federal/National

Chapter 1 discussed the infrastructure of public health, specifically dental public health. Figure 1-2 identified federal agencies with dental public health responsibilities, many of which offer opportunities for careers in public health (Table 4-1). One of the largest employers of dental personnel in the federal government is the **United States Public Health Service** (USPHS). The USPHS is under the jurisdiction of the **Department of Health and Human Services** (DHHS) and

TABLE 4-1 FEDERAL OPPORTUNITIES IN DENTAL PUBLIC HEALTH

AGENCY/DEPARTMENT	TYPE OF POSITION
USPHS Commissioned Corps	clinician, administrator, researcher, educator
Department of Justice Bureau of Prisons	clinician, administrator
Department of Veterans Affairs	clinician, administrator, researcher
Food and Drug Administration	researcher, consumer advocate
Centers for Disease Control and Prevention	researcher, administrator, consumer advocate
Department of Defense Military Installations	clinician, researcher, health educator
National Institutes of Health NIDCR	researcher, administrator
Migrant/Community Health Centers	clinician, administrator, educator

Indian Health Service
   Commissioned Corps
   Civil Service
	clinician, researcher
	health educator, consumer advocate

National Health Service Corps	clinician, administrator, health educator

provides support for the **Agency for Healthcare Research and Quality** (AHRQ), the **Agency for Toxic Substances and Disease Registry** (ATSDR), the **Centers for Disease Control and Prevention** (CDC), the **Food and Drug Administration** (FDA), the **Health Resources and Services Administration** (HRSA), **Indian Health Service** (IHS), **National Institutes of Health** (NIH), and the **Substance Abuse and Mental Health Services Administration** (SAMHSA). The USPHS offers careers in both the civil service and the **Commissioned Corps.** The Commissioned Corps of the USPHS is a non–arms-bearing branch of the Uniformed Services. Dental hygienists who join the Commissioned Corps must hold a bachelor's degree. They are provided the career benefits of uniformed service personnel, similar to the military branches of the Uniformed Services, including medical and dental benefits, vacation and sick leave, retirement, paid continuing education, and advanced training in dental public health and leadership.

Although the DHHS is the primary department responsible for public health activities, additional federal departments with public health opportunities include the **Department of Veterans Affairs, Department of Justice** (Federal Bureau of Prisons), **Department of Defense** (military), and the **Department of Education.** These agencies offer clinical, administrative, educational, or research positions. Many require a minimum of a bachelor's degree in dental hygiene or advanced degrees in public health. Indeed, many offer opportunities for repayment of college loans or for sponsored advanced education. Many positions may be through the Commissioned Corps of the USPHS. However, an alternative may be employment in a civil service position, which is employment by the United States Government, similar to a postal worker or other government position. The employee is provided benefits that include medical and dental, vacation and sick leave, and retirement, if employed in the system for the required period (Box 4-4) (Box 4-5).

State/Provincial/County/Local/City

As with federal opportunities, many choices are available at state or local levels, including positions in state or local oral health programs, state bureau of prisons, Maternal and Child Health (MCH) programs, **Women, Infant, and Children** (WIC) programs, and others. These positions can be clinical, educational, administrative, consultative, or even research oriented. They may be in migrant or community clinics, schools, Head Start programs, or tribal clinics (Table 4-2).

TABLE 4-2 STATE AND LOCAL OPPORTUNITIES IN DENTAL PUBLIC HEALTH

AGENCY/DEPARTMENT	TYPE OF POSITION
State/Local Dental Programs	administrator, clinician, consumer advocate, change agent, educator, researcher
Women, Infant, Child (WIC) Programs	educator, consumer advocate
Medicaid Programs	educator, consumer advocate, consultant, administrator, change agent
Maternal and Child Health Programs	consumer advocate, educator, change agent
Tribal Health Centers	clinician, educator, consumer advocate, administrator
State Bureau of Prisons	clinician, educator, consumer advocate

BOX 4-4 Federal Opportunities

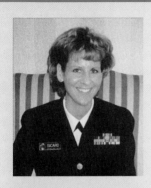

Karen Sicard, MPH, RDH
Lieutenant Commander (LCDR), U.S. Public Health Service, Indian Health Service, Crow Agency, Montana. Community Clinical Hygienist, Acting Dental Prevention Officer, Head Start Dental Consultant

Education: The position requires a bachelor's degree and licensure as a registered dental hygienist in at least one state.

Funding: The position is funded through federal Indian Health Service dental funds and the National Indian Health Service Head Start program.

Competencies that relate to your position: My job encompasses all AAPHD competencies, ADEA competencies, and ADHA dental hygiene roles.

Responsibilities:
- Provide training and technical assistance to the eight dental programs in the area.
- Collaborate with government and tribal entities.
- Develop, implement, and assess community intervention programs.
- Obtain funding.
- Develop training for area programs.

Describe your career path:
Like many dental hygienists in public health, my career path is unique. In 1987, I started as a dental tech in the Navy reserves. I worked as a dental practice manager from 1987–1991. I graduated from dental hygiene school in 1993 and worked in private practice from 1993–1997. I joined the U.S. Public Health Service in the fall of 1997. I chose to join due to my previous military experience, my desire to help people, and a sense of security.

I have had the opportunity to expand, grow, and develop. I've had a great time working with community programs. I work in a hospital setting with other health professionals, including public health nutritionists, physicians, nurses, mental health personnel, and physical therapists.

Describe the greatest challenges to public health for the next decade:
- Access to care for children from low-income families.
- The role of the dental hygienist in oral health care in the future.

What do you think is important to share with others considering a career in dental public health:
Do it! It's a great opportunity to utilize more than just clinical skills.

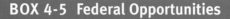

BOX 4-5 Federal Opportunities

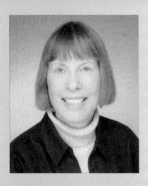

Alice Horowitz, PhD, RDH

Education Specialist, National Institute of Dental and Craniofacial Research, National Institutes of Health (NIH), Department of Health and Human Services

Education: The position requires at least a master's degree.

Funding: The position is funded with federal dollars; however, some initiatives are funded with nongovernmental funds.

Competencies that relate to your position: My work focuses on the ADHA roles for dental hygienists of administrator/manager, educator, researcher, consumer advocate, and change agent, all AAPHD competencies, and many ADEA Core Competencies.

Responsibilities:
- Conduct research and report findings through presentations and other mediums.
- Develop educational interventions for the public, health care providers, and the media.
- Work with communities, organizations, and other Institutes at NIH to promote oral health through symposia, lectures, workshops, publications, and other venues.
- Be a co-leader for the Healthy People 2010, Oral Health section.
- Contribute to Oral Health in America: A Report of the Surgeon General.

Describe your career path:
I knew before I finished dental hygiene school that I did not want to work full time in a clinical setting. I enjoyed a brief stint in academia where I thought I might return because I enjoy the students, but public health is really where it happens for me! I always knew I wanted a doctoral degree, or at least more than a master's degree. I considered dentistry and law, but my love is primary prevention, so I decided on a PhD in Health Education/Health Promotion. After becoming a registered dental hygienist, I worked in private practice for 1 year while I worked on a bachelor's degree. I also worked one summer in a hospital for disabled children. After earning my bachelor's degree, I began teaching full time in the College of Dentistry, University of Iowa, and worked part-time on a master's degree. Because I was on 9-month contracts, I worked during the summers in either private practice or on research projects for dental faculty. After earning my master's degree, I taught for 1 year and was then recruited into the U.S. Public Health Service where I have continued to work. I worked full-time while pursuing my PhD.

I have had numerous invitations to work with other countries, opportunities to work with researchers from other countries, and to have guest researchers work with me at the NIH. Because I enjoy working with students and guest researchers, I usually have one or more of each at any given time. We learn a lot from each other!

Describe the greatest challenges to public health for the next decade:
- Lack of dental public health infrastructure.
- Lack of money.
- Lack of information of the need for good oral health among decision makers and the general public.

- Lack of dental professionals trained in public health.

What do you think is important to share with others considering a career in dental public health?
There is never a dull moment! Public health offers excellent opportunities to be creative and help individuals and communities. Also, it provides excellent opportunities to try to get oral health integrated into general health—a very important concept.

In the United States in 2003, there were 10 states in which the state dental director was a dental hygienist.[5] In many states, dental hygienists fill key roles in state, county, and local oral health programs (Boxes 4-6, 4-7, 4-8). These roles may involve program management, clinical care, educational programs in schools and other institutions, fluoridation campaigns, sports injury prevention, or developing culturally appropriate educational materials.

BOX 4-6 State Opportunities

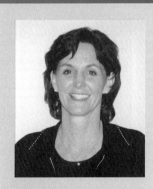

Mary E. Foley, MPH, RDH
Director of the Office of Oral Health, Massachusetts Department of Public Health (state dental director)

Education: The position requires a Master of Public Health degree

Funding: The position is funded through state appropriations and federal funding from the Health Resources and Services Administration (HRSA) and the Centers for Disease Control and Prevention (CDC).

Competencies that relate to your position: My job encompasses all AAPHD competencies, ADEA competencies, and ADHA dental hygiene roles.

Responsibilities:
- Plan, implement, monitor, and evaluate population-based oral health programs that promote oral disease prevention and access to dental care.
- Initiate and participate in partnerships with other organizations and state agencies to assure access to oral health education and dental care services for special population groups.
- Assure the provision of education and technical assistance to dental providers and other health professionals for the promotion of access to care and prevention of oral diseases.
- Coordinate multiple programs, including a school-based fluoride mouth rinse program and a Head Start fluoride supplementation program.
- Design and implement statewide oral health surveys.
- Provide technical assistance in the design of safety net dental clinics.

continued

- Promote the development of community coalitions to link communities in need of dental care to the three dental and seven dental hygiene schools throughout the state.
- Participate in partnerships with the Massachusetts Dental Society to: (1) provide treatment services for children who do not have access to a dental home; and (2) provide follow-up dental care for children identified through dental surveys to be in need of dental services.
- Provide technical assistance to the 135 communities in Massachusetts that fluoridate their water.
- Provide technical assistance and education to the boards of health on laws related to water fluoridation, including design, implementation, and maintenance of fluoridation programs.
- Educate community residents on the benefits of community water fluoridation.
- Partner with the Boston Public Health Commission (local health department) to integrate oral health into systems of care for underserved children.
- Work with dental schools to provide dental screenings, oral cancer detection programs, and dental care for targeted high-risk adult populations and seniors.
- Foster strong partnerships with dental insurers, including Delta Dental whose foundation provides millions of dollars each year to fund dental public health programs, such as school-based dental sealant programs, development of dental clinics, school-based/school-linked dental clinic programs across the state, and research.
- Provide technical assistance to agencies funded to implement oral health improvement programs.
- Partner with the state dental hygienists' association to implement train-the-trainer programs targeted at oral health needs for older adults.
- Provide educational seminars for WIC nutritionists.

Describe your career path:

I selected public health because I felt it would challenge me. Also, it was a way to practice my profession while allowing me to fulfill my role as a public servant, a role I felt strongly about as a health care professional. I have also found public health settings to be less restrictive than clinical practice.

I practiced clinical dental hygiene in a private practice for about 12 years. I returned to school part-time to complete my bachelor's degree while working part-time. I then became a dental hygiene clinical instructor and pursued a master's degree part-time.

After completing graduate school, I had opportunities to work in three different areas: (1) full-time faculty at a dental hygiene school, (2) director of a community health center dental clinic, and (3) public health dental hygienist for the Massachusetts Department of Public Health. I chose full-time employment in dental public health.

When I took the position at the Department of Public Health, I first managed a school-based fluoride mouth rinse program and the water fluoridation program. After being promoted to the directorship position, my duties and responsibilities increased substantially.

Presently, I teach a public health course at the Massachusetts College of Pharmacy in the Forsyth Dental Hygiene Program. Throughout my career, I have raised five children and continued to work in private practice at least one night a week.

I have had numerous and varied opportunities in public health including:

- Editor of the ASTDD newsletter

- ASTDD executive board
- AAPHD executive council
- Public health consultant to ADHA for the Future of Dental Hygiene Report
- ADHA Oral Health Institute member
- Participation in federal grant reviews
- Extensive travel
- ASTDD best practices committee chair
- Guest speaker in various national venues, including the National Conference of State Legislature and Oral Health America.

Describe the greatest challenges to public health for the next decade:
- Public health funding.
- Funding for necessary services so that oral health care services can be provided in an equitable way to all members of society.
- Qualified personnel to hire into public health programs.

What do you think is important to share with others considering a career in dental public health?
It's a dynamite idea because the sky is the limit! There are opportunities to really develop your skills and share passion with so many people while you are promoting oral health to large groups of people. Your impact will be with many more people than those you will have access to in a dental office. You will have an opportunity to help in ways new to you.

BOX 4-7 County Opportunities

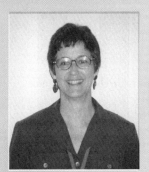

Susan M. Sanzi-Schaedel, MPH, RDH
Director of the School/Community Dental Health Programs, Multnomah County Health Department, Portland, Oregon

Education: The position requires experience and/or knowledge in public health dentistry; community education and health promotion; program planning; epidemiology, including collection and interpretation of data; quality assurance; clinical standards; and principles of supervision, training, and performance evaluation. A typical way to obtain knowledge and abilities would be 3 years of increasingly responsible, professional public health dental experience and a bachelor's degree in dental hygiene, community health or education, public health administration, or a related field.

Funding: The position and programs are funded by county general funds (county tax dollars) and grant dollars.

Competencies that relate to your position: Most competencies and roles apply to my position, with the exception of research. The clinical competencies are necessary for quality assurance,

continued

although I rarely provide clinical services. Although most of my routine duties are those of program planning (i.e., assessment through evaluation), most public health competencies are used.

Responsibilities: My work can be grouped into three categories: (1)school-based programs, (2) community-based programs, and (3) clinic-based programs. Most of the program activities I supervise are focused on tooth decay prevention. Through school programs, we provide fluoride in the form of mouth rinse or tablets to preschool, Head Start, and grade school children; deliver dental sealants through a school-based program; and provide oral wellness education to primarily grade school children. Through the community-based programs, we administer an early childhood cavity prevention program targeted at Early Head Start children, staff, parents, and pregnant women. Risk assessments, parent education, fluoride varnish applications, and referrals are provided in the clinic-based programs to children aged 9–24 months. Another clinic-based program is appointing pregnant women for preventive and restorative care, education about their oral hygiene, and anticipatory guidance on oral care for their babies. We are also planning a xylitol program for postpartum mothers.

As a program supervisor, I am engaged in all aspects of program planning, from community needs assessments, resource generation, implementation, and evaluation of program process and outcomes. I design quality assurance systems to monitor the quality of services and to ensure tax dollars are being spent in the most effective manner. I collaborate with organizations and agencies, such as school principals, nurses, and the dental society, to enhance the program's ability to provide preventive dental services in the community. I schedule programs with the schools and generate dentist volunteers. I support other agencies by participating on their advisory boards or committees. I participate on the dental division management team and health department committees, so that I can be a part of problem solving and policy development for both the department and division. I supervise professional and support staff. Technical assistance is also provided on a wide range of oral health topics and program implementation issues to health and dental professionals in Oregon. I currently work with a diverse group of individuals, including dentists, dental hygienists, health educators, dental assistants, community outreach staff, support staff, clinic operations managers, school principals and secretaries, registered nurses, students, and Medicaid program staff.

Describe your career path:

Even as a dental hygiene student, I knew I would seek opportunities outside the traditional dental treatment system. My concern was always for those who would never be able to access and be maintained in the traditional dental care system. I have always loved the evolving science of dentistry, but knew my role in bringing that science to the public would not be through my clinical skills. Public health practice has allowed me to provide services to broad targeted communities, rather than to individuals.

I received a bachelor's degree in dental hygiene and a master's degree in health education/ health behavior and dental public health. Additionally, I have participated in numerous continuing education and trainings in supervision, leadership, conversational Spanish, dental, and programmatic content areas.

Opportunities come serendipitously or are created. I have had both in my career. I have had opportunities to expand my roles through working with local, state, and national dental and public health organizations. I have held many positions of leadership within the Oregon Dental

Hygienists' Association, including president. I sat on the ADHA Council on Public Health; cochaired and participated on committees for Multnomah Dental Society; and participated in leadership and policy roles for both the Oregon Public Health Association and the American Public Health Association, including Chair of the Oral Health Section and Governing Council. I currently participate on a committee for the Association of State and Territorial Dental Directors. These opportunities have provided growth, both professionally and personally. I have also had the opportunity to chair a scholarship committee for second year dental hygiene students. Another opportunity has been in the area of mentoring dental hygiene, nursing, and dental students. My newest opportunity is to work on the Incident Command Team for the Health Department—a far cry from teeth, but an opportunity to learn a new approach for emergency response and to learn new skills.

Describe the greatest challenges to public health for the next decade:
- Loss of trained dental public health professionals.
- Loss of infrastructure supporting dental public health—diversion of funds to other state and federal initiatives.
- A widening gap in health disparities between the wealthy and the uninsured and working poor.

What do you think is important to share with others considering a career in dental public health?
It helps to be passionate about your work. You need to be flexible, have the ability to work collaboratively, be persistent in working toward your goals, be able to multitask, and to think outside the proverbial "BOX." It is an extremely fulfilling job, although one that requires me to set priorities and be realistic about what can be accomplished. It provides the opportunity to influence policy that can promote oral health of the community, allows for great creativity, and has a wonderful community of colleagues. And, best of all, the outcome of your work can improve the health of a diverse population. I still find it exciting and challenging after all these years!

BOX 4-8 State Opportunities

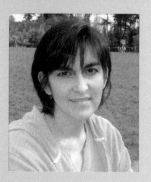

Rosa C. Sanchez-Dieter, BS, RDH
Child Oral Health Program Coordinator, Oregon Department of Human Services, Office of Family Health, Oral Health Section.

Education: The position requires a bachelor's degree and at least 5 years experience in public health, with preference to experience in the dental field.

Funding: The position is funded with Maternal and Child Health Block Grant dollars (federal).

Competencies that relate to your position: My job encompasses all AAPHD competencies, ADEA competencies, and ADHA dental hygiene roles.

continued

Responsibilities:
- Design, implement, and monitor dental health projects, including the school-based mouth rinse and chewable tablet program for school children in grades pre-K to 6 in Oregon.
- Facilitate and staff statewide interagency, multidisciplinary teams and assist them in developing or coordinating oral health programs at state and local levels (i.e., Early Head Start, Healthy Kids Learn Better, Tri-County Fluoridation Coalition).
- Facilitate staff meetings of the Early Childhood Cavities Prevention Coalition.
- Coordinate and provide public education, consultation, and technical assistance.
- Recruit, train, and supervise four part-time dental health consultants.
- Manage a budget.
- Write grant applications and initiate grant projects.
- Represent the Oral Health Section at meetings at the local, regional, state, and national levels regarding oral health issues.
- Seek support and buy-in from partners to promote oral health issues.

Describe your career path:
I worked as a certified dental assistant for 3 years and then as a clinical research assistant at a state university cancer center, working with Stage 3 and 4 cancer patients on investigational drug study protocols. During this time, I attended classes part-time to complete prerequisites for a dental hygiene program. After graduation, I worked as a clinical dental hygienist for a general practice and a periodontal practice. I then took my first position in public health coordinating the county school-based dental sealant program because it sounded like fun! My current position just followed by chance when my predecessor recommended me for the job. I now work half-time for the State of Oregon and have continued practicing clinical dental hygiene in a general practice 1 day per week.

Describe the greatest challenges to public health for the next decade:
- Funding.
- Decrease in dentist workforce.
- Expansion of the role of dental hygienists.

What do you think is important to share with others considering a career in dental public health?
I think there are many advantages and differences between public health and private practice including:
Advantages
- More flexibility with your time, not an hourly schedule like in a clinical setting.
- Reach a broader population with program development/implementation.
- Personal satisfaction of helping people who may not otherwise get help.
- County and state positions have good financial compensation, including paid holidays, vacation, and sick leave.
Differences versus private practice
- More administrative duties.
- Working with agencies and government programs versus individual patients can be frustrating!

In Native American communities, tribal clinics provide a wide variety of opportunities, based on the particular oral health needs of the tribal community. This setting often is a way to combine clinical services with community-based health education or health promotion activities. Providers in these settings may be hired from the USPHS Commissioned Corps or directly from the surrounding community. Tribes may also offer student loan repayment opportunities as an employment incentive.

Education

Public health opportunities in the educational setting include teaching and mentoring the next generation of dental professionals regarding their role in the community. It may also include managing an outreach program or clinic for the educational institution or developing educational opportunities in public health for student exploration. This can involve partnerships with other interested stakeholders to provide oral health care and education for the people of the region. In addition, the educational setting lends itself to research opportunities. Collaborative partners and populations for study may be readily available, and many faculty appointments require research to obtain tenure and for career growth within the institution. In many cases, advanced degrees in public health, health education, health promotion, or other related fields may be required (Box 4-9).

Research

Research opportunities are available in educational institutions, but they are also available with private industry, health departments, or philanthropic

---

BOX 4-9 Education Opportunities

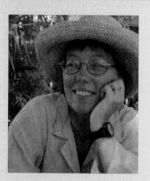

Charlotte J. Wyche, MS, RDH
Faculty in the Department of Periodontology and Dental Hygiene, University of Detroit Mercy School of Dentistry, Detroit, Michigan.

Education: The position requires being a registered dental hygienist and holding a Master of Science degree in a related field. I have been told that when I retire my position will be advertised for someone with a Master's in Public Health.

Funding: The position is funded by the University of Detroit Mercy.

Competencies that relate to your position: Because I teach community health, every AAPHD Competency, ADEA Competency, and ADHA role is integral to my present position. I not only teach them, but I need to remember that I am a role model for my students in each competency and role.

I teach my students about the Core Functions in classroom lectures. I think my teaching duties relate mostly to assessment—we teach about and provide dental screenings in various settings. I also teach students about their role as health professionals in legislative activity that can affect public health policy development.

Responsibilities:
• Coordinate the community health curriculum (three courses), a scientific presentation course, and lectures in the special patient care course for dental hygiene students.

continued

- Site director for a dental hygiene clinical rotation at a community-based free dental clinic located in a nurse managed health center.
- Coordinate the special patient care course for third-year dental students.

Describe your career path:

After graduating with my Dental Hygiene Certificate and receiving my license, I practiced in several private dental offices for nearly 10 years while completing course work toward my bachelor's degree. After receiving my master's degree, I taught clinical radiology to dental and dental hygiene students at the University of Michigan before being offered a position as a tenure track, full-time faculty member in the dental hygiene program at University of Detroit Mercy (UDM). Additionally, I have completed advanced continuing-education course work (via educational institutes) in special patient care, research, and service-learning.

Happenstance and my interest and previous community volunteer experience placed me in the role of teaching community health courses for dental hygiene students. The dental hygiene student's community health curriculum has expanded and become more integrated with the rest of the dental hygiene curriculum during the years I have taught. As I became trained in service-learning methodologies, our program has become stronger. For various reasons, including the Catholic traditions and the focus on service in our institution's mission, the community outreach at UDM and the broad and deep community experiences our students have each year have become a valued part of our program.

I regularly work with dentists (on campus), nurses and nursing students, and physicians at my community rotation site. My biggest joy has been the opportunities I have had over the years to place dental hygiene and nursing students together in some sort of community-based learning projects. Those experiences teach my students so much more about their role as broad-based community health educators than anything else I can arrange for them.

Describe the greatest challenges to public health for the next decade:

- Money is very much the limiting factor in improving access, minimizing disparities, and opening up all the possibilities for improving oral health that are called for in the Surgeon General's report.

What do you think is important to share with others considering a career in dental public health?

It's important that you really feel a passion for it. It isn't the same as private practice dental hygiene. It isn't easy; knowing that there is SO much need that you can't always address can burn you out. But there is nothing else so satisfying and nowhere else that you can feel that you have made SUCH a difference as when you are improving the oral health status of those who would not otherwise have access.

I love teaching community health because it gives me the opportunity to open the students' eyes to dental hygiene as a career that can open way up beyond the limitations most of us experience in the restrictive scope of practice available in most private practice settings. I think these possibilities will continue to grow.

organizations. Dental hygienists can participate as principle investigators, which may require an advanced degree (usually at the doctoral level) to compete in the world of research grants. However, a dental hygienist also can become involved as a study coordinator to oversee the process of the

TABLE 4-3 EDUCATION AND RESEARCH OPPORTUNITIES IN DENTAL PUBLIC HEALTH

AGENCY/DEPARTMENT	TYPE OF POSITION
Educational Institutions	educator, researcher, clinician, administrator
Student Health Centers	administrator, clinician,
Schools of Public Health	educator, researcher
Federal Opportunities	researcher, administrator

research or as a research associate who may be responsible for collecting data for the study (Table 4-3).

Industry/Corporate

Many dental product companies have educational divisions that target specific population groups for educational programs (Table 4-4). In addition to marketing a product or improving name recognition, these programs help improve the public's health. Employment of dental public health professionals to help target populations and develop culturally appropriate educational materials can be of great benefit to the public's oral health. In addition, as part of their corporate mission, companies may also provide avenues for giving back to the community. This is achieved by providing Web sites for consumer information, educational tools for college and university faculties, and classroom kits for teachers in elementary schools. All of these avenues promote oral health, and dental public health professionals are a natural fit for collaborating with corporations to accomplish this goal.

TABLE 4-4 INDUSTRY/CORPORATE/PRIVATE/VOLUNTEER OPPORTUNITIES IN DENTAL PUBLIC HEALTH

AGENCY/DEPARTMENT	TYPE OF POSITION
Dental Products Companies	educator, researcher, administrator, consumer advocate
Contractor/Consultant	educator, researcher
Health Policy	administrator, clinician,
Head Start	policy analyst, consultant
Nursing Home Program	change agent, consumer
Epidemiology	advocate
Volunteer	change agent, consumer advocate
Health Fairs	clinician, consultant, educator
Legislative Efforts	
Mobile Dental Vans	
Health Coalitions	
Special Olympics	
Schools	
National/International	

Private Contractor/Consultant

Many public health employment opportunities are created by a desire to solve a problem and find a creative approach to funding the solution. Many public health professionals create their own positions in this way, which requires initiative, skill at marketing an idea, and the patience to see it come to fruition. Are you self-directed, articulate, diplomatic, and productive? Do you have strong skills in scientific writing, public relations, marketing, and business management? Self-employed consultants and contractors have the opportunity to set their own hours, schedule, and remuneration and can decide with which projects they would like to be involved. However, the opportunities may not always provide a consistent paycheck or benefit package and there may be slack times.

Many states now are looking at alternatives to meet the oral health needs of their residents. Many have changed practice acts to allow dental hygienists to practice under general supervision or unsupervised in settings outside private practice. In these settings, dental hygienists have started their own businesses and are developing innovative ways to facilitate care for those who are un-able to receive treatment or who are unlikely to seek care in a dental office. In these settings, dental hygienists must be their own business manager and public relations person. Good marketing and communication skills are a necessity. Also, good collaboration with local oral health providers is important to facilitate care that cannot be provided by the dental hygienist.

Many public health professionals work as consultants to federal, state, or local agencies. Agencies may be able to provide short-term support for a specific program, develop an educational program, or research a particular problem and develop policy statements relating to the issue. Consultants may have several concurrent projects and may choose projects according to their particular expertise or interest. For example, an oral epidemiologist may focus on performing oral health surveys to determine the oral health status of specific communities or groups. An oral health policy analyst may focus on how the state can best manage Medicaid funding to provide the most services with limited funds. An oral health education consultant may help a school system develop an oral health education program for the school district (Box 4-10).

BOX 4-10 Private Contractor/Consultant/Researcher Opportunities

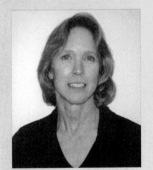

Kathy Phipps, MPH, PhD, RDH
Associate Professor at Oregon Health & Science University; Independent Consultant.

Education: The position of Associate Professor requires a doctoral degree and experience in the development and management of oral health research projects. A master's degree is required to be successful as an oral health consultant, together with extensive experience in dental public health.

Funding: The position at Oregon Health & Science University is funded by grants, mostly from the National Institutes of Health. The consultant positions are usually individual contracts with federal, tribal, state, and nonprofit organizations. Most contracts are for a set amount during a defined period—usually 1 year.

Competencies that relate to your position:
- Select interventions and strategies for the prevention and control of oral diseases and promotion of oral health.
- Incorporate ethical standards in oral health programs and activities.
- Evaluate and monitor dental care delivery systems.
- Design and understand the use of surveillance systems to monitor oral health.
- Communicate and collaborate with groups and individuals on oral health issues.
- Critique and synthesize scientific literature.
- Design and conduct population-based studies to answer oral and public health questions.
- Assess the oral health needs of the community and the quality and availability of resources and services.
- Evaluate the outcomes of community based programs and plan for future activities.
- Identify individual and population risk factors and develop strategies that promote health-related quality of life.

In my duties as an oral health surveillance consultant, I help state and tribal organizations monitor their progress toward meeting the Healthy People 2010 goals. As an oral health researcher, I am attempting to develop methods that will reduce oral health disparities in high-risk population groups.

Responsibilities:
- Oral epidemiologist for two NIH funded research projects. The first study evaluates the association between skeletal bone loss and oral bone loss in older men. The second study is designed to assess the feasibility of fasting plasma and saliva for the evaluation of total body burden of fluoride. As the epidemiologist for these projects, I provide input into methods for collecting data, data analysis, and manuscript preparation.
- Consultant for the Association of State and Territorial Dental Directors, Northwest Portland Area Indian Health Board, The Dental Health Foundation, and the Indian Health Service. As a consultant to these organizations, I provide a wide range of services, focusing on oral health surveillance, oral health policy, data collection, and data analysis.

Describe your career path:
I started my career as a clinical dental hygienist in a rural practice, but soon realized that I was more interested in public health than clinical practice. As a clinical hygienist, I felt that I was unable to provide service to those most in need. After practicing for about 1 year, I pursued a Master's in Public Health (MPH) at the University of Michigan. After graduation, I took a position as the health administrator for a tribal organization and then moved on to a position as social service manager for an organization providing services to the frail and elderly. Although I enjoyed both positions, I soon realized that I was more interested in research than administration. I returned to the University of Michigan to pursue a doctorate in oral epidemiology.

After earning my DrPH, I have been a faculty member at Oregon Health & Science University and an oral health consultant. I have enjoyed all of my careers, but find research, epidemiology, and consulting the most rewarding.

continued

A career in public health has afforded me the opportunity to continually learn and change my day-to-day work routine. I have had many opportunities that would not have been possible in clinical practice. I have worked with various high-risk groups, including the frail elderly, minority populations, and institutionalized adults. I have traveled to places most people have only heard of, including rural Alaskan villages and the Soviet Union (before its fall). I have met people from all over the world and have friends and colleagues on most continents.

I routinely work with various health professionals, including dental hygienists, dentists, physicians, epidemiologists, statisticians, public health educators, environmental health professionals, and public health administrators.

Describe the greatest challenges to public health for the next decade:
• Funding is always an issue in public health. State programs are often targeted for reductions, but there are still positions in various settings. If research is an interest, funding is tight but available for a bright and dedicated individual.

What do you think is important to share with others considering a career in dental public health?
When I was a dental hygiene student, I had a "feeling" that I might not really enjoy clinical practice. After practicing for a short time, I realized that clinical practice was not my first career choice. Rather than leaving the field of dentistry, I decided to pursue a graduate degree that allowed me to be involved in dentistry while doing more than just clinical dental hygiene. If you feel that you may want something other than a career in a private office, talk to hygienists in public health positions and volunteer in public health settings. Some of you will really love it and want to pursue a career in public health.

Volunteer

Volunteer opportunities abound and provide a way to learn about public health, network with other professionals, and develop skills without a major time or monetary commitment. Time commitment is flexible—1 day per month on a volunteer van, a few hours per week or month at a school, or 1 to 2 weeks per year in another country can all provide variety and increased career satisfaction. In addition, these activities can increase flexibility in your long-term career progression. There is no limit to possibilities in local, regional, or international arenas. Local, national, or large regional organizations are a good place to look for volunteer opportunities. The **Special Olympics Special Smiles** program holds events in many areas throughout the United States. Different levels of participation are available—from local coordinator to a few hours volunteering with the athletes.

Prevent Abuse and Neglect through Dental Awareness (PANDA) provides opportunities for training dental and other health professionals about dental and orofacial signs of abuse and neglect. If your interest is in preventing tobacco use, the **National Spit Tobacco Education Program** (NSTEP) is a place to begin finding information about that health promotion effort.

There are also large regional medical and dental nongovernmental organizations (NGO) that provide opportunities both locally and internationally for professionals to contribute expertise (see Resources). Opportunities may be with children, teens, or adults. Bilingual health care providers are especially in demand for these organizations. When considering volunteering with an organization, it is advisable to investigate its philosophical background, history, and expectations and also the cost to the volunteer. Often, travel costs are borne by the volunteer; however, the rewards are traditionally much greater than the cost!

Many communities have nursing homes, health fairs, free clinics, homeless shelters, and other sites that welcome the participation and input from oral health providers. This is a way to network with other health care providers in your local area.

ADVANCED EDUCATION OPPORTUNITIES

There are many opportunities to obtain advanced education in dental public health, with many more appearing on the Internet. It is important to use your assessment and critical evaluation skills to determine which opportunity for advancement is of the type and quality to lead you successfully down your chosen path. Talking to public health professionals can also aid you in this endeavor.

Available programs include limited or full coursework online, programs that can be pursued while working by attending intensive courses at a university, or programs that require full-time attendance on campus for the specific time it takes to complete the degree. There is certainly great flexibility in pursuing advanced education in public health. Some resources to begin your search are listed in the resource section of this chapter.

SUMMARY

There are many varied opportunities for dental hygienists to contribute to the public's oral health and build a satisfying career in public health. Many entry-level and clinical positions in public health settings do not require advanced education; however, positions for career dental public health professionals with higher authority and responsibility may require advanced training in dental public health. Whichever path leads to a public health career or whether you use volunteerism to improve the oral health of the community, it is a rewarding and satisfying experience.

 Learning Activities

1. Research an employment setting in dental public health.
2. Interview a public health dental hygienist about their job (e.g., qualifications, responsibilities, funding, percentage of time in different activities, and competencies and skills needed). This can be done online by e-mail if the public health professional is not local.
3. Shadow a public health professional for a day.
4. Compare and contrast the skills needed for a public health dental hygienist and a private practice dental hygienist.
5. Compare and contrast the different sets of competencies/skills developed by the various organizations in dental public health.
6. Shadow or work on a mobile dental van for a day.
7. Visit a foreign country with a dental team.
8. Create a classroom game based on the ability to link an acronym with a public agency and the role it has in public health. Include the agency's mission and location and other details.
9. Investigate a local dental public health agency or program to identify the funding sources.

RESOURCES

Competency Documents (see References):

Educational Opportunities:

Dental hygiene programs (e.g., degree completion, related master's degrees). Available at: http://www.adha.org/careerinfo/dir_education.htm.

Schools of public health. Available at: http://www.apha.org/public_health/schools.htm.

Search words: school of public health, master's in public health, and doctorate in public health

Volunteer Opportunities (National and International):

American Cancer Society. Available at: http://www. cancer.org.

American Dental Association Web site. Search "volunteer" for local, national, and international volunteer opportunities. Available at: http://www. ada.org.

American Dental Hygienists' Association. Available at: http://www.adha.org.

International Federation of Dental Hygienists (IFDH). For international dental hygiene clinical opportunities. Available at: http://www.ifdh.org/ workabroad/.

Mercy Ships—International. Available at: http:// www.mercyships.org.

National Smokeless Tobacco Education Program (NSTEP). Available at: http://www.nstep.org.

Northwest Medical Teams International—National and International. Available at: http://www.nwmti. org.

Prevent Abuse and Neglect through Dental Awareness (P.A.N.D.A.). Search P.A.N.D.A. for local affiliates.

Special Olympics Special Smiles (SOSS). Available at: http://www.specialolympics.org.

World Health Organization. Available at: http:// www.who.int.

Review Questions

1. The primary difference between public health practice and private practice is:
   a. assessing the patient's/client's oral health needs.
   b. planning an appropriate intervention.
   c. implementing a treatment plan.
   d. evaluating outcomes of an intervention.
   e. the community is the client, rather than an individual.

2. Which organization has developed competency statements specifically for the newly graduated dental hygienist?
   a. American Association of Public Health Dentistry
   b. American Dental Education Association
   c. American Dental Hygienists' Association
   d. American Board of Dental Public Health
   e. Council on Linkages Between Academia and Public Health Practice

3. What is the primary department of the federal government that oversees public health activities at the national level?
   a. American Association of Public Health Dentistry
   b. Association of State and Territorial Dental Directors
   c. United States Public Health Service
   d. Department of Health and Human Services
   e. Commissioned Corps of the United States Public Health Service

REFERENCES

1. American Dental Education Association. Competencies for entry into the profession of dental hygiene, Exhibit 7. J Dent Educ 2003;67(7):1–5. Available at: http://www.adea.org/cepr. Accessed February 2004.

2. Types of dental hygiene careers. American Dental Hygienists' Association Online. Available at: http://www.adha.org/careerinfo/types.htm. Accessed January 2003.

3. Council on Linkages Between Academia and Public Health Practice. Core Competencies for Public Health Professionals. Washington, DC: Public Health Foundation, 2001.

4. American Association of Public Health Dentistry/American Board of Dental Public Health. Competency Statements for Dental Public Health. J Public Health Dent 1998;58(Suppl. 1):119–122. Available at: http://www.aaphd.org.

5. Association of State and Territorial Dental Directors. 2003 Membership Data.

PROGRAM PLANNING
AND EVALUATION

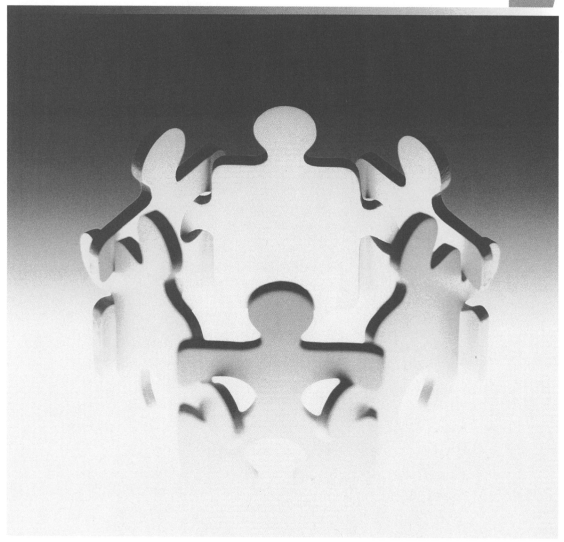

Effective Community Programs

5

Objectives

After studying this chapter and completing the study questions and activities, the learner will be able to:

- Compare and contrast community program development with individual patient care.
- Describe the crucial aspects of effective program development.
- Identify potential community partners for addressing a local oral health issue.

KEY TERMS

APEX-PH	Healthy People 2010 Toolkit	PATCH
ASTDD Seven-Step Model	Leveraging resources	Planning models
Coalitions	Logic model	Precede-Proceed
Common risk factor approach	Mobilizing for Action through	Resources
Cost-effectiveness	Planning and Partnerships	Stakeholders
Efficacious	Needs	Target group
Healthy Communities 2000: Model	Partners	Targeting
Standards	Partnerships	

The American Dental Education Association competencies addressed in this chapter include[1]:

HP.4:   Identify individual and population risk factors and develop strategies that promote a health-related quality of life.

CM.1:   Assess the oral health needs of the community and the quality and availability of resources and services.

CM.3:   Provide community oral health services in various settings.

CM.4:   Facilitate client access to oral health services by influencing individuals and/or organizations for the provision of oral health care.

CM.6:   Evaluate the outcomes of community-based programs and plan for future activities.

Introduction

A basic characteristic of dental public health professionals is the ability to assess oral health needs and then develop, implement, and evaluate effective programs aimed to improve the oral health of target populations. This chapter describes the criteria for effective program development and highlights the similarities and differences between the process of individual patient care and community program development. Several planning models are available to guide the development process; selected models will be described.

THE ROLE OF PROGRAM DEVELOPMENT IN PUBLIC HEALTH

Program development is the heart of dental public health. It is integral to effectiveness at the local, state, regional, national, and international levels. Program development incorporates the three core functions of public health—assessment, policy development, and assurance. Many of the essential public health services described in Chapter 1 are used in the development process, including:

- monitoring health status to identify community health problems.
- diagnosing and investigating health problems and health hazards in the community.
- mobilizing community **partnerships** to identify and solve health problems.
- evaluating effectiveness, accessibility, and quality of personal and population-based health services.
- developing policies and plans that support individual and community health efforts.

- researching for new insights and innovative solutions to health problems.[2]

Public health dental hygienists must appreciate their role as health professionals at the local, state, and national levels. This role requires the graduate dental hygienist to assess, diagnose, plan, implement, evaluate, and document programs and activities to benefit the general population. In this role, the dental hygienist must be prepared to influence others to facilitate access to care and services."[1]

The program development cycle, as shown in Figure 5-1, is a continuous loop. Assessment occurs first, followed by diagnosis, planning, implementation, evaluation, and documentation. Information gleaned from the evaluation feeds back to the planning cycle. Each step builds to the next, with the evaluation leading to program improvements. This cycle is integral to all planning models.

COMPARISON OF COMMUNITY PROGRAM DEVELOPMENT TO INDIVIDUAL PATIENT CARE PROCESS

Community program development in public health parallels the individual patient care process. However, in community-based programs, a **target group** is the patient, the "big picture" is even bigger, and the process is more complex (Table 5-1). Just as it is important to involve the patient in planning their individual care, it is important to involve the community in every step of the program development process.

An oral health provider first collects information to assess the **needs** of the patient. Needs can be defined as those things that are lacking but that are necessary for people to be in a healthy state. Similarly, the public health professional collects or

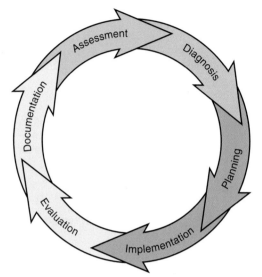

FIGURE 5-1 Program Development Cycle. Assessment, Diagnosis, Planning, Implementation, Evaluation, and Documention.

uses information to identify the needs of a community or group. In both the individual patient and community levels, the assessment of needs leads to a diagnosis. The patient's values, priorities, financial ability, health status, and many other factors are considered in prioritizing the needs and then developing a treatment plan to address and alleviate the patient's needs. In public health, **resources,** community priorities, politics, the environment, and other factors are considered in developing a plan to alleviate the identified needs. In private practice, an individual's treatment is implemented, the results are reevaluated periodically, and the patient is retreated as necessary to improve and maintain health. Public health programs are implemented, monitored, evaluated, and adapted to improve and maintain the health of the community. In both settings, careful planning ensures that the right interventions are provided effectively and efficiently. Evaluation provides accountability to those with a vested interest and guides effective individual patient care, as well as program improvements at the community level. Lastly, the individual patient care provider documents in a

patient's chart and shares the information with patients, other providers, and third-party payers. Similarly, the public health provider documents the results of programs to share with interested parties, government agencies, and funding sources.

CRITERIA FOR EFFECTIVE COMMUNITY PROGRAM DEVELOPMENT

Programs must meet several criteria to be effective in improving the public's health. They must be designed to meet a community recognized need, based on sufficient community resources, cost-effective, targeted toward identified needs, and accepted by the community. A proactive approach should be used rather than a reactive approach, and a common risk factor approach should be used as much as possible.

Community Recognized Need

The community must consider problems serious and relevant. "Public health professionals and policy makers must understand that oral health is essential to general health and well-being at every stage of life."[3] Ownership and commitment to the success of the program are especially important. For example, if parents view high tooth decay rates in children as serious enough to interfere with their health, wellness, and ability to learn, they will be more likely to endorse a school-based fluoride mouth rinse program.

Sufficient Community Resources

Sufficient resources, including people power, money, time, facilities, supplies, equipment, and legislative authority, must be available to support the start-up and continuation of a program. To start a program without the necessary resources is potentially worse than doing nothing at all; the recognized unmet needs could result in frustration and mistrust. Most funding agencies are interested in knowing how a program will sustain itself after initial pilot funding. Although it can be a challenge to obtain funding for new and innova-

TABLE 5-1 COMPARISON OF INDIVIDUAL PATIENT CARE PROCESS TO COMMUNITY PROGRAM DEVELOPMENT

INDIVIDUAL PATIENT CARE PROCESS	COMMUNITY PROGRAM DEVELOPMENT
Assessment • dental and medical history • intraoral and extraoral examination • periodontal health • caries status • oral hygiene • related factors (social, behavioral, psychological, cultural, economic)	**Assessment** • community oral health needs • demographics • related factors (social, cultural, economic, political, environmental, common risk factors, stakeholders) • community resources (people power, funding, services available, possible partnerships)
Diagnosis • caries status • periodontal status • other oral needs	**Diagnosis** • analyze and prioritize community needs • include partners, stakeholders, and advisory group
Planning • determine services to be rendered (preventive, periodontal therapy, restorative, esthetic, referral for specialty services, nutrition or tobacco counseling) • select appropriate provider to provide care (dental hygienist, dental therapist, assistant, general dentist, or specialist) • obtain informed consent	**Planning** • determine priorities and alternatives • gather resources • develop goals and objectives • select appropriate activities and interventions to meet goals • select appropriate personnel (dentist, dental hygienist/therapist, assistant, teachers, health care personnel, social workers, health educators, WIC counselors) • obtain community acceptance
Implementation • provide patient care (scaling, root planing, fluoride, tobacco counseling)	**Implementation** • provide intervention (clinical services, education, legislation, advocacy) • formative/process evaluation
Evaluation • post-treatment oral health • compare pretreatment and post-treatment data • appropriateness of care • patient satisfaction • determine next phase of treatment	**Evaluation** • attainment of goals and objectives • cost-effectiveness of program • appropriateness of activities • community satisfaction • summative/outcome evaluation
Documentation • provide thorough chart entries • inform patient • report to other health professionals • report to third party payers	**Documentation** • report to funding agencies • report to stakeholders (program participants, decision makers, partners, interested parties)

tive programs, it can be much more difficult to obtain funding for an existing program.

Most programs need various resources, including: people (time, skills, and talent), communication (printing, postage, telephones, copying), equipment (dental equipment, furniture, computers), supplies (sealant material, disposables, fluoride, pencils, paper, food), space (meeting places, offices, storage), transportation (airplanes, buses, cars), and special or miscellaneous needs (child care, security).[4] A community's assets can potentially support a program for a long time. Service clubs, insurance companies, hospital foundations, and dental organizations may serve as potential long-term funding sources. Service clubs, parents, and dental professionals may provide volunteer support; car dealers may volunteer the use of vehicles; and dental supply companies may donate supplies.

A change in policy may also help program sustainability. For example, if a state's practice act does not allow dental hygienists to be directly reimbursed for services, the practice act could be changed. Or, possibly a nonprofit community health center or county clinic could serve as the "provider" to be reimbursed by Medicaid or insurance to cover the dental hygienist's services.

Oral health programs frequently function in isolation from other public health efforts although multiple programs may be striving to achieve the same results while competing for limited funds. The concept of **leveraging resources** is emerging in response to the difficulty of trying to provide programs dependent on limited government funds. A program's potential can be greatly expanded by combining resources with other programs, working in **coalitions** or with **partners** to accomplish mutual goals. For example, oral hygiene education can be offered by Women Infant Children (WIC) counselors, oral health assessments and fluoride varnish applications can be incorporated into well-baby visits or immunization appointments, and comprehensive nutrition programs can include oral health applications. Further, insurance companies may be interested in reducing treatment costs by working with local or state health departments to cosponsor education and prevention programs.

Cost-Effectiveness

Cost-effective programs deliver enough benefit to justify their cost. Community-wide water fluoridation is considered one of the most cost-effective preventive measures available, costing approximately 50 times less than restoring teeth. It may seem obvious that a program that costs less but has high impact is more desirable to funding sources than a program that costs more with the same or lower impact. However, less effective programs may be more popular. Because of local political climates, water fluoridation may be less popular than school fluoride mouth rinse programs even though it is more effective.

Because of recent research linking oral health with general health, benefits can be compared to reductions in the cost of treating diabetes, heart disease, and low-birth-weight infants. Many oral health programs may be cost-effective based solely on their reduction in systemic diseases and related economic burden.

Targeted Interventions

Oral health promotion programs must match current needs and health priorities and use resources wisely by **targeting** efforts toward at-risk populations.[5] This means that high-priority populations are targeted with appropriate **efficacious** interventions. Interventions should be science-based and proven appropriate for individuals and communities.[3] The *Guide to Community Preventive Services* and the *Guide to Clinical Preventive Services* provide criteria and guidance for evaluating scientific literature and promoting effective interventions.[6]

For example, if a program goal was to reduce dental caries in children aged 6–12 years, it would not be enough to just teach a class on toothbrushing methods at every school in a community. Multiple age-appropriate interventions might be recommended, including fluoride, oral hygiene measures, school-based sealants, and healthy snacks in vending machines.

Preventive interventions also should be culturally appropriate or developed in consideration of language, health beliefs, dietary practices, child rearing practices, and other factors that influence health practices. Additionally, assessments showing that low-income minority children are dispropor-tionately affected means that those schools in low-income and/or ethnic neighborhoods would re-ceive priority over schools in mid- to high-income neighborhoods.

Community Acceptance

Stakeholders' acceptance is crucial to the success of programs. Stakeholders are people who have the potential to be affected by a program and could include community and organization deci-sion-makers, dental health professionals, and tar-geted end users (community members and taxpay-ers).[7] Broad representation should be included during initial program development and contin-ued during all stages. It is not safe to assume that a program's ability to improve health will automati-cally lead to various parties' commitment, support, and acceptance. However, groups are motivated by the recognition that programs will have a direct benefit to them. For example, policy makers are motivated by saving taxpayer money and by voter approval. Dental/dental hygiene school faculty may be interested in providing students with qual-ity community experiences.[8]

Proactive Approach

Health promoting interventions are most effective if they strategically predict, plan, and prevent po-tential crisis rather than react to problems. For ex-ample, it would be preferable to promote the use of mouth guards, helmets, and seat belts than to spend valuable resources on the treatment of pre-ventable injuries.

Common Risk Factors

Factors that increase oral disease risk often in-crease the risk for other diseases as well. Smoking increases oral cancer risk and also increases the risk for heart disease and many other diseases. Frequent high-sucrose snacking often leads to dental caries and can also lead to obesity and affect diabetes. Programs such as tobacco cessation, diet

counseling, and health education that address these common risk factors can effectively reduce the risk for many diseases and at the same time use funds efficiently in a fiscally responsible way.

It is more common to integrate oral health with general health programs in European countries than in the United States.[9] A **common risk factor approach** shares resources and improves effec-tiveness.[10] This approach makes sense. Tobacco, unhealthy diet choices, and poor oral hygiene are behaviors that contribute to many diseases. Through general health programs, oral health can be improved, coinciding with diabetes control, re-duced heart disease, and improved birth outcomes. The ways to plan for sustainability of programs are infinite.

Seven criteria for effective program develop-ment have been described. If any criteria are miss-ing, the initial program may be adapted to im-prove weak areas. Suppose a plan to decrease early childhood caries is proposed and that plan includes assessment, education, and placement of fluoride varnish. Initial development reveals that there are not enough oral care providers or a state practice act does not support an activity such as the application of fluoride varnish by a dental hy-gienist if children have not had a dental exam by a dentist. A program could then train nurses, physi-cian assistants, and nurse practitioners to include an oral assessment and fluoride varnish applica-tion in their regular well-baby visits, increasing the actual available assets or resources to carry out a program. The program could also, at the same time, advocate for changes in the dental practice act to provide more flexibility.

DISCUSSION OF PLANNING MODELS

Planning models can be thought of as structured guides or tools that are used when developing com-munity programs. There are several planning mod-els used by oral health programs and general health programs. Six selected models will be illustrated, followed by a discussion of their similarities and dif-ferences. These models include Assessing Oral

MODEL ORAL HEALTH NEEDS ASSESSMENT

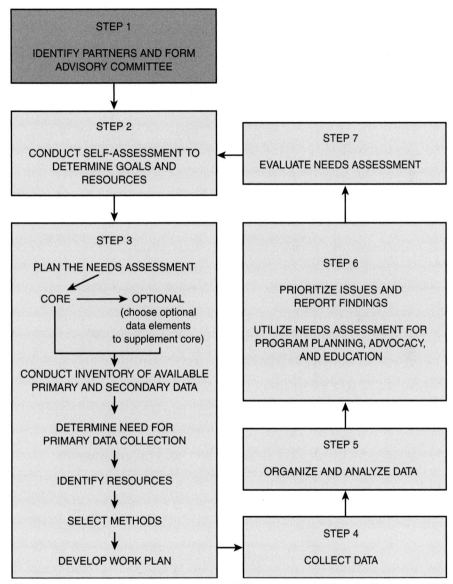

FIGURE 5-2 Seven-Step Needs Assessment Model (Source: Assessing Oral Health Needs: ASTDD Seven-Step Model [1995]. Available at: http://www.astdd.org. Accessed January 2004.)

Health Needs: ASTDD Seven-Step Model, logic models, Healthy People 2010 Toolkit, Precede-Proceed, Healthy Communities 2000: Model Standards, and Mobilizing for Action Through Planning and Partnerships.

Assessing Oral Health Needs: ASTDD Seven-Step Model

Assessing Oral Health Needs: Association of State and Territorial Dental Directors (ASTDD) Seven-Step Model is a needs assessment tool that can be accessed through the Association of State and Territorial Dental Directors Web site. It is used by many states, although many modify it to meet their needs. Figure 5-2 illustrates the seven steps involved.[5]

Logic Models

A **logic model** is a concise way to show how a program is designed and will make a difference for a program's participants and a community. It shows the relationship between the program's ultimate

LOGIC MODEL FOR LEARNING
Adding Additional Evaluation Components

PROGRAM		OUTCOMES	EVALUATION AND LEARNING
DESIRED RESULTS			**DATA SOURCES AND METHODS** Where the data needed to track the indicators and performance measures will come from.
MOTIVATING CONDITIONS AND CAUSES	◄►	INDICATORS	**EVALUATION QUESTIONS** Questions, based on indicator data and movement that will determine whether the strategy needs to be modified. Questions, based on the performance measures, that determine whether the project is working as intended, what lessons have been learned, and how the project may need to be modified to get better results.
STRATEGIES	◄►	PERFORMANCE MEASURES	**STAKEHOLDERS** The funders, collaborators, and other individuals or organizations with a vested interest in the program who need to be involved in learning from the data being collected.
ACTIVITIES			**MECHANISMS FOR LEARNING** The opportunities for stakeholders to come together and learn from and make decisions based on the data about the program.

FIGURE 5-3 Logic Models for Learning. (Reprinted with permission from Harvard Family Research Project. Learning from logic models in out-of-school time. Cambridge, MA: Author, 2002.) (Logic model is adapted from: Watson S. Using results to improve the lives of children and families: A guide for public-private child care partnership. Washington, DC: Child Care Partnership Project, 2000.)

aim and the strategies and activities used to get there, together with an outline of how progress will be measured along the way.[11] Displayed graphically, it is customized according to defined health issues and identified risk factors.[12] Figure 5-3 illustrates an example of a logic model.

Healthy People 2010 Toolkit

Healthy People 2010 Toolkit provides guidance, technical tools, and resources to help states, territories, and tribes develop and promote successful, state-specific Healthy People 2010 plans. It may be helpful as a resource for similar planning activities. It is organized around seven major action areas derived from national Healthy People initiatives. These areas are:

- Building the foundation: leadership and structure
- Identifying and securing resources
- Identifying and engaging community partners
- Setting health priorities and establishing objectives
- Obtaining baseline measures, setting targets, and measuring progress

- Managing and sustaining the process
- Communicating health goals and objectives.

The Healthy People 2010 Tool kit is available in a Web-based version.[13]

Precede-Proceed

Dr. Lawrence W. Green and colleagues developed the **Precede-Proceed Model** of health promotion program planning illustrated in Figure 5-4. The goals of the model are to "explain health-related behaviors and to design and evaluate the interventions designed to influence both the behaviors and the living conditions that influence them and their sequelae." It is founded on many disciplines and emphasizes that (1) multiple factors influence health and health risks; therefore, (2) multidimensional or multisectorial efforts are needed, and will be explored further in Chapter 9. It has been used to plan various health education programs.[14]

Healthy Communities 2000: Model Standards

Healthy Communities 2000: Model Standards is a guidebook and tool for planning public health efforts. Local public health agencies used it to work

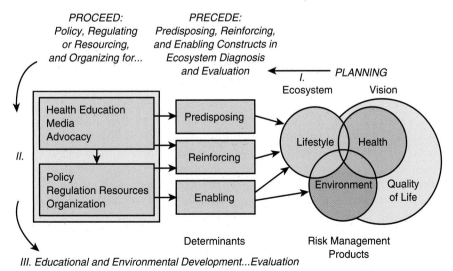

FIGURE 5-4 Precede-Proceed Model of Health Promotion Program Planning (Source: Green LW. Available at: http://www.ihpr.ubc.ca/ProcedePrecede.html).

toward Healthy People 2000 objectives. It has not been updated for the 2010 objectives and was instead replaced by the Healthy People 2010 Toolkit described earlier. It does not incorporate behavioral and social dimensions or diversity issues. It includes two planning tools: **APEX-PH** (Assessment Protocol for Excellence in Public Health) and **PATCH** (Planned Approach to Community Health).[15]

Mobilizing for Action Through Planning and Partnerships

Mobilizing for Action through Planning and Partnerships (MAPP) is a community-wide strategic planning tool for improving community health that builds on Healthy Communities 2000: Model Standards. It emphasizes community ownership and community-driven initiatives. This model includes phases that start with Organizing for Success and Partnership Development and follows with Visioning, Assessments, Identifying Strategic Issues, Formulating Goals and Strategies, and an Action Plan. Key content areas drive the process. Detailed information, guidance, tools, and vignettes can be found about the model from the National Association of City and County Health Officials.[16]

Comparison of Models

All of the models provide useful insight into the stages and framework involved in the community program development process. Commonalities exist among them. In some form, all of the models use the steps of assessment, diagnosis, planning, implementation, evaluation, and documentation. Older models can be criticized for not considering the sociocultural, political, and environmental context of health or the lack of community involvement in the process.[17]

Some planners feel that Greene's Precede-Proceed model is highly theoretical and cumbersome. ASTDD's-seven step has proved helpful in planning and evaluating assessments but not for

program implementation and evaluation stages. In addition, professionals from other health disciplines are not familiar with this model, and its use may encourage the perception that dental public health practice is isolated from other public health programs. Some experts consider APEX-PH and PATCH models outmoded because of current issues of interest such as diversity, geomapping, bioterrorism, and community empowerment. MAPP stresses community capacity and is considered to be more powerful than APEX-PH and PATCH because it has built on the lessons learned with the previous model. The strength of the logic model is its ease of understanding use and customization. The advantages and disadvantages of selected models are outlined in Table 5-2.

No single model may be sufficient for all situations. Models are continuously being adapted as new factors arise that influence programs. Elements of different models may be combined to apply to a new situation or need.

COMMUNITY PARTNERS

It is vital to involve many community partners through coalitions and collaborative approaches. Performance is optimized through shared or leveraged resources and responsibility.[18] Partners or stakeholders can be involved as advisory groups, key decision makers, or working groups. Their involvement increases their acceptance of the program. Broad community representation should be sought and can include members from the groups listed in Box 5-1.[18]

The smart planner includes all parties throughout the program development process, from assessing the needs of the community through documentation, in a celebration of successes. It is important not to overlook the roles and contributions of every individual and group. Presentations and certificates of appreciation recognize each group's contribution to sustain excitement for the shared process.[16]

TABLE 5-2 COMPARISON OF PLANNING MODELS

MODEL	PURPOSE	ADVANTAGE	DISADVANTAGE
Precede-Proceed	Plan health education programs based on analysis of multiple health and risk factors	Familiar to many professionals	• Cumbersome • Highly theoretical
Healthy Communities 2000 Model Standards/APEX-PH and PATCH planning tools	Guidebook and toolkit to plan programs to meet HP 2000 objectives	• Internet resources available • APEX-PH adaptable and easy to use	• Not updated • Lacks behavioral, cultural, and social dimension
MAPP	Strategic community-wide planning tool	• Comprehensive • Emphasizes community involvement	Requires numerous resources
Healthy People 2010 Toolkit	Help communities meet Healthy People 2010 Objectives	• Current • Available on the Internet	Cumbersome for small programs
Assessing Oral Health Needs: ASTDD Seven-Step Model	Plan assessments	Available on the Internet	Requires using additional sources for program development pieces
Logic Model	Custom-designed plan to address various health issues and identified risk factors	Easy to use and understand	Assumes user has previous knowledge

BOX 5-1 Community Partners

- Professional oral health organizations
- Oral health providers
- State or local oral health departments
- State maternal and child health programs
- Women, Infants, and Children (WIC) Program
- Medicaid program
- Early and periodic screening, diagnosis and treatment (EPSDT)
- Public and private school systems, including dental and dental hygiene schools
- Advocacy health organizations (eg, Children's Defense Fund)
- Other health professional associations and their members
- Organizations advocating for special populations
- Civic groups, trade unions, and local businesses
- Consumer groups
- Mass media
- Decision makers and community leadership
- Dental and related industries
- Insurance agencies and companies
- Athletic organizations
- Faith organizations[18]

Source: Cohen LK. Promoting oral health: guidelines for dental associations. Int Dent J 1990;40(2):79–102.[18]

SUMMARY

The activities involved in public health program development parallel the assessment, diagnosis, planning, implementation, evaluation, and documentation activities of individual patient care. In the same way that a dental provider assesses a patient's needs prior to planning and implementing care and then evaluates the outcomes, a public health planner must also have a guiding process. It is helpful to use a standard planning approach, as do the models presented in this chapter. All of the models have elements that are useful, and the learner should recognize and have a basic understanding of different models and be prepared to contribute to the program development process. Programs are much more effective when planning is accomplished with the input and acceptance of the community and when there are sufficient resources to conduct a program. Effective programs use appropriate targeted interventions, have recognized benefit to all stakeholders and, in today's world, may use the common risk approach and leverage resources to optimize their effectiveness.

 Learning Activities

1. Refer to the list of essential public health services in Chapter 1. Peruse the local newspaper for articles about local public health efforts. Identify how essential public health services are or could be applied in the local public health efforts.
2. Contact a local community health center or nonprofit organization. Request a list of advisory board members. Identify how the program may benefit or be of interest to each party.
3. Interview the director of a local program, asking questions related to the seven criteria for effectiveness to see if each is met by the program.
4. Identify a public health initiative in a neighboring country (i.e., Mexico or Canada) and identify key stakeholders.

RESOURCES

PROGRAM PLANNING WEBSITES:

The Precede-Proceed Model of Health Promotion: Available at: http://www.ihpr.ubc.ca
Healthy Communities: Model Standards. Available at: http://www.apha.org/ppp/science/TheGuide.htm
Healthy People 2010 Toolkit. Available at: http://www.health.gov/healthypeople/state/toolkit
Arizona Prevention: Available at: http://www.Resource Centerazprevention.org
Logic Model: Available at: http://www.azprevention.org
Association of State and Territorial Dental Directors (ASTDD). Available at: http://www.astdd.org

Centers for Disease Control and Prevention (CDC). Available at: http://www.cdc.gov/eval/resources.htm

Review Questions

1. All of the following are required for effective program planning EXCEPT for:
   a. sufficient time and resources.
   b. prompt reaction to a crisis.
   c. community recognition of a need.
   d. behavioral, cultural, environmental, and political influences addressed.
   e. community input and ownership.

2. The most important consideration when creating effective public health programs is to:
   a. have a Master's degree in public health.
   b. discuss problems with key stakeholders.
   c. increase the public's awareness.
   d. get the community's input prior to planning programs.
   e. hire a program evaluator.

3. The best time to get community input when developing dental public health programs is:
   a. during the evaluation stage.
   b. during implementation.
   c. during needs assessment.
   d. during the writing of the goals and objectives.
   e. during the grant writing phase.

4. Determining the cost-effectiveness of a community dental program is most similar to what element of the individual patient care process?
   a. Setting a patient payment plan
   b. Obtaining the patient's informed consent
   c. Evaluating the effectiveness of treatment
   d. Documenting the results of treatment
   e. Diagnosing treatment needs

5. Sufficient resources are necessary for effective programs. The creative planner will use which of the following methods to make the best use of resources?
   a. Leveraging resources
   b. Considering common risk factors
   c. Working in coalitions
   d. Developing partnerships
   e. All of the above

REFERENCES

1. American Dental Education Association. Competencies for entry into the profession of dental hygiene, exhibit 7. J Dent Ed 2003 July;67(7):1–5. Available at: http://www.adea.org/cepr. Accessed January 2004

2. Essential Public Health Services. Public Health Foundation. Available at: http://www.phf.org/essential.htm. Accessed January 2004.

3. A national call to action to promote oral health: A public-private partnership under the leadership of the office of the Surgeon General. DHHS NIH Publication No. 03-5303, May 2003. Available at: http://www.nidcr.nih.gov. Accessed January 2004.

4. Promoting oral health: interventions for preventing dental caries, pharyngeal cancers and sports-related craniofacial injuries. MMWR November 2001 SO (RR21)1–13. Available at: http://www.cdc.gov/mmwr. Accessed January 2004.

5. Assessing oral health needs: ASTDD seven-step model. 1995. Available at: http://www.astdd.org. Accessed January 2004.

6. U.S. Preventive Services Task Force Guide to Clinical Preventive Services. 2nd Ed. Baltimore, MD: Williams and Wilkins, 1996.

7. Watson MR, Horowitz AM, Garcia I, Canto MT. A community participatory oral health promotion program in an inner-city Latino community. J Public Health Dent 2001;61(1):34–41.

8. DeAngellis S, Warren C. Establishing community partnerships: providing better oral health care to underserved children. J Dent Hyg 2001;75(4):310–315.

9. Homan MS. Promoting Community Change: Making It Happen in the Real World. Pacific Grove, CA: Brooks/Cole, 1993.

10. Edhag O. Quality assurance in prevention. Adv Dent Res 1995;9(2):89–90.

11. Harvard Family Research Project. Learning from logic models in out-of-school time. Cambridge, MA: Author, 2002. Logic model is adapted from: Watson S. Using results to improve the lives of children and families: A guide for public-private child care partnerships. Washington, DC: Child Care Partnership Project, 2000. Available at www.hfrp.org. Accessed January 2004.

12. Arizona Prevention Resource Center: Guide to a Healthy Arizona. Available at http://www.azprevention.org. Accessed January 2004.

13. Healthy People 2010 Toolkit: A Field Guide To Health planning. Public Health Foundation. Available at: http://www.health.gov/healthypeople/state/toolkit. Accessed January 2004.

14. Green LW, Kreuter MW. Health Promotion Planning: An Educational and Ecological Approach, 3rd ed. Mountain View, CA: Mayfield Publishing, 1999. Available at: http://www.ihpr.ubc.ca/ProcedePrecede.html Accessed January 2004.

15. A guide to implementing model standards. American Public Health Association. Available at: http://www.apha.org/ppp/science/theguide.htm. Accessed January 2004.

16. Mobilizing for action through planning and partnerships. National Association of City and County Health Officials. Available at: http://naccho.org/. Accessed January 2004.

17. Watts R, Fuller S. Approaches in oral health promotion. In: Pine CM, ed. Community Oral Health. Boston, MA: Reed Education and Professional Publishing Ltd, 1997. p 238–251.

18. Cohen LK. Promoting oral health: guidelines for dental associations. Int Dental J 1990;40(2):79–102.

Planning for Community Programs

Objectives

After studying this chapter and completing the study questions and activities, the learner will be able to:

- List the types of data that should be included in a community assessment.
- Identify relevant data sources.
- Differentiate between primary and secondary data sources.
- Describe the parts of the program plan.
- Develop mission statements, goals, and objectives.
- Provide examples of interventions and activities.
- Develop a sample time line.
- Develop a sample budget.

KEY TERMS

Activities
Community needs assessment
Community profile
Cost-benefit ratio
Direct activities
Flow charts
Indirect activities

In-kind support
Interventions
Job descriptions
Mapping
Mission statement
Needs analysis
Organizational diagram

Pilot test
Primary data
Program goals
Program objectives
Secondary data
Time line
Work statement

The American Dental Education Association competencies addressed in this chapter include[1]:

C.3:   Provide dental hygiene care to promote patient/client health and wellness using critical thinking and problem solving in the provision of dental hygiene care.

C.4:   Use evidence-based decision making to evaluate and incorporate emerging treatment modalities.

CM.1:   Assess the oral health needs of the community and the quality and availability of resources and services.

CM.3:   Provide community oral health services in a variety of settings.

HP.1:   Promote the values of oral and general health and wellness to the public and organizations within and outside the profession.

HP.4.   Identify individual and population risk factors and develop strategies that promote a health-related quality of life.

Introduction

This chapter discusses the first three phases of the basic program development process described in Chapter 5, including assessment, diagnosis, and planning for community-based programs. Specific evaluation methods will be discussed in Chapter 7; however, it is important to consider evaluation strategies throughout development of the program plan. Each part is interrelated and integral to the success and effectiveness of programs. The methods for program development incorporate the common steps included in the various planning models presented in Chapter 5. The entry-level learner, who understands these steps, is prepared to contribute to the program development process.

It is important to include an advisory group into the program development process. The advisory group described in Chapter 5 can provide input into identifying relevant problems, considering alternative solutions, developing a plan for making effective and efficient use of resources, identifying resources necessary for implementation and evaluation and, finally, fostering ownership for the plan and commitment to its success.[2]

THE COMMUNITY NEEDS ASSESSMENT

The **community needs assessment** (Box 6-1) has several purposes. This step in program plan-

ning helps determine to what extent the needs exist and their salience when compared with other problems and needs. The needs assessment phase includes the collection, analysis, and interpretation of information and is the foundation for effective program planning and successful program development. The planning models discussed in Chapter 5 illustrated various methods for the collection and organization of data.

Collecting Facts

The first step in needs assessment is to collect facts to build a community assessment or **community profile.** The information includes demographic data, knowledge, attitudes and practices, oral health status, and the impact of current oral health levels.

Demographic data help the planner understand the makeup of the community. This data may include information about age, gender, education, occupation, income, ethnicity/language, geographic area, length of residence, and school enrollment.

BOX 6-1 The Community Needs Assessment

- Collection of Facts
- Identification of Needs
- Analysis of Needs
- Prioritization of Needs

The collection of knowledge, attitudes, and self-care practices leads to an understanding of the level and type of health promotion interventions that are indicated. Data may include the community's knowledge and attitudes and practices concerning oral health, such as frequency and values regarding visits to oral health care providers; reasons and expectations for oral health services; knowledge about water fluoridation, plaque removal, use of fluoride regimens; frequency of consumption of sweets and other highly refined carbohydrates; tobacco and alcohol use; and use of oral-facial protection.

Oral health status indicators for the community can be compared with state and national data. These may include the percentage of people with decay experience, percentage of untreated decay, percentage of children with sealants, percentage of edentulousness, and the percentage of tobacco users.

The impact of current oral health levels is needed to understand the costs of disease and the potential benefit of programs. This data may include time lost from school and work and expenditures for dental services.[2,3]

Facts about dental resources and existing programs are also included in a needs assessment. These may include number, type and distribution of dental providers; number and type of low-cost clinics; and percentage and type of providers who accept Medicare/Medicaid patients. It is also help-ful to collect data about barriers such as the percentage of people without dental insurance. Finally, information about the environment, including schools, water systems, transportation services, other health care facilities, and laws and regulations regarding oral health, are also important. Working with other interested agencies and an advisory group of key leaders and stakeholders is invaluable to effectively identifying needs and community assets.

Information relating to the community may be readily available. Data that is already available is referred to as **secondary data.** In other situations, it is necessary to collect information directly by means of a survey or dental screening method. Data collected specifically for use in a program is referred to as **primary data.** The collection of secondary data, prior to collecting any primary data, will save time and money, depending on how well the data fits the information needs. For this reason, it is important to search for secondary data carefully and thoroughly. Table 6-1 lists the advantages and disadvantages of primary and secondary data.

There are many ways to collect useful secondary data. Sources may include federal, state, and local health agencies; other public health programs; and the state dental board. A research librarian can be tremendously helpful in this process. In addition, the Internet presents a useful tool. Table 6-2 illustrates examples of Internet sites that contain secondary data.

TABLE 6-1 COMPARISON OF PRIMARY AND SECONDARY DATA

TYPE OF DATA	TECHNIQUE/TYPE	ADVANTAGE	DISADVANTAGE
Primary	• Survey/questionnaire • Interview • Observation • Experiment	• Current Information • Answers specific question • Known source	• Expensive • Time consuming
Secondary	• Computerized database • Bibliographic database • Numeric database	• Inexpensive • Readily available • Enhance existing data	• May not match needs • Definitions may not be useful • May be out of date • May be difficult to assess credibility

TABLE 6-2 WEB SITES FOR SECONDARY DATA

TYPE OF DATA	WEB SITE
Federal data	http://www.fedstats.gov
Census data	http://www.census.gov
National opinion poll data	http://www.gallup.com
National Oral Health Surveillance System	http://www.cdc.gov/nohss/
National Center for Health Statistics	http://www.cdc.gov/nchs/products.htm
Bureau of Labor Statistics	http://stats.bls.gov/
Healthy People 2010 Objectives	http://www.healthypeople.gov
Examples of state data	http://www.hs.state.az.us/ http://www.chawisconsin.org/oralhealth.htm http://www2.cdc.gov/nccdphp/doh/synopses/index.asp http://www.cdc.gov/OralHealth/data_systems/index.htm

Survey Methods

After an exhaustive search for secondary data, the planner can consider methods for collecting primary data. There are advantages and disadvantages of different types of measurement to consider before embarking on a survey, questionnaire, or screening. The type of information needed also determines the type of data collection that is necessary. Focus groups, surveys, and individual interviews can determine attitudes, knowledge, behaviors, and values. Oral health status information, including oral hygiene, dental caries, and periodontal disease levels, requires a screening using a dental index with standardized methods and calibrated examiners. Chapter 13 addresses the dental indices useful for community health programs.

It may be useful to consult with experienced personnel, for example, the state department of health or a regional office of the U.S. Public Health Service. A statistician can help with sampling, records, data analysis, and presentation of findings. Problems with questions can be identified and solved in advance by using a **pilot test.** A pilot test is a method of checking to make sure the survey is useable and to determine if people interpret questions as intended and to make sure that given answers include all possibilities. Finally, it helps to work out all of the "bugs." For example, a survey is planned to assess Head Start parents' knowledge, attitudes, and behaviors regarding oral health. A small group of Head Start parents from a different community could take the survey as the pilot test and offer feedback on misleading or unclear questions.

Table 6-3 shows a comparison of survey methods. The type of survey is determined by comparing the pros and cons of each and by considering the type of information needed. A random phone survey would be an appropriate way to assess the

TABLE 6-3 COMPARISON OF SURVEY METHODS

	MAIL	TELEPHONE	PERSONAL
Quantity of Data	Good	Fair	Excellent
Control of Interviewer	Excellent	Fair	Poor
Control of Sample	Poor	Excellent	Good
Speed	Poor	Excellent	Good
Flexibility	Poor	Good	Excellent
Response Rate	Poor	Good	Good
Cost	Good	Fair	Poor

percentage of people who wanted water fluoridation. A personal open-ended interview may be the best choice to collect information about cultural patterns that impact disease. A mailed survey may be a good choice for collecting information about dental providers.

The Community Profile

All of the primary and secondary information collected create a factual picture or community profile. The community profile will help assess the feasibility of the planned program and help determine whether there are sufficient resources to provide the program. A program is likely to fail if there are neither enough nor the right resources available. The community profile is a demographic description of a community, including the total population, number of households and size, age distribution, household income, marital status, racial/ethnic composition, education geographic boundaries, the political and economic atmosphere, and dental and medical resources.

Analyzing and Displaying Information

After primary and secondary data are collected, they are tabulated, organized, and interpreted to present an accurate and overall view. Complex data are easier to understand if presented graphically. Tables and charts should be simple and clear with matching formats (e.g., pie charts all in the same color scheme).

It may be helpful to use **mapping** as a tool to identify trends, patterns, and opportunities. This technique, borrowed from the business world, uses geographical information systems to provide analysis and display of health-related data sets on maps. Relationships between variables can become easily apparent and intervention efforts can be targeted to areas where they are most needed. For example, dental disease indices can be combined with census and postal codes. This could illustrate clusters of such oral problems as injuries, oral cancer, or dental decay related to demographic or socioeconomic factors. It is also an ef-

fective way to identify mismatches between dental services and population needs.[4]

Prioritizing Needs

The **needs analysis** helps determine whether a problem is caused by a lack of service or a lack of use of existing services. The planner wants to demonstrate that the problem takes priority over other concerns and that money spent solving the problem will save money in the long term. When setting priorities, it is important to consider the emergency nature of the problem, the number of people affected, the public's perception of its importance, the availability of resources, the degree to which the conditions can be prevented or controlled, and the availability and acceptance of effective technologies.[2] An advisory group can help determine how needs should be prioritized.

Epidemiologic indices demonstrate the prevalence of a problem. Local data can be compared with state and national data to show how a local problem compares with the national average or relevant marker. The severity of the problem and consequences if the program does not exist can be strong motivators for acceptance. A hypothetical example: Orange County data screenings and surveys reveal a severe dental problem. In comparison, among Orange County 6–8 year olds, 49% have untreated dental decay compared with 37% in California and 39% in the United States. School nurses report that more children miss school as a result of dental problems than for any other health complaint. If this dental disease is not treated, the dental caries will progress and the children's learning and overall well-being will be affected. Their untreated dental disease will become more expensive to treat.

The success rates for similar programs may motivate communities to give increased priority for the program. An estimated **cost-benefit ratio** is also helpful. This is the difference between the cost of providing the program versus the cost of not providing the program. For example: water fluoridation costs about as much as one filling per person per lifetime. It prevents 50% of future decay. Or, one dollar spent on water fluoridation annually saves $38 in dental bills.[5]

Finally, support letters from stakeholders can be collected and included to demonstrate recognition of the problem by many agencies and respected citizens or leaders in the community. These will be much easier to solicit if these stakeholders are involved from the beginning.

DEVELOPING THE PROGRAM

Program development begins with assessing needs, diagnosing and prioritizing the problem, and then drafting the mission statement, program goals, program objectives, program interventions, and program activities. These are the building blocks to a strong and effective program (Box 6-2). The data from the needs assessment and the community profile are used to develop a solution for the problem. The needs analysis may have revealed multiple factors. High decay rates in a community could be influenced by a multitude of factors, including lack of fluoride in the water supply, low utilization of dental care, culturally related patterns related to snacking, and people's attitudes. Most state and some local programs set key indicators against which they measure the success of their programs. They may come from Healthy People 2010 objectives or other sources. These indicators may be helpful reference points for the development of goals and objectives.

The Mission Statement

There are many ways to write program mission statements, goals, and objectives. One such system is presented here. These statements are used to focus the program, clarify expectations, provide a framework for evaluation of the program, and provide a guide for all personnel in the program.

A **mission statement** is a single statement that expresses a broad, overarching purpose for the program's existence. It serves as a broad, long-term program guide and should not include any

---

BOX 6-2 Goals and Objectives

- The Mission Statement
- Program Goals
- Program Objectives
- Program Interventions
- Program Activities

---

goals, objectives, activities, or interventions. It is written as follows:

To + directional statement + quality of life or category of service area + target group

Program Goals

Program goals address identified needs and are more specific than the mission statement. Although there is only one mission statement, there can be more than one program goal supporting the mission statement. Goals are broad-based statements of desired long-term or short-term changes that, if achieved, will alleviate identified needs. They are numbered and written as follows:

To + directional statement + need area + target population

Program Objectives

Program Objectives are designed to meet goals and are more specific than goals, because they guide program interventions. Objectives are designed to address needs and reasons for needs that were identified by focus groups or interviews during the needs assessment. For example, the needs assessment may have shown that Miami males develop oral cancer because they chew tobacco. Focus groups noted that professional baseball players encourage the action by chewing tobacco during major league games, that children imitate major league baseball players, and that tobacco companies target children in spit tobacco advertising. Objectives define a desired change in the clients or the environment. Often, there are multiple objectives for each goal. Program objectives also are identified with a number to match each goal and include an extension. They are written using this formula:

To + directional statement + change in client or environment + target population

It is critical that objectives be developed with the consideration of how they will be evaluated. A common guide for writing objectives is the SMART formula. This formula has been adapted in different ways by program developers, but is extremely useful for creating objectives focused on the program goals. Objectives should be:

Specific: Focus and precision are essential in setting objectives. This eliminates confusion and allows easier measurement.

Measurable: They must be easily assessed to gauge progress of the program.

Appropriate: Needs of the population group should be the central focus in the objectives of any intervention. The end result should be reasonably attainable.

Realistic/Related: Achievable, yet challenging, objectives help motivate those involved in delivering the intervention. They should also be directly related to expected outcomes.

Time Bound: It is essential that a timescale be specified to assess changes achieved. Time frames can be for intermediate or end of program outcomes.[6]

Program Interventions

Program **interventions** are task-oriented and designed to answer the explanation of the problem or identified need. They are matched to goals and identify what the program will actually provide. Needs are more effectively impacted with multiple levels and types of interventions. There are four types of program interventions:

- Educational (provision of information to target group)
- Direct service (provision of services)

- Organizational (changes in organizational infrastructure)
- Power (can involve litigation or law forming)

Program interventions are written as follows:

To + action term + units of service + target population

It is important to draw on the successes of others. The effectiveness of various oral health promotion interventions was evaluated and summarized by Watt el al. in 2001 (Box 6-3).[6]

Program Activities

Program **activities** are the component steps required to carry out an intervention. They are the program building blocks. For example, a fluoride mouth rinse program might include sending out and then collecting permission slips, ordering supplies, scheduling, reporting, and many other steps. Time frames are indicated for the completion of each activity. There are two types of activities, direct and indirect.

Direct activities are those steps directly involved in the delivery of the intervention. These activities involve the actual steps necessary in an intervention. An educational session could involve such steps as reviewing materials, drafting a lesson plan, developing and printing handouts, scheduling a pilot test, running a pilot test, evaluating the lesson, revising the lesson, scheduling the lessons, and many more.

Indirect activities are the "behind-the-scenes activities" required to carry out the intervention. They are supportive in nature and not necessarily numbered. They may include record keeping, secretarial support, or equipment maintenance. A sample goals and objectives section of a hypothetical program is shown in Table 6-4.

THE WORK STATEMENT

The **work statement,** or action plan, explains what, where, and when the program activities are accomplished. It includes a time line for comple-

BOX 6-3 Effectiveness of Oral Health Promotion Interventions

- Water fluoridation is effective at preventing dental caries. Fluoride toothpaste is another effective method of delivering fluoride.
- Improving an individual's knowledge of oral health can be achieved through oral health promotion, but the clinical, behavioral, and health significance of this is unknown.
- Information alone does not produce long-term behavior changes
- Oral health promotion on an individual level is effective for reducing plaque levels. However, these produce only short-term changes. School-based toothbrushing campaigns aimed at improving oral hygiene are not effective.
- Few studies have assessed the effect of oral health promotion on sugar consumption. Those studies that have attempted to alter sugar consumption have used self-reported outcome measures that have limited validity.
- Health education studies, which target the entire population, may increase inequalities in oral health.
- Little evidence on cost-effectiveness has been assessed in oral health promotion. However, traditional oral health education using health professionals is relatively costly.
- Mass media campaigns are ineffective at promoting either knowledge or behavior changes, although they may increase awareness.
- Limited evidence exists on the effectiveness of screening for the early detection of oral cancer.

Source: Watt RG, Fuller S, Harnett R, Treasure ET, Stillman-Lowe C. Oral health promotion evaluation—time for development. Comm Dent Oral Epidemiol 2001;29:161–166.[6]

tion of each activity and a narrative that describes the activities. It may be helpful to organize the plan in a chart similar to the one shown in Table 6-5. Another professional should be able to pick up the work statement and understand it well enough to run the program.

Time Lines and Narrative

A **time line** is a chart that depicts target dates for completion of program activities (Fig. 6-1). Various styles are effective, depending on the complexity of the program. The time line helps staff to complete activities and see the "big picture" with concurrent activities. The aim is to keep on time and ahead of budget. A narrative details the activity steps. For example, for Step 1, the narrative might say: August 05: Contact county immunization clinic, Head Start, and WIC staff to

determine the most efficient way to see children. Pilot test the assessment form and complete edits of the form.

ORGANIZATION

The organization of the program plan provides details about the networking of the program and includes job descriptions, an organizational diagram, flow charts, and a program budget.

Job Descriptions

Job descriptions are written for use in hiring staff and for dividing necessary activities. They also clarify each person's role in the program. Job descriptions generally include four parts. (1) Job title, which should be simple and descriptive. (2) Job qualifications, including a description of the minimal level of education and skills needed to

TABLE 6-4 GOALS AND OBJECTIVES

LEVEL	FORMULA	EXAMPLES
Mission Statement	To + directional statement + quality of life or category of service area + target group	To improve the oral health of Miami, FL, citizens.
Goals	To + directional statement + need area + target population	1. To decrease oral cancer in males living in Miami, FL.
Objectives	To + directional statement + change in client or environment + target population	1.1 To decrease the initiation of tobacco chewing among youth in Miami, FL.
		1.2 To decrease tobacco advertising targeted toward youth in Miami, FL.
		1.3 To discourage youth imitation of major league players' chewing tobacco.
		1.4 To increase the opportunities for tobacco cessation support in Miami, FL.
		1.5 To increase the early detection of precancerous oral lesions.
Interventions	To + action term + units of service + target population (the types of interventions are shown in parentheses)	1.11 To provide 50 educational sessions to little league baseball teams. (educational)
		1.21 To sue the tobacco industry for targeting children in spit tobacco advertisements. (power)
		1.31 To provide tobacco-free professional baseball player role models. (organizational)
		1.32 To promote tobacco-free youth baseball teams.
		1.41 To provide a tobacco user's helpline. (direct service)
		1.51 To provide oral cancer screenings to 200 little league baseball players. (direct service)
Direct Program Activities	Activity + due date	1.111 Review educational materials used by other programs by December 1.
		1.112 Develop educational program by March 1.
		1.113 Pilot test educational program by April 1.
Indirect Program Activities	Administrative	fiscal control, record keeping, supervising
	Support	secretarial support
	Maintenance	equipment repair and maintenance, computer service contracts
	Risk management	insurance, safety procedures

TABLE 6-5 ACTION PLAN

IMPLEMENTATION	INTERVENTION	MARKETING	WHERE	WHAT	WHO	WHEN	REINFORCEMENT	MONITORING
Goal One								
Objective one:								
Objective two:								
Objective three:								
Goal Two								
Objective one:								
Objective two:								
Objective three:								

perform the job. (3) Job responsibilities, including a description of the necessary duties and activities expected in the position, direct and indirect activities, as well as record keeping. (4) Job compensation, which is a description of the salary or wage offered, as well as direct and indirect benefits. Salary is often listed as a range. A description of any unusual travel, any late hours, and preference for sec-

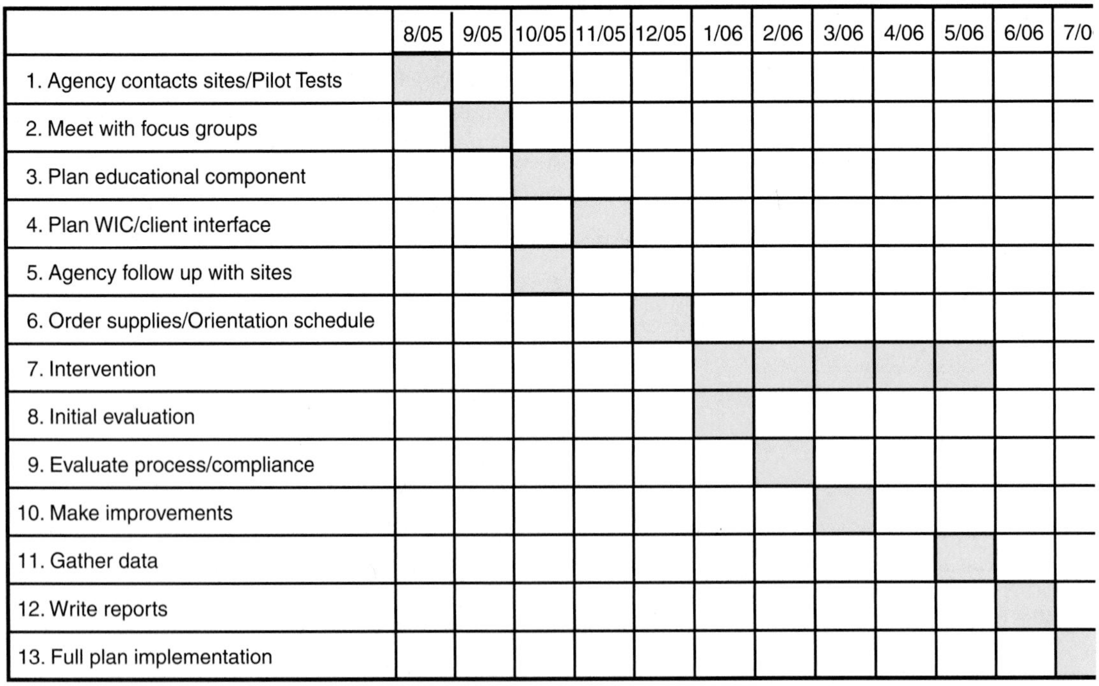

	8/05	9/05	10/05	11/05	12/05	1/06	2/06	3/06	4/06	5/06	6/06	7/0
1. Agency contacts sites/Pilot Tests	■											
2. Meet with focus groups		■										
3. Plan educational component			■									
4. Plan WIC/client interface				■								
5. Agency follow up with sites				■								
6. Order supplies/Orientation schedule					■							
7. Intervention						■	■	■	■			
8. Initial evaluation						■						
9. Evaluate process/compliance								■				
10. Make improvements									■			
11. Gather data										■		
12. Write reports											■	
13. Full plan implementation												■

FIGURE 6-1 Community Program Time Line. A graphic time line helps visualize the flow of the program through a time period. A narrative would accompany the time line to clarify each step.

ond language should be included. It may be wise to consult with agency personnel or the human resource department for help writing the job description to ensure meeting legal requirements (Equal Employment Opportunity/ Affirmative Action).

Organizational Diagram

The **organization diagram** (Fig. 6-2) details the chain of command and explains how information flows through a department, agency, or work group. Software programs are available to help draw organizational diagrams.

Client Flow Charts

Although the organizational diagram illustrates how information flows through the system, information **flow charts** illustrate how clients or patients flow through the system. They offer checkpoints for decision-making, documentation, and data collection. Geometric figures guide the reader through the chart. The planner can draw flowcharts by hand or use a computer application designed specifically for flowcharts. Figure 6-3 demonstrates a flow chart designed for an Early Childhood Caries program.

Program Budget

Inadequate funding, along with lack of resources, is one of the major reasons for program failure. Ineffective programs can result from trying to create a program with inadequate funds. Ideally, a program is planned with all the necessary funding, resources, supplies, equipment, and facilities to operate. In reality, public health programs are often, by necessity, planned around predetermined and limited funds. However, creative program planners use leveraged resources by working with other programs/players toward common goals.

There are several budget items to consider:

- **In-Kind Support** is provided by the agency or other entity to illustrate a match for a portion of the funds. Many grant sources require an in-kind match. It is not usually required to be cash; instead it can be the estimated value of an agency's contribution. Community based programs can include volunteer time, travel expense, office space, and staff support in their in-kind estimate.
- Personnel expenses include salary and employee related expenses (ERE). If employees are contracted, ERE may not be included. ERE is usually a percentage in addition to the salary. Agency personnel can estimate a percentage based on insurance costs, workmen's compensation, social security tax, retirement contributions, and other employer expenses.
- Rent is budgeted by the cost per square foot per month times the number of months of the program or funding cycle.

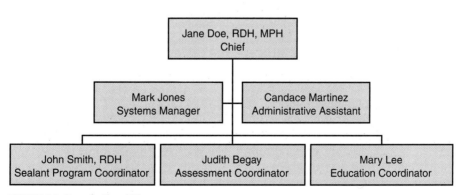

FIGURE 6-2 Organizational Diagram

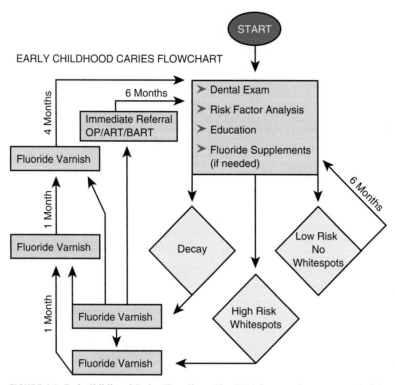

EARLY CHILDHOOD CARIES FLOWCHART

FIGURE 6-3 Early Childhood Caries Flow Chart. The OVAL denotes the start or end of the flow chart with the words *Start* or *End* inside the oval. The RECTANGLE conveys actions or steps. DIAMONDS are used for decisions or questions. CIRCLES are the "Go To" symbols, used when charts get too big for one sheet of paper or when flow charts are complicated (to avoid crossing arrow lines). BRANCHING is used for options in decision-making. ARROWS connect the shapes.

- Telephone cost is budgeted by the cost per month times the number of months.
- Supplies are budgeted at full retail price, but often can be purchased at discount to allow for unforeseen price increases. It is wise to plan generously.
- Equipment may include computers, office equipment, or dental equipment. It is best to lease computers and include maintenance contracts on all purchased equipment.
- Insurance may include liability, renters, automobile, or any other necessary for the program and not included in the ERE.
- Travel may include cost per mile of a private vehicle or the daily fee plus mileage for a fleet

or rented vehicle. It may also be necessary to include per diem for food and lodging when a program requires travel outside of a reasonable distance.

Table 6-6 demonstrates a hypothetical budget for an Early Childhood Caries prevention project.

EVALUATION

Program evaluation is an important component of the planning process. From the beginning of planning, it is important to consider how program goals and objectives will be evaluated. A more specific and detailed guide to program evaluation is presented in Chapter 7.

TABLE 6-6 BUDGET FOR EARLY CHILDHOOD CARIES PREVENTION PROJECT

IN-KIND SUPPORT	
Office Equipment	(estimate value of each)
Phone	
Office Space/Storage	
Mirrors and Explorers	
Use of Private Vehicle	
CONTRACT PERSONNEL	
Project Director: $30.00/hour, 4 hours/week x 36 weeks	$4,320.00
Dentist: $50.00/hour, 4 hours/month x 6 months	$1,200.00
Assistant: $18.00/hour, 4 hours/month x 6 months	$432.00
TOTAL FOR PERSONNEL	**$5,952.00**
DENTAL SUPPLIES	
Toothbrushes: $8.00/dozen x 50	$400.00
Fluoride varnish: $20.00/tube x 100 tubes	$2,000.00
Disposable application brushes: $19.00/box of 144 x 100	$190.00
Disposable dappen dishes: $35.00 per box of 1000 x 2	$70.00
Incentives: $1.00 x 1200	$1,200.00
TOTAL FOR DENTAL SUPPLIES	**$3,860.00**
PROGRAM TOTAL	**$9,812.00**

SUMMARY

Developing a community program is a cyclical process and is designed to meet community-recognized needs. Measurable goals and objectives drive program interventions with appropriate activities to accomplish the plan. These same goals and objectives guide the evaluation of programs. Many community oral health programs begin on a small scale and later expand the program after working out any logistics during the implementation and evaluation.

RESOURCES

Fink A, ed. The Survey Kit. 2nd Ed. Thousand Oaks, CA: Sage Publications, 2003.

INTERNET RESOURCES FOR PROGRAM DEVELOPMENT

Surveys: Available at: http://www.irss.unc.edu/irss/shortcourses/wigginshandouts/questionhandout0400.pdf

Job Descriptions: Available at: http://www.ruf.rice.edu/~humres/Training/HowToHire/Pages/4.shtml
http://www.hronline.com
http://www.culpepper.com/infor/jd/default.asp

Organizational Charts: Available at: http://www.smartdraw.com/resources/centers/orgcharts/index.htm

Sample Budgets: Available at: http://www.npguides.com/guide/budget.htm

http://www.nfconline.org/main/info/cnm/ budget_guidelines.htm

Mission statements: Available at: http://www.nonprofits.org/npofaq/03/21.html

Flow chart symbols: Available at: http://deming.eng.clemson.edu/pub/tutorials/ qctools/ flowm.htm
http://www.patton-patton.com/ basic_flow_chart_symbols.htm

 ## Learning Activities

1. The second-year dental hygiene class at Best College has generally poor study habits. A focus group revealed that students only skim reading material, cram for tests at the last minute, and party too much. Design a small program to change this behavior.
   a. Write a mission statement.
   b. Write a goal for the program.
   c. Write two or more objectives for the program.
   d. List possible interventions that could be implemented.
2. Design a flow sheet to track patients' flow through a dental clinic.
3. Design an organizational chart for a school department or place of employment.
4. Collect demographic data about a target group.
5. Design a survey instrument to collect community information.

Review Questions

1. The reasons for conducting a needs assessment include all of the following EXCEPT:
   a. gathering data to publish a paper.
   b. identifying the extent and severity of a need.
   c. assessing the cause of a problem.
   d. determining the resources needed for a program.
   e. establishing priorities.

2. Which of the following is an example of an indirect program activity?
   a. Toothbrushing education
   b. Data collection
   c. Convening a task force
   d. Repairing equipment
   e. Developing a lesson plan

3. The heart of the program plan is:
   a. the goals and objectives.
   b. the management information system.
   c. the flow chart.
   d. the needs assessment.
   e. the organizational diagram.

4. The mission statement is a broadly based statement of desired changes that should occur to alleviate the needs that have been identified.
   a. True
   b. False

5. To save time and money, secondary data should be collected before any primary data are collected.
   a. True
   b. False

6. "To improve the oral health of Anytown citizens" is an example of a:
   a. mission statement.
   b. program goal.
   c. program objective.
   d. program intervention.

7. "To decrease the consumption of high-sugar beverages at Anytown public schools" is an example of a:
   a. mission statement.
   b. program goal.
   c. program objective.
   d. program intervention.

8. "To decrease dental caries of Anytown citizens" is an example of a:
   a. mission statement.
   b. program goal.
   c. program objective.
   d. program intervention.

9. "To ban soft drinks at Anytown public schools" is an example of a:
   a. mission statement.
   b. program goal.
   c. program objective.
   d. program intervention.

REFERENCES

1. American Dental Education Association. Competencies for entry into the profession of dental hygiene. Exhibit 7 J Dent Ed 2003;67(7):1–5. Available at: http://www.adea.org/cepr. Accessed January 2004.
2. Cohen LK. Promoting oral health: guidelines for dental associations. Int Dent J 1990;40(2):79–102.
3. Assessing oral health needs: ASTDD seven-step model (1995). Available at: http://www.astdd.org. Accessed January 2004.
4. Gordon A, Womersley J. The use of mapping in public health and planning health services. J Public Health Med 1997;19(2):139–147.
5. Griffin SO, Jones K, Tomar SL. An economic evaluation of community water fluoridation. J Public Health Dent 2001;61(2):78–86.
6. Watt RG, Fuller S, Harnett R, Treaure ET, Stillman-Lowe C. Oral health promotion evaluation—time for development. Community Dent Oral Epidemiol 2001;29:161–166.

Program Evaluation

7

Objectives

After studying this chapter and completing the study questions and activities, the learner will be able to:
- Describe why program evaluation is important.
- Identify and describe the types of program evaluation.
- Define evaluation terms.
- Design a program evaluation instrument.

KEY TERMS

Attitudes	Postprogram	Program evaluation
Behaviors	Preprogram and postprogram	Qualitative
Efficiency	Preprogram and postprogram with	Quantitative
Formative evaluation	a comparison group	Reliable
Impact	Preprogram and postprogram with	Stakeholders
Knowledge	a control group	Summative evaluation
Management information systems	Process evaluation	Valid
Outcome evaluation		

The American Dental Education Association competencies addressed in this chapter include[1]:

HP.5:   Evaluate factors that can be used to promote patient/client adherence to disease prevention and/or health maintenance strategies.

C.8:   Provide quality assurance mechanisms for health services.

CM.6   Evaluate the outcomes of community-based programs and plan for future activities.

Introduction

This chapter introduces the learner to program evaluation and enables participation in the process. It covers the purpose, focus, and value of program evaluation. An overview of evaluation design, data collection methods, and management information systems is described.

PURPOSE OF PROGRAM EVALUATION

It is natural for humans to evaluate their actions. A cook tastes a dish to decide whether to add more seasonings, athletes watch videotapes to analyze and improve their performance, and students check grade reports. **Program evaluation** is simply an extension of this common sense practice to organized settings or programs. Public health professionals strive to improve health. They design programs and interventions, such as tobacco cessation classes, fluoride mouth rinse programs, and sealant programs. How do we know if these well-intentioned efforts are effective? Are the programs worth the effort, the time, or the money? These are questions asked by funding sources, administrators, and stakeholders; evaluation provides the answers. A combination of both qualitative and quantitative methods lends the answers to questions like how much, why, and who cares? Finally, thorough documentation provides quality assurance to all interested parties.

The most important purpose for program evaluation is the contribution to the provision of quality services to people in need.[2] Evaluation is important for several additional reasons: as a means to developing good practice, to make the best use of scarce resources, to provide feedback to staff and participants, and to shape policy development.[3] The results of the interventions are measured against the program objectives that were developed.[4] The evaluation answers whether the program was successful in reducing or eliminating the identified need or problem.

Questions one might ask about programs are:

- Did the program accomplish what it was designed to do?
- Did the program work better than other similar programs?
- Did the program reduce health costs?
- How could the program be improved?
- Should the program be continued?
- Does the program merit continued funding?
- Should the program be expanded?

EVALUATION TIMING

Ideally, evaluation decisions and tools are designed during the program development phase and prior to any implementation, not at the conclusion of a program. If this piece is not designed until the conclusion, the opportunity to collect pretest data is missed, and the evaluation can be biased by knowledge of program operations.

There are two types of evaluation that occur at different times. **Formative evaluation** (also referred to as **process evaluation**)[4] occurs during the implementation process, and **summative evaluation** (also referred to as **outcome evaluation**)[4] occurs after the intervention. Formative evaluations help point out problems and identify opportunities to make improvements. This is similar to evaluating instrumentation technique and deposit removal during the scaling appointment in individual patient care. This type of program evaluation is tied to routine operations with practical, ongoing measurement of processes and outcomes involving program staff and stakeholders. Formative evaluation may answer several questions, such as: What is the nature of the people being served? Is the program operating as expected? Do the activities match the plans for the program? In a summative evaluation, the results of the program are compared with the goals and objectives and used to determine the **impact** of the program on the community's health. This is similar to reevaluating an individual patient posttreatment to determine the effectiveness of scaling on the health of the tissue. Summative evaluation answers questions such as: Has oral disease been reduced? Has tobacco use changed? How many dental sealants have been placed? Summative evaluation helps all interested parties make decisions about the value and possible continuance of programs.

EVALUATION FOCUS

Evaluation methods are directly tied to the attainment of goals and objectives. It is important to judge a program by what it was designed to do. It is also important to examine why a program succeeds or fails, to consider unexpected positive or negative effects, and to examine whether the goals were appropriate for the clients served. The most appropriate focus for most evaluations is on improvement of processes, implementation, **efficiency,** or anything that makes a program more organized and cost-effective. Scheetz and Gholston[5] use an evaluation model that asks several questions (Box 7-1).

A combination of **quantitative** and **qualitative** methods is best used to specify and measure identifiable objectives. Together, they lend numbers and traits to tell stakeholders whether, and by how much, a program had an impact. Qualitative methods are helpful when long-term changes are expected. They are more likely to tell us why something changed, what factors are involved and, finally, they lend to program improvement more readily than quantitative methods. For example, quantitative methods may tell us that a certain proportion of people in a population received fluoride varnishes. Qualitative methods could tell us what people liked or did not like about the prod-

---

BOX 7-1 Evaluation Questions

How important was the problem toward which the program was directed? Is the ultimate goal important to responsible individuals? Answering this question involves the values of key players.

How much of the problem was solved? People may have different opinions of what constitutes a successful outcome.[2] Some may consider changes in plaque levels a successful outcome; others may consider decreased bleeding successful. Some may consider a 25% improvement a success; others may consider this a failure.

To what extent did the activities attain the objectives? It may be difficult to establish a cause-effect relationship because the causes of change are sometimes difficult to establish.[2] Certain factors not related to the program could be influencing the outcomes. A close dialogue between patients and planners may be helpful.[2] As much as possible, it is important to determine whether the program is making a difference.

What was the cost in resources to attain the objectives? The cost analysis is an important piece. It is important to measure efficiency outcomes, cost-effectiveness, and cost-benefit. This answers: What is the cost per unit of achievement? For example, what was the cost in labor and supplies per sealant? Examples of resources that affect costs include provider wages or salary, the nature of an intervention, the conditions, and the materials.

What desirable and undesirable adverse effects occurred? It is important to analyze any unexpected effects because this will offer valuable information for future planning. For example, medications that solve problems usually create undesirable adverse effects. On the positive side, learning new skills can increase self-esteem.

Sources: Posavac EJ, Carey RG. Program Evaluation: Methods and Case Studies, 5th ed. Upper Saddle River, NJ: Prentice Hall, 1997[2]

Scheetz, JP, Gholston LR. Applying an evaluation model to a dental public health program. J Public Health Dent 1985;45(3):187–192.[5]

uct or process and lend information that leads to better processes, acceptance, and outcomes.

Evaluation methods should fit the nature and timescale of the intervention.[6] Intermediate outcomes might be a better measure for educational programs than long-term health outcomes. Educational programs could lead to health behaviors that, when sustained over a long-term, would lead to reduced risk and better health. It takes a long time to realize those health benefits. Therefore, it might make more sense to measure intermediate variables, such as changes in **knowledge, attitudes,** and **behaviors,** than long-term changes in disease rates or health. Intermediate outcomes could be intentions to quit smoking, improvements in plaque levels, agreement to receive sealants, or decreased sugar consumption. Unfortunately, it cannot be assumed that the desired long-term health outcomes will occur. Although positive health changes may have occurred over a short-term, they may be superficial and dissolve over time.[2]

STAKEHOLDERS

The involvement of all **stakeholders** is essential to the evaluation process, just as it was during the program development and implementation stages. If only providers or other limited parties are involved, the scope and value of the evaluation is reduced. The participation of policy makers, funding agents, and community representatives increases the relevance and credibility of the results, as well as the likelihood of long-term participation.[7]

ASSIGNING VALUE TO PROGRAM ACTIVITIES

Programs are judged on several criteria, including their merit or quality, worth or cost-effectiveness, and significance or importance. A program can have merit but not be worth its cost. Before assigning value and making judgments regarding programs, the following questions must be answered:

- What will be evaluated?
- What aspects of the program will be considered when judging a program's performance?

- What standards must be reached for the program to be considered successful?
- What evidence will be used to indicate how the program has performed?
- What conclusions regarding program performance are justified by comparing the available evidence to the selected standards?
- How will the lessons learned be used to improve public health effectiveness?

FRAMEWORK FOR PROGRAM EVALUATION

The Centers for Disease Control and Prevention describes six steps in public health program evaluation.[8,9] Table 7-1 summarizes those steps. Figure 7-1 illustrates the interrelationships of the steps.[9]

The first step in an evaluation is to involve the stakeholders.[8] Previously described in Chapter 5, those are the people who are personally involved in the program, who derive income from it, whose future career might be affected by it, or who are clients or recipients of its services.[2]

Next, the evaluator describes the program in enough detail for others to understand such as-

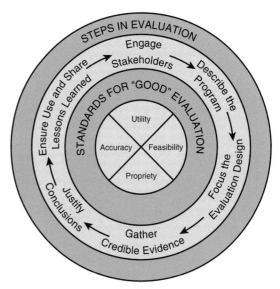

FIGURE 7-1 Steps in Evaluation (Source: Centers for Disease Control and Prevention. Practical Evaluation of Public Health Programs. PHTN Course VC-0017. Workbook.)[9]

TABLE 7-1 FRAMEWORK FOR PROGRAM EVALUATION

STEP	DESCRIPTION	DETAIL
1	**Engage stakeholders**	Persons or organizations having an investment in what will be learned and what will be done: • Those involved in program operations • Those served or affected by the program • Primary users of the evaluation
2	**Describe the program**	Convey the mission and objectives of the program being evaluated: • Statement of need • Expected effects • Activities • Resources • Stage of development • Context • Logic model
3	**Focus the evaluation design**	The evaluation must assess the issues of greatest concern to stakeholders while using time and resources efficiently • Purpose • Users • Questions • Methods • Agreements
4	**Gather credible evidence**	The information collected should convey a well-rounded picture of the program that is credible: • Indicators • Sources • Quality • Logistics
5	**Justify conclusions**	Conclusions are justified because they are based on evidence: • Standards • Analysis and synthesis • Judgments • Recommendations
6	**Ensure use and share lessons learned**	Deliberate action is taken to make sure evaluation process and findings are used and disseminated: • Design • Preparation • Feedback • Follow-up • Dissemination • Additional uses

Adapted from Morbidity and Mortality Weekly Review. Available at: http://www.cdc.gov/mmwr/preview/mmwrhtml/rr4811a1.htm[8]

pects as how the program works, where it is conducted and who is served, when it occurs, what is expected, what supplies and resources are used, how clients/patients interface, and the nature of clients served.

The third step is to focus the design of the evaluation on the issues most important to stakeholders. The design of the evaluation is tied to whether or not the program is resolving unmet needs; providing services; improving health; reducing risk; or changing attitudes, knowledge, or behaviors. An evaluation might be measuring whether one intervention or approach works better than another. Before an evaluation is designed, it is important for all stakeholders to agree on what constitutes a successful outcome.

Fourth in the framework of program evaluation is the need to gather credible evidence. To be meaningful, measurement must be **reliable,** meaning that different observers look at the same phenomenon and report similar levels. Reliability also means that a particular technique applied repeatedly yields the same result each time. An instrument that is **valid** helps measure variables objectively.[10] A valid measure accurately measures a variable. An instrument can be reliable but not valid and vice versa. A flexible tape measure that is stretched will measure the same way repeatedly and so is reliable but not valid because it is not a true measure of length.

Fifth is the justification of conclusions. It is important to base recommendations and conclusions on the weight of real evidence and to consider all the conditions and variables that might have affected change.

Finally, an evaluation is not good to anyone unless the process and findings are used and disseminated. Evaluations present valuable feedback to improve programs. Sharing the lessons learned helps others who are providing similar programs.

EVALUATION DESIGNS

Four commonly used evaluation designs are shown in Table 7-2[11]: postprogram only, preprogram and postprogram, preprogram and postprogram with a comparison group, and preprogram and postprogram with a control group. The purpose and type of information needed determines the selection of the design. The selection of the design also impacts the usability of the information and the ability to draw conclusions.

Postprogram Only

In **postprogram** only design, the outcomes are assessed after the program is completed. This is the least useful design because it is difficult to assess the amount of change that occurs. There is no baseline measurement taken before the program to compare with outcomes at the end of the program. This design is useful only when it is more important to ensure that participants reach a specific desired outcome than it is to know the degree of change. When this design is used, it is impossible to judge the amount of change that occurs or the influence of other factors on the change.

Preprogram and Postprogram

The **Preprogram and Postprogram** evaluation design enables an assessment of the amount of change. Baseline measurements taken prior to the program are compared with measurements taken at a program's conclusion. The same measurement is completed in the same way before and after a program. This type of evaluation is an improvement over the postprogram only design, but still may not offer complete confidence that the program was responsible for the outcomes because it does not account for changes in the target group that are not related to the program.

Preprogram and Postprogram With a Comparison Group

A **Preprogram and Postprogram with a Comparison Group** evaluation design includes the assessment of a group similar to the target group but who did not receive the program. Both the target and the comparison groups are assessed prior to the program, the program is delivered to the target group, and then both groups are assessed at the conclusion of the program. The comparison group must be as similar as possible to the target group demographically (e.g., gender, race/ethnicity, socioeconomic status, age, education) and in a similar situation as the target group.

TABLE 7-2 EVALUATION DESIGNS

DESIGN	METHODS				
Postprogram Only				Implement program to Target Group	Assess Target Group after the program
Preprogram and Postprogram	Assess Target Group before the program			Implement program to Target Group	Assess Target Group after the program
Preprogram and Postprogram with a Comparison Group	Assess Target Group before the program			Implement program only to Target Group	Assess Target Group after the program
	Assess Comparison Group before the program				Assess Comparison Group after the program
Preprogram and Postprogram with a Control Group	Randomly assign people from same population to Group A or B	Group A	Assess Program Group	Implement Program only to Group A	Assess Group A
		Group B	Assess Control Group		Assess Group B

Adapted from Arizona Program Design and Evaluation Logic Model: Resource Packet. Available at: http://www.azprevention.org/Downloadable_Documents/logicresourcepacket.pdf. Accessed January 2004.[11]

The more the two groups are alike, the more confidence there is that the program was responsible for the outcomes. An example would be two same grade-level classes at the same school whose participants had plaque levels measured. Only one group receives an intervention, such as tooth-brushing education. Both classes are again measured afterward and their preprogram and postprogram scores are compared.

Preprogram and Postprogram With a Control Group

The **Preprogram and Postprogram with a Control Group** evaluation design provides the greatest prospect to claim that the program was responsible for the outcomes. People are randomly assigned from the same overall target population to either a control or target group. In random assignment, each person has an equal chance of being selected for either group, so that the con-

trol group is as close as possible to the comparison group.

DATA COLLECTION METHODS

The information needs time, resources, skills, and available expertise to determine the selection of the type of data used to measure program outcomes. There are advantages and disadvantages to the many different ways to collect data. Table 7-3 compares data collection methods. Generally, it is best to use various techniques, as each method has its weakness. The use of several methods is complementary and, when each yields the same results, it strengthens the conclusions.[11]

Surveys fit the needs for descriptive data and can describe, explain, or explore. For example, a survey would fit the need to know about dental practice patterns.

Experiments fit the need for testing hypotheses. For example, a dental index used in a

TABLE 7-3 DATA COLLECTION METHODS

METHODS	PROS	CONS	COSTS	TIME TO COMPLETE	RESPONSE RATE	EXPERTISE NEEDED
Self-administered surveys (pen and pencil)	Anonymous; inexpensive; easy to analyze; standardized; easy to compare to other data	Results are easily biased; misses information; attrition is a problem for analysis	Moderate	Moderate, depending on system (mail, in-person delivery	Moderate, depending on system (mail is lowest)	Little to gather; moderate for analysis and use
Telephone surveys	Same as self-administered; increased ability to clarify responses	Same as self-administered; requires more staff time; misses those with no phone (low income)	More than self-administered	Moderate to high	More than self-administered	Some to gather; moderate for analysis and use
Face-to-face structured surveys	Same as self-administered; ability to clarify responses	Same as self-administered; requires more staff time	Moderate to high	More than self-administered; same as phone	Moderate to high	Some to gather; moderate for analysis and use
Archival trend data	Fast; inexpensive; extensive data available	Comparison can be difficult; may not show changes	Inexpensive	Quick	Usually good, depending on the original collection method	None needed to gather; some needed to analyze and use
Observation (i.e., dental indexes)	Can see a program in operation	Requires much training; can influence participants	Depends on staff time and costs	Quick; depends on the number of observations	Not an issue	Some needed to devise coding scheme and calibrate examiners
Record review	Objective; quick; does not require program staff or participants; pre-existing	Can be difficult to interpret; data often incomplete	Inexpensive	Can be time consuming	Not an issue	Little needed; coding scheme may need to be developed
Focus groups	Can quickly get information about needs, community attitudes and norms; information can be used to generate survey questions	Can be difficult to analyze data; need a good facilitator	Inexpensive, depending on location; can be expensive to hire facilitator	Groups themselves last about 1.5 hours	Good; people usually agree to participate, depending on schedule	Good interview/conversation skills; technical aspects can be easily learned

TABLE 7-3 DATA COLLECTION METHODS (continued)

METHODS	PROS	CONS	COSTS	TIME TO COMPLETE	RESPONSE RATE	EXPERTISE NEEDED
Unstructured interview/narratives	Gather in depth, detailed information; information can be used to generate survey questions	Takes much time and expertise to conduct and analyze; potential interview bias possible	Inexpensive if using current staff; can be expensive to hire interviewers and/or transcribers	Varies by length of interview; analysis can be lengthy, depending on method	People usually agree to participate if it fits their schedule	Good interview/conversation skills; formal analysis methods are difficult to learn
Open-ended questions on a written survey	Can add more in-depth detailed information to a structure survey	People often do not answer them; may be difficult to interpret meaning of written statements	Inexpensive	Adds a few more minutes to a written survey	Moderate to low	Content analysis skills
Participant observation	Can provide detailed information and an "insider" view	Observer bias common; can be a lengthy process	Expense based on time	Time consuming	Participants may not want to be observed	Data analysis skills
Archival research	Can provide detailed information about a program	May be difficult to organize data	Expense based on time	Time-consuming	Documents may not be able to be reviewed	Data analysis skills

Adapted from Data collection methods at a glance. CSAP and NCAP. Getting to Outcomes. Arizona Program Design and Evaluation Logic Model Resource Packet. Available at: http://www.azprevention.org.[11]

preprogram and postprogram with a comparison group would test whether a certain product was more effective at removing plaque.

MANAGEMENT INFORMATION SYSTEMS

Management information systems (MIS) help organize the data necessary to manage a program and make decisions. It may be necessary to track such information as numbers and types of services performed, sealants retained over a specified amount of time, numbers of attendees at an educational forum, or responses to evaluation forms. A state sealant program may use several forms, including a medical history, permission slip, form for diagnosis of teeth to be sealed, and a record of sealants provided. Standard instruments enable a comparison within and between programs. Evaluators should develop tracking forms that are simple and user friendly. Information from forms is entered into a database to track a program's production, such as numbers per provider or children served at a school. Paper spreadsheets or computer spreadsheets are often used. Finally, information must be tabulated, summarized, and displayed graphically to make it useful and understandable.

SUMMARY

This chapter outlines the purpose, timing, focus, and value of program evaluation. Additionally, it introduces the learner to a basic framework, data collection methods, and management information systems, and offers additional resources. Examples of evaluated information are described. The learner should be able to design a simple evaluation tool, as well as understand and contribute to the program evaluation process.

RESOURCES

Internet resource for health promotion and community development: Community toolbox Available at: http://ctb.lsi.ukans.edu/.

Centers for Disease Control and Prevention. Evaluation Working Group: Resource List. Available at: http://www.cdc.gov/eval/index.htm.

Program Development and Evaluation. Available at: http://cecommerce.uwex.edu/pdfs/G3658_1. PDF. [Taylor-Powell E, Steele S, Douglah M. Program development and evaluation, planning a program evaluation. University of Wisconsin —Extension, 1996 Feb(G3658-1).]

Centers for Disease Control and Prevention— Evaluation Workbook. Available at: http://www.

 Learning Activities

1. In the learning activities in Chapter 6, the learner was asked to design a small program to improve the study habits of students at Best College.
   a. Describe a way to evaluate whether the program made a difference.
   b. Give examples of survey questions.

2. Write an objective to change oral cancer screening rates.
   a. Identify an intervention to accomplish the objective.
   b. Describe how you would evaluate the success of the intervention in accomplishing the objective.

3. Select an article about a public health intervention and
   a. Identify the evaluation methods,
   b. Discuss whether the methods are summative or formative, and
   c. Discuss the implications for public health practice.

4. List possible formative and summative evaluation methods for a fluoride mouth rinse program.

phppo.cdc.gov/phtn/Pract-Eval/workbook.asp. (Centers for Disease Control and Prevention. Practical evaluation of public health programs. PHTN Course VC-0017. Workbook.)

Guide for community-based programs. Available at: http://www.horizon-research.com/reports/1997/taking_stock.php. (Bond SL, Boyd SE, Rapp KA. Taking stock: A practical guide to evaluating your own programs. Horizon Research, 1997.)

Handbook. Available at: http://www.ed.gov/ PDF Docs/handbook.pdf. (Muraskin LD. Understanding evaluation: The way to better prevention programs. U.S. Dept of Education. Contract #LC89089001; Task Order #LC900940, 1993.)

Review Questions

Anytown has 10 public elementary schools. It does not have fluoridated community water. One half of the schools are in middle- to upper-income neighborhoods and one half are in low-income neighborhoods. The children in the low-income neighborhoods represent a more diverse ethnic background than their counterparts in the higher income schools. The state health department completed screenings demonstrating higher dental caries rates and high rates of untreated dental caries in the lower-income schools.

1. The county hygienist has been asked to plan a program to address these unmet needs. Which of the following would be the first step in program planning?
   a. Interview the parents
   b. Meet with the school nurses
   c. Form an advisory group
   d. Rescreen the children
   e. Recruit dentists to provide services

2. With limited funds to implement a program, which of the following is recommended?
   a. Develop coalitions or partnerships
   b. Write a grant

   c. Combine resources with other health programs
   d. Target only high-risk populations
   e. All of the above.

3. If the goal of the program is to reduce dental caries rates in the school children, which of the following would be the most effective intervention?
   a. Toothbrushing education in the schools
   b. Nutrition education in the schools
   c. School-based treatment programs
   d. Community water fluoridation
   e. School fluoride rinse program

4. What is the most appropriate basis for evaluating an intervention that addresses these identified needs?
   a. A survey of children's oral health knowledge
   b. The goals and objectives
   c. A survey of local dental offices
   d. A defs survey of the children
   e. Program activities

5. Who should be involved in the evaluation process?
   a. Health promotion practitioners
   b. Policy makers
   c. Funding agencies
   d. Community representatives
   e. All of the above.

6. When should the evaluation methods be determined?
   a. At the conclusion of the program
   b. After consultation with the state health department
   c. During the development of the program
   d. During focus group sessions
   e. During the summative evaluation process

7. The best example of a summative evaluation for a sealant program would be:
   a. the number of permission slips returned by school children.
   b. a 1-year assessment of sound surfaces compared with decayed surfaces on previously sealed teeth.

c. an assessment of patient flow through a sealant program.

d. an assessment of infection control procedures.

e. a staff meeting to determine if activities are being accomplished.

8. To make the best use of limited funds, how would the dental hygienist determine the criteria for sealant placement?

a. All children should be targeted for sealant placement.

b. Children with deep pits and fissures at specific grades and schools should be targeted.

c. Children with no access to dental care should be targeted.

d. Children who do not receive a fluoride mouth rinse should be targeted.

e. Dental sealants should not be used.

REFERENCES

1. American Dental Education Association. Competencies for entry into the profession of dental hygiene, exhibit 7. J Dent Ed 2003 July;67(7):1–5. Available at: http://www.adea.org/cepr. Accessed January 2004.

2. Posavac EJ, Carey RG. Program Evaluation: Methods and Case Studies, 5th Ed. Upper Saddle River: Prentice Hall, 1997.

3. Blinkhorn A. Evaluation and planning of oral health promotion programmes. In: Schou L, Blinkhorn A, eds. Oral Health Promotion. Oxford: Oxford University Press, 1993, p 249–270.

4. Cohen LK. Promoting oral health: guidelines for dental associations. Int Dent J 1990;40(2):79–102.

5. Scheetz JP, Gholston LR. Applying an evaluation model to a dental public health program. J Public Health Dent 1985;45(3):187–192.

6. Watt R, Fuller S, Harnett R, Treasure E, Stillman-Lowe C. Oral health promotion evaluation—time for development. Community Dent Oral Epidemiol 2001;29:161–166.

7. Health Promotion Evaluation: Recommendations to Policy Makers. Copenhagen, Denmark: World Health Organization, 1998.

8. Framework for program evaluation in public health. MMWR: Recommendations and Reports, September 1999;48 9RR11:1–40.

9. Centers for Disease Control and Prevention. Practical Evaluation of Public Health Programs. PHTN Course VC-0017. Workbook.

10. Babbie E. The Practice of Social Research. 7th Ed. Belmont, CA: Wadsworth Publishing, 1994.

11. CSAP and NCAP. Getting to Outcomes. Conference Edition (June 2000). Arizona Prevention Resource Center. Available at: http://www.azprevention.org. Accessed 2004.

HEALTH PROMOTION AND ORAL HEALTH EDUCATION

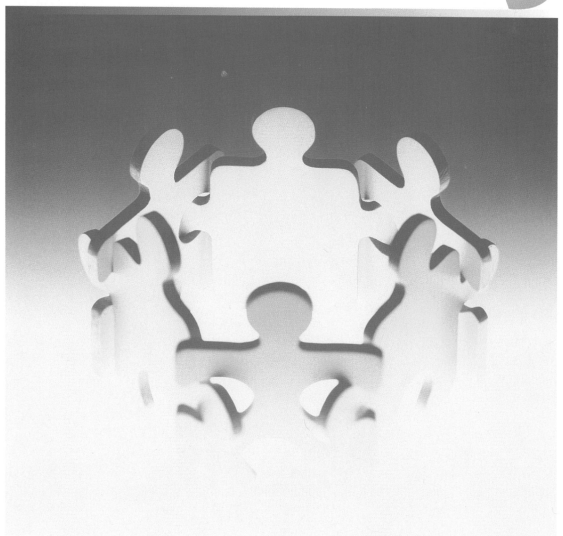

Oral Health Promotion

Objectives

After studying this chapter and completing the study questions and activities, the learner will be able to:

- Define oral health promotion.
- Identify the features that cause water fluoridation to be considered one of 10 top health promotion programs of the 20th century.
- Plan, implement, and evaluate an oral health program using the components of an effective oral health program and address appropriate level(s) of influence.
- Analyze how changes in society may influence the future of oral health promotion.
- Accept the role and responsibility of the oral health professional in oral health promotion.

KEY TERMS

Access to care	Fluoride tablets	Health promotion
Barriers	Fluoride varnish	Initiative
Community water fluoridation	Health disparities	Interdisciplinary
Extrinsic motivation	Health habits	Intervention

Intrinsic motivation

Macro level

Meso level

Micro level

Milk fluoridation

Multifactorial

Ottawa Charter for Health Promotion

Pit and fissure sealants

Prevention

Primary prevention

Quality of life

Quantity of life

Referendum

Risk factors

Salt fluoridation

School-based programs

School water fluoridation

Secondary prevention

Social factors

Socially equitable

Target population

Tertiary prevention

Xylitol

The American Dental Education Association competencies addressed in this chapter include[1]:

HP.1: Promote the values of oral and general health and wellness to the public and organizations within and outside the profession.

HP.2: Respect the goals, values, beliefs, and preferences of the patient/client while promoting optimal oral and general health.

C.3: Provide dental hygiene care to promote patient/client health and wellness, using critical thinking and problem solving in the provision of evidence-based practice.

C.4: Assume responsibility for dental hygiene actions and care based on accepted scientific theories and research, as well as the accepted standard of care.

C.5: Continuously perform self-assessment for lifelong learning and professional growth.

C.6: Advance the profession through service activities and affiliation with professional organizations.

C.7: Provide quality assurance mechanisms for health services.

C.8: Communicate effectively with individuals and groups of diverse populations, both verbally and in writing.

C.9: Provide accurate, consistent, and complete documentation for assessment, diagnosis, planning, implementation, and evaluation of dental hygiene services.

Introduction

This chapter is designed to assist the learner in understanding general health and oral health promotion and the significance on local and global health and **health disparities.** The chapter is divided into three separate sections: Health Promotion, Oral Health Promotion, and Model Programs. Health promotion, the process of enabling people and groups of people to increase control over and to improve their health through change in policy and law, is explored. The focus of this section is on community oral health promotion, with an introduction to individual general and oral health promotion and professional and patient self-responsi-

bility. Individual health promotion focuses on the health of one individual at a time. Community health promotion is promoting health in society as a whole through policy change and program planning and implementation.

The reader will learn to identify appropriate audiences and approaches for oral health promotion programs by studying **risk factors** for oral disease, health behaviors, determinants, and disparities in oral health. Also included are descriptions and examples of effective oral health promotion programs, including community water fluoridation and school-based pit and fissure sealant programs to assist the professional in planning, implementing, and evaluating oral health promotion programs. The learner will acquire the skills needed to participate in a fluoride intervention and to evaluate oral health promotion endeavors for populations at risk. The section concludes with recommendations for oral health programs and their promotion.

It is the author's desire that the learner will become passionate about oral health promotion through this unit. And this unit will inspire professionals to continually be involved in interventions and educational programs for their communities. Although community projects are arduous, they are, by far, some of the most rewarding activities in which oral health professionals can participate. There are numerous interventions, such as community water fluoridation, that impact the entire community's general and oral health.

HEALTH PROMOTION AND ORAL HEALTH PROMOTION

Health promotion is the science and art of helping people and society change their lifestyles to attain optimal health. It places an emphasis on improving quantity and quality of life for all and enables people to improve their health. Health promotion includes the use of any preventive, educational, administrative policy, program, or law to achieve this outcome. Oral health promotion is aimed at four preventable oral diseases: dental caries, disease of the supporting structures, oral pharyngeal cancers, and craniofacial injuries. The poor, minorities, and the elderly share a disproportionate amount of preventable oral disease. Prevention is vital to health promotion. The goal of any oral health program should be to empower people to attain equity in health and to reduce the incidence and prevalence of oral disease through education and interventions.[2] Some examples of this multipronged effort in dentistry are Community Voices: Healthcare for the Underserved

Initiative, Pipeline, and the National Spit Tobacco Education Program.

General Health Promotion

The World Health Organization (WHO) defines health promotion as "the process of enabling people to increase control over and to improve their health."[3] WHO continues to state, "Health promotion goes beyond health care. It puts health on the agenda of policy makers in all sectors and at all levels, directing them to be aware of the health consequences of their decisions and to accept their responsibilities for health. Health promotion policy combines diverse but complementary approaches including legislation, fiscal measures, taxation, and organizational change. It is a coordinated effort toward creating supportive environments and strengthening community action. Health promotion works through concrete and effective community actions in setting priorities, making decisions, and planning and implementing strategies to achieve better health. Community development and empowerment draws on existing human and material resources in the community to facilitate self-help, social support, participation, and ownership."[4] Although individual health promotion focuses on the health of one individual at a time, community health promotion has the much broader purpose of promoting health in societies as a whole.

Traditional Western medicine focuses on the treatment of disease in an attempt to improve quantity of life. **Quantity of life** refers to the number of years an individual lives. **Quality of life** is how meaningful a given life is, which is partially dependent on an individual's overall health. However, health care is evolving from disease treatment to disease **prevention** and, more recently, to promotion of health. Disease treatment and disease prevention are centered on quantity of life, while health promotion places an emphasis on improving quantity and quality of life for all.[5]

Because individual behaviors and thinking are not easily altered, health promotion must employ an **interdisciplinary** approach, involving clinical care, health education, research, public policy, social science, and public health, with the overarching objective to eliminate health disparities. To achieve this objective, health promotion must address factors within society, private organizations, government agencies, and policy makers to ensure access to preventive measures, appropriate health behaviors, and a healthy environment. Organizations and governmental agencies that impact health promotion are listed in Box 8-1.

Health professionals are presented with several **barriers** to the promotion of health. Those involved in health promotion must recognize that health and health-related issues are subject to decisions made by governmental agencies and organizations. Further, attempts at health promotion are not always successful because of the complexity of individual human motivation and other barriers, such as public policy.

The WHO has outlined strategies of health promotion in an attempt to overcome barriers to promoting health. WHO's five core strategies of health promotion are: to (1) create supportive environments, (2) build healthy public policy, (3) strengthen community action, (4) develop personal skills, and (5) reorient health services.[6] The WHO's focus is on removing barriers to health by working with people. At the **Ottawa Charter for Health Promotion,** the WHO delineated prerequisites for health for all as follows:

1. Advocate: Health promotion action aims at making conditions favorable through advocacy for health.
2. Enable: Heath promotion action aims at reducing differences in current health status and ensures equal opportunities and resources for all to achieve health.
3. Mediate: Health promotion aims at involving people in all walks of life as individuals, families, and communities. Strategies should be adapted to the local needs of countries and regions to consider differing social, cultural, and economic systems.

BOX 8-1 Organizations and Agencies Impacting Oral Health Promotion

- Clubs
- Churches
- Schools
- Places of employment
- Political parties
- Community action groups
- Federal, state and local health agencies
- Health insurance agencies

---

4. Build Healthy Public Policy: Public policy and policy makers at all levels should consider the health consequences of their decisions and accept responsibility for the same.
5. Create Supportive Environments: Make global decisions that are conducive, not detrimental, to health.
6. Strengthen Community Action: Set priorities, make decisions, and plan and implement strategies to achieve health through community action.
7. Develop Personal Skills: Provide information through education to individuals that enhances life skills that ultimately increase health options.
8. Re-orient Health Services: Health professionals and organizations must move in the direction of health promotion.[7]

Health is of primary concern to many because of its effect on quality of life. The United States has begun to address this concern through the drafting of Healthy People 2010, which outlines specific goals, objectives, and outcomes that target health disparities.

The goal of Healthy People 2010 is to achieve health equity through improving health education, housing, labor, justice, transportation, agriculture, and the environment.[8] Objective 13 of Healthy People 2010 focuses on oral disease. The Healthy People Toolkit, a companion document, provides communities with tools for planning interventions.[9] A Canadian document, *New Perspective on the Health of Canadians,* has challenged traditional views about health. Four main elements—human biology, environment, lifestyle and health care organization—have contributed to the knowledge and development of health promotion, health protection, and health care.[10,11]

Oral Health Promotion

There is no single indicator of oral health. However, there are health determinants and risk factors that impact health, such as genetic constitution, individual and group behavior, social and physical environment, and policy and interventions.[8] Health depends on a complex interaction between determinants of health. Thus, health outcomes are dependent on health habits, environment, and host susceptibility. The four common, preventable oral diseases have modifiable risk factors that health professionals can target when developing an oral health promotion program.

Recent studies have elucidated links between general health and oral health, making the importance of oral health more significant than previously thought. For many years, oral health professionals, especially dental hygienists, have focused their care and philosophy of care on prevention. These current findings make that philosophy even more relevant. Numerous diseases or disease processes are related to oral health and many systemic diseases have oral manifestations that may be the initial signs of the disease. The oral cavity is the portal of entry and site of disease for bacterial infections that affect general health. The function of the oral cavity can be adversely affected by medications and treatments, which may have a negative effect on the patient's treatment. Oral infections increase the morbidity rate for immunocompromised and hospitalized individuals. For example, individuals with diabetes are at greater risk for periodontal disease. Further, association between cardiovascular disease, stroke, and adverse pregnancy outcome has been found in animal studies and some human studies.[12-14]

The biologic and social relationship between general and oral health challenges oral health professionals to focus their efforts on oral health promotion to have a positive influence on general health. However, community health professionals have discovered that education alone will not prevent disease; a more global approach is needed.

Oral health promotion includes educational programs, such as tobacco prevention and cessation programs, and public school oral hygiene instruction. Social programs include water fluoridation and school sealant programs. Legislative activities include creating laws and funding for programs that promote oral health.

Oral disease is a biologic, psychological, and social phenomenon. Inasmuch as traditional Western medicine has attempted to make disease a biologic problem, it is necessary to reframe health and disease as **multifactorial.** Effective oral health promotion strategies should focus on the structure of assuring the availability of and access to appropriate oral health services, particularly preventive technology. The oral health professional has a responsibility to promote health and to encourage individuals and society to take responsibility for their oral health. Oral health professionals must take an active role in changing the perceptions related to oral health by being involved in local and state initiatives that promote health so that oral health becomes an integrated part of general health. The perception of the public, policy makers, and other health care providers must be influenced so that public policy can support overall health.[14,15] Health care providers have a social obligation to promote the health of the community through community action, community service, or political action.

PREVENTION AND ORAL HEALTH PROMOTION

Prevention is an essential aspect of oral health promotion because most oral diseases are preventable. Although prevention is a critical part of health promotion, it is not by itself sufficient to improve the quality of life. The purpose of prevention should be to ensure that a disease process never starts or is curtailed at an early stage. Early interventions are central to preventing many oral diseases.[16] United States Surgeon General, Dr. David Satcher, reports, "safe, effective disease prevention measures exist that everyone can adopt to improve oral health and prevent disease.[14] Dental caries; diseases of the supporting structures, including gingivitis and periodontitis; many oral pharyngeal cancers; and sports-related craniofacial injuries can be prevented.

Three levels of disease prevention—primary, secondary, and tertiary—have been identified. **Primary prevention** is the intervention in disease before it occurs. Primary preventive interventions include community water fluoridation, fluoride varnish, pit and fissure sealants, and preventive education. **Secondary prevention** is the treatment or control of disease early in the process. Examples of secondary preventive measures are conservative amalgam restoration, remineralization of early caries, and conservative periodontal therapy. **Tertiary prevention** is limiting a disability from a disease or rehabilitation of an individual. Examples of tertiary prevention are dentures or other prosthetic dental devices and periodontal surgery.

In the past, preventable diseases have been treated after they occur; in contrast, health promotion is intended to reduce the incidence of these diseases. One way that health promoters reduce disease incidence is through influencing social factors.

SOCIAL FACTORS IN ORAL HEALTH PROMOTION

Social factors, including customs, values, social networks, and ethnicity, are associated with oral disease. Social factors that impact general health include exposure to conditions that contribute to illness, susceptibility of disease, habits and values, and general social changes that alter resources.

Sociologists and anthropologists have found that oral health has extensive social implications. Well-being and quality of life are related to oral health. Untreated oral disease diminishes the quality of life through lack of sleep, limited eating, and depression. Oral disease has further negative impact, affecting the ability to chew and swallow foods and, therefore, limiting the quality and selection of foods. Individuals with craniofacial dysfunction report that oral conditions limit communication, social interaction, and intimacy as a result of loss of self-image, limited self-esteem, and increased anxiety and depression. Conversely, oral disease and pain place a burden on society through loss of work and school days.[13]

Social factors may operate on the **micro level,** influencing the individual; the **meso level,** involving institutions, organizations, and social networks; or the **macro level,** impacting social, cultural, and political agencies.

Micro Level: Individual. Characteristics, such as age, gender, socioeconomic position, ethnicity, and race may dictate one's place in a culture, community, society, or family group. Age is correlated with the occurrence of oral disease and conditions, as well as the use of dental services. The young and the elderly often have limited access to care as a result of transportation needs. Yet, there is little evidence that aging itself causes changes in host resistance to oral diseases or disorders. Rather, accumulated exposures to systemic disease, trauma, and adverse environmental and social conditions result in a cumulative impact.[17] An example of the micro level of influence can be seen in family income levels. Family income has a direct impact on health and oral health. A disproportionate number of minorities are at lower socioeconomic positions and have poorer oral health.

Socioeconomic position has an influence on oral health; the lower socioeconomic groups have lower access to health knowledge and care. The cost of health care, whether real or perceived, is a barrier for those of lower socioeconomic position.

Meso Level: Institutional. Institutions, organizations, and social networks sustain individual behavioral norms and health practices. Social networks extend from the family as the primary unit, to small groups and larger organizations, from which health habits arise from the family. The family is the most powerful social determinant in oral health; values, beliefs, and knowledge stem from the home and may be based in cultural traditions. Moreover, the family acts as a social network, influencing norms throughout life. A mother who was taught by her mother to dip her baby's pacifier in honey to appease her fussing infant is an illustration of the role that family and culture play in the oral disease process. In that culture, it is believed that a child should be happy and the mother has an obligation to assure the child's satisfaction. Mothers from this culture learn very early how to calm a crying child. This mother is convinced that she is being a good parent and may not realize the damage she is causing her child. Health professionals may recognize that the child will likely develop Early Childhood Caries, but the mother may not. Even if the mother realized the ill effects of the honey, she may find it more important, based on cultural values, to appease the child. The cultural habit of the sugary food on the pacifier contributes to the disease process, whereas the baby may not develop carious lesions without the honey.

Groups and organizations, such as athletic associations, parent-teacher associations, and professional organizations, reflect social norms that influence oral health. For example, professional athletes are powerful role models for youth. Young athletes imitate professional athletes. When professional athletes use tobacco, young people aspiring to be like them are more likely to use tobacco. Another example is a fluoride rinse program. If a parent-teacher organization is supportive of a fluoride rinse program, it is much easier to implement. However, if they are not in favor of the program, it becomes a greater challenge to provide school children with fluoride. These organizations can also act as a source of health information, as in some of the tobacco education programs that will be discussed later.

Macro Level: Agencies. Culture and society have control over oral health at the macro level. Evolving values and beliefs in large institutions and government influence their policies. These policies reflect society's beliefs, which define the missions and purposes of institutions.[18] One example of the impact that values have on health is Medicaid dental coverage for adults. Until recently, oral health was not viewed as important and, therefore, individuals and, more specifically, politicians did not value oral health. Individuals who did not understand the importance of dental services formed Medicaid policy and, therefore, many states do not offer dental coverage for adults. This can also be seen in the number of total Medicaid dollars allocated for all dental care. One study, conducted by Milbank Memorial Fund, reports Medicaid underfunds dental care for children. Dental care is 25 to 27% of total health care spending for children, but only 2.3% of Medicaid spending for children.[19] In addition, states experiencing budgetary shortfalls often elect to eliminate all state-funded dental care for adults while maintaining other health care, demonstrating the value that policy makers ascribe to oral health.

PSYCHOLOGICAL FACTORS IN ORAL HEALTH

If positive health behaviors lead to staying healthy and negative health behaviors lead to disease, why is it that those involved in health promotion do not simply tell their patients to brush and floss daily, not use tobacco, stay out of the sun, wear a seat belt in a car, and wear a helmet when they ride their bike? Adopting these positive health behaviors would result in a dramatic reduction of oral disease prevalence.

Changing a behavior is difficult even if the change is important in maintaining health. Behaviors depend on the individual's knowledge, beliefs, and values and require compliance.[20] Although oral health professionals can educate, they cannot change an individual's behavior. The patient must value and have access to preventive measures to adopt positive health behaviors. It is not enough for individuals to value prevention if they do not have access to preventive agents. Conversely, it is not enough for individuals to have access to preventive agents. An illustration of this: if a patient has dental floss, but they do not understand or believe that they are susceptible to disease or value oral health, they are not likely to use the floss on a regular basis. Likewise, if the individual understands and values oral health yet cannot afford dental floss, they are still unlikely to change the behavior.

Social, cognitive, and emotional factors such as stress, values, attitudes, self-esteem, helplessness, vulnerability, isolation, emotional poverty, family modeling and beliefs, and the influence of the media play a role in health behaviors.[21] Positive health behaviors that promote general health also contribute to oral health. One of these behaviors—eating a diet high in fiber and low in fat to promote cardiovascular health and reduce certain type of cancers—has also been found to reduce the incidence of oral cancer. Eating a diet low in simple carbohydrates helps reduce the incidence of obesity and helps control dental caries. Health behaviors that improve oral health include regular toothbrushing and use of interdental cleaning devices, regular self-oral exams, and the use of oral protective mouth guards and protective gear during sports activities. The lines between the social and psychological factors become fuzzy and overlap in the discussion of health habits. Psychological habits can be influenced by an individual's environment. For example, if a person is attempting to stop smoking when their partner continues to use tobacco, the environment is such that it is much more difficult for the person to quit.

Health Habits. Health habits can influence health either positively or negatively. Regular exercise, adequate rest, and proper nutrition have a positive effect on health and wellness. In contrast, negative health habits, such as poor diet, excessive stress, and alcohol abuse, contribute to disease. Negative oral health habits, such as tobacco use (pipes, cigarettes, smokeless chew, and snuff), anorexia, bulimia, and drug abuse, have a deleterious effect on oral health. On the other hand, positive habits of regular flossing and brushing and self-oral cancer screening promote oral health.

Health habits are developed in early childhood because of social and cultural norms. Although habits are formed at a young age, they can be changed with new information and individual motivation. The goal of patient motivation is to assist the person to move from a state of unawareness to a positive oral health habit.

Human Motivation. Motivation is complex, yet it is necessary to bring about behavioral changes that promote health. There is a saying, "Getting between the teeth is easy. It is getting between the ears that is difficult." Individual performances are based on the degree to which they are motivated. Individual expectations, ideas, feelings, desires, hopes, attitudes, and values shape motivation. Motivation is either **intrinsic** (from within oneself) or **extrinsic** (from an outside source). A man who sees the dental hygienist because his wife told him that his breath smells bad is motivated extrinsically. He is motivated by the hope that his breath will no longer offend his wife. Intrinsic motivation comes from within one self. A woman who stops smoking because she believes it is bad for her health is an example of intrinsic motivation. This woman may have gained new knowledge or had a change in values that resulted in a behavior change. Intuitively, it makes sense that intrinsic motivation is more powerful. The will to change because of belief in something is much stronger than the influence of another person.

Reinforcement and punishment support behavior change. Effective motivators recognize their patient's values, expectations, feelings, and ideas, and direct the patient to reinforce positive behavior. Models and theories of behavioral change and motivation will be discussed in greater detail in Chapter 9.

Behavioral Change: A Psychosocial View. Volumes have been written on the nature of behavioral change. Psychologists have been studying behavior and how to bring about changes in behavior for years.

Behavioral change is complex, and humans must be viewed in their social context. Viewing people in their social context means seeing how they live, what their daily life is about, and understanding what dynamics might support or interfere with positive health behaviors. The following example illustrates the difficulty of trying to motivate a young mother to change her behavior. Maria, an 18-year-old single parent, works at night at the local minimarket to support herself and her 1-year-old daughter. The absent father does not provide emotional or financial support. Maria's family disowned her when they found out she was pregnant. When she was kicked out of her parents' house, she rented a small, one-bedroom, downtown apartment. Because she is determined to provide a good life for her daughter, Maria is attending the local community college during the day and working 12-hour shifts at night. Maria is struggling to keep up with her studies while working long hours and caring for her daughter. When she gets home from work, the baby is awake, and Maria is exhausted. She rocks the baby for a few minutes and puts her to bed with a bottle of milk so she will quickly fall asleep. Maria was told that giving a baby a bottle with milk at bedtime can cause cavities, but she is just too tired to listen to her baby cry.

Recognizing how complicated life is at times and trying to understand how life's complexity can interfere with doing what someone knows is best, is important in any health promotion program. The professional must consider the life and lifestyle of individuals in the target population to develop an effective oral health promotion program.

ACCESS TO CARE AND UTILIZATION OF SERVICES

Access to care and utilization of services are important factors in determining the oral health of certain groups of individuals.[15] Access to dental care varies with gender, race/ethnicity, income, and education levels. More than 108 million children and adults living in the United States do not have dental insurance, 2.5 times the number without medical insurance.[14] Only 42% of individuals aged 25 years and older with less than a high school education visited the dentist one or more times in the previous year compared with 74% of those with at least some college education.[14] Only 68% of the U.S. population reported visiting a dentist or dental clinic within the past year.[22] The Surgeon General's Report on Oral Health states that women use dental services at a higher rate than men; Hispanic individuals had the lowest use; and Whites had the highest use. Nearly twice as many individuals living above the poverty level visit their oral health care provider as individuals below the poverty level.[14] Further, many families with income levels above the poverty level cannot afford dental services.

COMPONENTS OF AN EFFECTIVE ORAL HEALTH PROMOTION PROGRAM

The complexity of human nature, our society, and oral diseases demands that effective oral health promotion programs have specific components. An effective program is well planned, outlining the **target population,** in its objectives and goals. Aspects of effective health promotion programs are listed in Box 8-2.

Interventions. An **Intervention** is defined as any health action—any promotive, preventive, curative or rehabilitative activity—in which the primary intent is to improve health.[4] All activities that occur between baseline assessment and final evaluation are termed interventions. Interventions that have multiple activities are more likely to succeed than those that employ only a single activity. Interventions should be effective and efficient and based on sound rationale. Activities such as communication, education, community advocacy, health status evaluation, incentive and disincentive, and behavior modification may be used as part of an intervention.

Cultural competence, the process of effectively working within a cultural context of an individual or community from a diverse background, is an integral part of intervention and education. See Box 8-3 for considerations in selecting an appropriate intervention.[23]

Education. Education alone is not effective in preventing diseases.[24] Personal values must be

BOX 8-2 Aspects of an Effective Health Promotion Program

- Not dependent on compliance
- Cost-effective, cost-benefit analysis
- Assurance of correct use
- Adequate funding
- Available to those in need
- Effective in reducing disease incidence
- Feasible
- Safe
- Evaluated frequently
- Based on partnership
- Centered on pluralist methodologies.

Adapted from Gift HC. Prevention of oral diseases and oral health promotion. Curr Opinion Dent 1991; 1:337–347.[16]

BOX 8-3 Aspects to Consider When Selecting Appropriate Interventions

- Fit between the goals, objectives, and activity
- Fit between target population and activity
- Level of influence desired
- Activities based on theory
- Adequate resources to support the activity
- Proven effective program
- Single or multiple activities.

Adapted from Mckenzie JF, Smeltzer JL. Planning, implementing, and evaluating health promotions programs: A primer. 3rd Ed. Needham Heights, MA: Ally and Bacon, 2001.[23]

changed and interventions must be accessible. Education is another health promotion activity that has been determined effective if used with other techniques. Health promoters have defined education as any combination of learning experiences or educational interventions designed to help individuals or groups learn new health information and develop new health behaviors.

Education should be specific to the target audience. For example, a tobacco education program that targets sixth grade children should include age-appropriate information, activities, and reading materials that are entertaining and easy to understand. The health promoter should capitalize on what many sixth grade teachers recognize; for example, school children are captivated by interactive computer programs. Fun, interactive computer activities for classrooms or adjunct education that centers on oral health promotion should be developed. For more specific information on health education principles, see Chapter 9, Community Oral Health Education.

Model Programs

The Task Force on Community Preventive Services, an independent, nonfederal group, was formed to evaluate oral health interventions. The Task Force made recommendations to those starting, planning, and implementing programs as follows:

1. Assess goals in light of the national goals and objective.
2. Assess the current burden of oral health conditions in their populations.
3. Review the current status and history of intervention activities.
4. Identify opportunities for improving intervention effectiveness and oral health status.[25]

UNITED STATES

The Task Force conducted a systematic review of interventions to promote and improve oral health. The interventions were aimed at preventing dental caries, oral pharyngeal cancers, and sports-related craniofacial injuries.[25-28] Educational programs, such as statewide tobacco education projects, were not evaluated.

The Task Force strongly recommended community water fluoridation and school-based sealant programs among the interventions aimed at preventing or controlling dental caries, stating that these programs proved to be effective oral health promotion programs.[25-28] Further, the Centers for Disease Control and Prevention (CDC) strongly recommends the same two community-based interventions, community water fluoridation and school dental sealant programs.[29] These interventions were evaluated on:

- Effectiveness: Did the intervention reduce dental caries prevalence?
- Applicability: What population is the intervention useful for?
- Positive or negative effects: Were there any added benefits or ill effects caused by the intervention?
- Economics: Was the intervention cost-effective to deliver?
- Barriers: What might interfere or prohibit the delivery of the intervention?[26]

School-Based Pit and Fissure Sealant Programs. School-based programs deliver **pit and fissure sealants** at schools or in private practices to children unlikely to receive dental care. These programs may partner with the local schools, the CDC, the National Institute of Dental and Craniofacial Research, Health Resource and Services Administration, and the Indian Health Service to target children at risk for dental caries. The CDC reports that school-based pit and fissure sealant programs reduce dental caries as much as 60%. One exemplary school-based pit and fissure sealant program is Healthy Smiles for Wisconsin. This coalition of 25 agencies was organized to place sealants in 3,000 school-age children during the 2000–2001 academic year.[30]

Partnerships. Effective oral health education and interventions rely on partnerships. School-based sealant programs are one example of partnering to create effective interventions. Many philanthropic organizations are joining with universities, community health agencies, and the federal government to make the objectives of Healthy People 2010 a reality. The Robert Wood Johnson Foundation is providing support to various oral health initiatives, including Pipeline and Profession and Practice: Community-Based Dental Education. Pipeline has three areas of concentration: (1) recruitment and retention of low-income and minority dental students, (2) establishment of community-based practices for senior dental students in areas of high need, and (3) development of dental curricula that support service delivery.[31] The W. K. Kellogg Foundation has formulated Community Voices: Healthcare for the Underserved Initiative to improve access to oral health for vulnerable populations. These initiatives are founded on the premise that oral health care must be integrated within a primary care system, accessible, acceptable, and available to all. Community Voices partners with local schools, dental schools, and community health organizations to support early interventions. Community DentCare, a partner with Community Voices, is considered a model for community-based care that uses schools to provide preventive and basic services to children and community members.[32] The National Spit Tobacco Education Program (NSTEP) partners with baseball star Joe Garagiola, the Major League Baseball Players Association, the Professional Baseball Athletic Trainers Society, the American Coaches Association, and Little League Baseball Incorporated. NSTEP provides educational resources to schools, community members, and health professionals through a Robert Wood Johnson Foundation grant. This program excels at recruiting professional baseball players as role models to educate young athletes about the harms of spit tobacco.[33]

Community Water Fluoridation. The CDC stated that **community water fluoridation** was one of the 10 most significant public health measures of the 20th century.[34] Community water fluoridation is the upward adjustment of natural fluoride levels in a community's water supply to prevent caries. Communities have been optimizing the level of fluoride in water systems for more than 50 years. More than five decades of research has proven the safety of water fluoridation.[35] The benefits of fluoride in strengthening tooth enamel, reducing sensitivity of exposed roots, and remineralizing teeth has been so thoroughly documented that it is generally accepted as a fact within the dental community.[36,37] The CDC recommends an optimal concentration of 0.7–1.2 ppm, depending on the average maximum daily air temperature of the area.[38] The American Dietetic Association strongly reaffirms its endorsement of the use of systemic and topical fluorides, including water fluoridation as an important health promotion measure.[39] The 2000 Dietary Reference Intakes also established recommendations for fluoride intake.[40]

Why Is Community Water Fluoridation Successful? Water fluoridation is a model oral health promotion intervention. It is **socially equitable;** community members who have access to public water receive the benefits of fluoridated water regardless of age or socioeconomic position. The fluoride levels are adjusted at the water treatment plant, based on the naturally occurring concentration. Those in need receive the benefits of the fluoride without concern for using it correctly or the costly service of a health professional. Water fluoridation strengthens the host, the tooth enamel, without requiring individual behavior changes; no active participation is required.

Water fluoridation is cost-effective and much less expensive than restoring a single tooth. It is estimated that the range of cost to optimize the fluoride levels in community water supplies is $0.40 to $2.70/person/year.[26] This can be compared with the dietary fluoride supplement; estimated cost of $37/person/year. A cost-benefit analysis revealed that for every dollar spent on fluoridation, $80 are saved in treatment costs.[38] Local, state, and federal agencies partner to support the optimization of fluoride in community water supplies. It is easily funded through local,

state, and federal budgets. The CDC recently supported communities with the initial installation of the fluoridators and monitoring devices. Community water fluoridation is not difficult to implement and monitor through standard community water systems.

Community water fluoridation decreases tooth decay in adults by nearly 35%.[41,42] Children who lived in fluoridated communities had 50 to 60% fewer decayed, missing, and filled permanent tooth surfaces in comparison with those children living in nonfluoridated communities.[43] The impact that fluoridation has on caries can frequently be evaluated by oral health surveys. One of the most significant benefits of water fluoridation is the multiple mechanism of action; it acts as both a topical and a systemic agent, as well as demonstrating antimicrobial activity to reduce dental caries. The primary mode of action is topical, in that it promotes remineralization and inhibits demineralization by continually bathing the teeth in saliva with low concentrations of fluoride.

In spite of the benefits of water fluoridation, only 66% of the U.S. population received fluoridated water through public water supply systems in 2000.[38] Only California, Connecticut, Delaware, Georgia, Illinois, Minnesota, Nebraska, Nevada, Ohio, South Dakota, District of Columbia, and the Commonwealth of Puerto Rico legislate mandatory statewide fluoridation.

Water Fluoridation—Public Policy Change. Water fluoridation is the only community health issue that is voted on by the public. The community does not vote on immunization, water purification, or air contaminate levels. Although it may be evident to health professionals that water fluoridation improves health for all, for voters, it is a social, economic, and psychological issue. Voters have heard propaganda from those opposed to fluoridation about the ill effects of water fluoridation, such as the unfounded claims that it lowers the IQ or causes cancer.

Oral health professionals have an obligation to promote water fluoridation. For example, dental hygienists adhere to the America Dental Hygienists' Association ethics code that describes benefi- cence, "We have a primary role in promoting the well-being of individuals and the public by engag- ing in health promotion/disease prevention activi- ties."[44] Water fluoridation is clearly an effective health promotion intervention, establishing an ethical obligation to be involved.

Fluoride Campaigns. Although fluoridation can be legislated at the local or state levels, local enactment is most common. Local health officials in many communities have the authority to imple- ment water fluoridation but rarely execute this authority. Instead, water fluoridation is more commonly implemented through a public **initia- tive** or **referendum.** Voter initiative is the process whereby an action is placed on the ballot by request of a citizen group. Voter referendum is the process whereby an action by public officials is placed on the ballot for voter support. For example, in 2001, the Flagstaff, Arizona, city council voted to optimize the fluoride levels in community water. Because a group opposed to community water fluoridation wanted "pure wa- ter," they gathered enough signatures for a refer- endum vote to overrule the city council's authority. The issue was placed on the ballot and, unfortu- nately, the public voted not to implement water fluoridation. Requests could have been made to place the water fluoridation on the ballot without a city council decision, which would have been an initiative.

A target goal for Healthy People 2010 is for fluoridation of 75% of U.S. community water sup- plies.[8] To achieve this goal and to avoid devastat- ing defeats, community readiness must be assessed. Recall the components of a needs assessment from Chapter 6, including taking a proactive approach, obtaining community buy-in, creating targeted in- terventions, designing cost-effective interventions, identifying sufficient resources, and assessing com- munity-recognized need.

Taking a proactive approach to initiating com- munity water fluoridation requires assessing the readiness of the community by determining public opinion, political climate, media influence, com- munity apathy, demographics, external forces, public awareness and perception of fluoride, and health professional politics.

Considerable preparation is necessary prior to a water fluoridation campaign. Those involved must be committed to an endeavor that may take years to come to fruition. One of the first steps in a com- munity water fluoridation campaign is to identify available resources. Educating the public, engag- ing an experienced campaign manager, and form- ing a political action committee are expensive and should be considered prior to beginning a cam- paign. Frequently, organizations such as the CDC, American Dental Association, or the American Dental Hygienists' Association set aside funds to support public health initiatives such as water fluoridation. Creativity is in order to find funds— it will not be easy or inexpensive.

Community education should start before an- nouncing an official campaign and should con- tinue until well after water fluoridation is imple- mented. The education should focus on the positive scientific data, speaking to the safety, cost- benefit, and efficacy of fluoride. The multilevel approach should be used in education, including in-office education; walking initiatives; get-out- and-vote drives; and TV, radio and newspaper ads. Activities should concentrate on safety, cost-bene- fit, and efficacy and should avoid negative cam- paigns. Negative campaigns do not work. Instead, they raise voter doubt. Education projects should present the facts, not argue or debate with so- called experts opposed to fluoride. Enlist trusted community leaders to get involved in education. Community leaders have built trust with citizens and are not perceived by individuals as "the authority," telling them what is best for their health.

Background knowledge and preparation are es- sential prior to initiating a campaign. See Box 8-4 for information on preparing for a campaign.

It is critical to know the position of the local media prior to initiating a campaign. The local me- dia have a powerful influence in politics and can be a best friend or a worst enemy. It is critical to know the local media's position on water fluoridation prior to initiating a campaign. Using the media can backfire on a campaign if they are not in support of community water fluoridation. It is also important to know what type of media the voters use as their source for information. Older, educated people are more likely to read the newspaper. Local newspapers are more likely to investigate and report the issue more completely than other forms of media. Younger, busy individuals use television as a source of information. Television reports are typically short, brief bits of information. A rapidly growing source of information is talk radio. Nine of ten talk radio listeners are registered voters, compared to six of ten in the general population.[45] Talk radio is an outlet for many who otherwise do not have a platform; antifluoridationists frequently use this form of media to send their message. The Internet is also a rapidly growing source of information, although some sites are accurate and scientific and others are not, and the public may not necessarily know how to evaluate them.

Knowing who votes and when is beneficial in planning a fluoride campaign. It is also important to know if your community demonstrates voter apathy, as low voter turnout is not positive for water fluoridation. Low voter turnout generally has a negative impact because a contingent that always votes and always "no" regardless of the issue exists

---

BOX 8-4 Preparing a Water Fluoridation Campaign

- Know the history of previous local water fluoridation attempts.
- Determine the sentiments of city council members.
- Get to know your city council members.
- Consider the political climate.
- Understand the process, timing, paperwork, water policy, and local budgets.
- Follow local politics.
- Know your area's natural fluoride levels.
- Do not expect to be the absolute authority on fluoride.
- DO NOT PARTICIPATE IN A DEBATE.
- Be prepared.
- Have a plan.
- Develop a strategy and tactics.
- Recruit outside experts.
- Include local or national celebrities.
- Have a wide base of support.
- Form a citizen's political action committee (PAC) when appropriate (donations to a PAC are tax deductible).
- Research, READ, READ, and READ, both the supporting and the opposing information.
- Form a speaker's bureau of trained speakers. Toastmasters' is a good place to get experience speaking. The ADA may also conduct training.
- If asked to speak at a public forum, assign individuals to address specific topics. For example, assign one speaker to address safety. This speaker should read and know both the supporting and opposing safety information.

in most communities. With low turnout, this group can sway the outcome of the election. Voter turnout is higher during mayoral elections. The typical voter, according to the U.S. Census Bureau, is well-educated, middle class, urban, White, female, and a homeowner. To ascertain local voter information, it may be beneficial to conduct a public opinion poll, determining how many people will vote and how they will vote on the fluoride issue.[24]

Ethics of Community Water Fluoridation. Research has proved that fluoridation is safe and effective, yet opposition argues the ethics of adding an element to community water. Professor of Philosophy John Harris successfully argues the ethics of community water fluoridation stating, "The issue of the ethics of fluoridation seems to me to be both simple and straightforward. The issue depends on establishing that fluoridation is both harmless and beneficial. Relying on evidence from a number of sources, there is no reason to suppose that fluoridation of the public water supply, to the level of one part per million that is envisaged, is anything but safe."[46]

Harris argues the civil rights of water fluoridation by stating, "In short, not all constraints on free choice are constraints on liberty. Citizens living in a community that adds fluoride to their water are no less free than those living in a community that does not."[46]

GLOBAL PROGRAMS

FLUORIDES

Fluoride is considered one of the most effective anticaries methods developed to date. Fluoride is being widely used on a global scale, with much benefit. More than 500 million people use fluoridated toothpaste, about 210 million people benefit from fluoridated water, some 40 million people benefit from fluoridated salt, while other forms of fluoride applications are administered to about 60 million people.[4] Several national and international organizations and governments are in favor of water fluoridation where it is practical. In areas where there is no community water source, salt and milk fluoride programs are promoted.[47-50] However, populations in many developing countries do not have access to fluoride for prevention of dental caries for practical or economic reasons.[4]

Community Water Fluoridation Worldwide. Water fluoridation has proved safe and effective in worldwide research conducted for more than 50 years. Currently, 39 countries worldwide provide artificially fluoridated water supplies, serving millions of people. In addition, about 40 million individuals drink naturally fluoridated water. Australia, Canada, Israel, New Zealand, Singapore, Spain, Switzerland, and the United Kingdom are a few countries that provide community water fluoridation. In New Zealand, 57% of the population has access to fluoridated water through community water supplies; in Israel, 50%. Approximately two thirds of the Australian population resides in communities that fluoridate community water. Mandatory legislation requiring all water systems to fluoridate was enacted in South Africa, and Israel requires all cities with more than 5,000 residents to provide fluoride in the water.[46] About 10% of the U.K. population receives fluoridated water.[50]

Federation Dentaire International (FDI), or World Dental Federation, with representation from Belgium, France, Germany, Israel, Latvia, Netherlands, Spain, Sweden, U.K., and the U.S., amended their Fluoride Position Statement as follows: "Fluoridation of water supplies, where possible, remains the most effective public health measure for the prevention and treatment of dental decay."[48] The National Alliance for Equity Dental Health, composed of 75 organizations, is coordinated by the British Fluoridation Society, the British Dental Association, and the British Medical Association. The Alliance, committed to reducing health inequalities, concluded that water fluoridation is the "great equalizer."[49,50] This means that everyone, regardless of age, race, or socioeconomic position, can access community water fluoridation as a preventive agent.

The WHO, in support of water fluoridation, has set requirements for its use:

- Areas with moderate or high risk of dental caries.
- Areas where the economy can support it and the technology is available.
- Areas where water supplies are well organized, used by the public, and appropriately funded.
- Equipment in the water plant should be of a high standard.
- Fluoride chemicals should be available and trained personnel should be available to manage the system.[51]

In addition, the WHO made the following recommendations for future water fluoridation:

- It should be maintained and expanded where feasible.
- The fluoride levels in the water should be continuously monitored.
- Further research is needed to examine the appropriate fluoride levels in water, taking account of other sources of fluoride and changing patterns of water consumption.

School Water Fluoridation. Other fluoride programs have been attempted with less success than community water fluoridation. One such alternative to community water fluoridation is fluoridating a school's water supply system. This method can be used if the school has a stand-alone water system that is not connected to the community water supply. Because children are only at school part of each weekday, the recommended concentration is 4.5 times the optimal concentration for a community system.[52]

School water fluoridation systems present several concerns. Maintaining school systems that are smaller than typical community fluoridation systems creates difficulties, which can result in higher than recommended fluoride concentrations in the drinking water. Although these higher concentrations present reason for concern, they have not resulted in lasting effects among children.[52]

Fluoride Rinse Programs. Approximately 3 million children in the United States participated in school-based fluoride mouth rinsing programs during the 1980s. A study conducted by the National Preventive Dentistry Demonstration Program (NPDDP) reported that these fluoride mouth rinses had little effect among schoolchildren, either among first-grade students with high and low caries experience or among all second- and fifth-grade students.[53]

Fluoride rinse programs implemented through school programs have demonstrated limited success. The school programs depend on teacher and/or school nurse compliance and individual parental consent. The teacher must set aside time for students to participate in the rinse program.[53] In addition, individual consent by parents often results in children at high risk for caries not being included in the program. Therefore, it is difficult for a school rinse program to truly target the children who could benefit most.

Fluoride Varnish. Fluoride varnish programs are being implemented as community health programs to assist in reducing the incidence of dental caries, particularly in the very young. High-concentration fluoride varnish is painted directly onto the teeth. The varnish is not intended to adhere permanently. Instead, it holds a high concentration of fluoride in contact with the teeth for several hours. Fluoride varnish has several advantages, including ease of application, a nonoffensive taste, and use of smaller amounts of fluoride than required for gel applications. Fluoride varnish is considered the most effective professional fluoride treatment for primary caries.[54]

Fluoride varnish has been widely used in Canada and Europe since the 1970s to prevent dental caries. The Food and Drug Administration's Center for Devices and Radiological Health has not approved fluoride varnish as an anticaries agent, but lists it as a medical device to be used as a cavity liner and root desensitizer. The CDC states that "Caries prevention is regarded as a drug claim and companies would be required to submit appropriate clinical trial evidence for review before this product could be marketed as an anticaries agent.[52] However, a prescribing practitioner can use fluoride varnish for caries prevention as an "off-label" use, based on professional judgement."[55]

Fluoride varnish programs appear to be most effective when integrated into an existing program such as Woman Infant Child (WIC) or Head Start or well-child checkups with a trained health care professional. The Nevada Healthy Smile, Happy Child program has developed training materials for health professionals to start a fluoride varnish program.[54]

Salt Fluoridation. Fluoridated salt is an alternative in areas where water fluoridation is not possible. France, Germany, Switzerland, and certain South American countries use **salt fluoridation.** The recommended concentration is 400 mg/kilogram of salt. The WHO has established the following criteria for salt fluoridation:

- Where water fluoridation is not possible
- Where there are low levels of fluoride
- Where the political will to introduce water fluoridation is absent
- Where there is a centralized salt production with strong technical support.
- Additionally, appropriate labeling of the salt packages is essential.[51]

Milk Fluoridation. Milk fluoridation delivered through school-based programs has proven to effectively reduce caries in children. In spite of its efficacy, milk fluoridation is limited as an oral health promotion intervention.[55] Milk is difficult to deliver, as it must be continuously refrigerated.

Fluoride Tablets. Fluoride tablets were originally designed to be dissolved in water and given to a child throughout the day. Eventually, the pill-oriented society evolved into giving a tablet to be chewed up and swallowed once a day. Currently, several countries have established recommended dosage schedules for fluoride tablets. These dosage schedules differ among countries, but all are based on assessing risk factors for dental caries for the individual person.

XYLITOL

Xylitol is a five-carbon sugar alcohol used in many foods and snack items. It prevents *Streptococci mutans* from metabolizing other sugars and inhibits enamel demineralization. It is an important method of dental caries control in many countries, including Finland, where it is distributed with college lunches and in military survival packs.

RECOMMENDATIONS FOR THE FUTURE

The world is changing more rapidly than ever before. It is estimated that the population will be much more culturally diverse in the near future. These changes bring new challenges to those working to promote health and prevent diseases. Oral health professionals must provide culturally appropriate services in a cost-effective manner.

The major challenges to the future will be to translate knowledge and experiences of disease prevention into action programs.[4] This will require the use of technology, development of an appropriate professional workforce, and use of evidence-based interventions.

Using Technology

Technology can be used to meet the growing need for preventive and educational services.[56,57] The Internet was used during the terrorist attacks of September 11, 2001, and in ensuing events, as an educational tool for health care providers. Information was available in a matter of minutes for those providing health services to injured or sick individuals. Previous dissemination of health information to a broad audience took days or even months; the Internet can deliver information in a matter of hours. One proactive Web site is the CDC home page. This resource should be expanded and health care professionals should be taught, as a regular part of their education, to evaluate Web sites as sources for scientific information. More information on evaluating Internet content is in Chapter 15.

The Internet can also be used in training health care providers to: (1) deliver oral health promotion, (2) present continuing education in rural communities, and (3) provide opportunities for dental hygienists to complete their bachelor's degree. For example, some schools offer a bachelor's degree completion program that is delivered completely online. Practicing professionals can stay in their hometown when taking courses. This is especially beneficial for rural communities that have a shortage of health providers and limited access to educational opportunities.

The Internet can also be used in creative ways to provide educational programs through community centers, schools, and public libraries. Technology can be used when face-to-face interventions are impractical.[58] Today's children expect to use interactive software, Web sites, and games as a part of everyday life. Oral health education software can be developed and distributed to schools and after-school programs. Games that are based on eliminating the "tooth bug" and conquering tooth decay can be fun and educational.

Oral Health Professional Workforce

The burden of need for effective oral health promotion initiatives can be reduced by better use of oral health professionals. One example is developing alternative models of care by using nondentist oral health care providers as described in Chapter 3. Most dental hygienists are competent to place pit and fissure sealants, as well as evaluate the need for such sealants. However, many dental practice acts do not allow the placement of sealants without the supervision of a dentist. Few board certified public health dentists and fewer dentists in private practice can take time away from their practice to supervise dental hygienists outside of private practice.

A second example was revealed in a systematic review of oral cancer screening programs. The authors concluded that there is a need for other health care providers to assume more responsibility to ensure that the public receives oral cancer examinations.[59]

The Task Force on Community Preventive Services was charged with determining interventions to promote and improve oral health. It determined that it is time to for dentists and politicians to think seriously about educating other oral health professionals who encounter populations at high risk for oral disease.[58] Increased use of other oral health care providers, in many cases, requires educating politicians. Politicians must understand the need for more oral health professionals who will provide care to those with health disparities. To bring about policy changes and amend practice acts, public health professionals must be actively involved in educating state representatives. Politicians should be continuously informed of emerging data on oral health and oral health interventions.

Evidence-Based Research

Evidence-based practice must be a standard part of all oral health promotion interventions and educational programs.[60-62] Quality evaluations need to be included in every part of the oral health promotion program, starting with planning. Watt suggested that 10% of a program's total budget be set aside for evaluation.[63] The reason the Task Force did not strongly recommend most of the evaluated promotion programs was not because of ineffectiveness but because they lacked supporting data. It is important to recognize that interventions that work in private practice may not be equally effective for high-risk groups.

To promote more evidence-based research in oral health promotion, Congress authorized the Health Promotion and Disease Prevention Research Centers Program, administered by the CDC. The program's key features are multidisciplinary faculty, knowledge of community needs, and collaboration with new and traditional health partners. The 26 centers involved focus on reducing priority health risks and promoting health behaviors.[64]

SUMMARY

In summary, oral health promotion, the process of enabling people to increase control over and to improve their health, is directed at four preventable oral diseases—dental caries, diseases of the supporting structures, oral pharyngeal cancers, and sports-related craniofacial injuries. Prevention or stopping disease before it occurs or in its early stages is central to health promotion. Amelioration of health inequities also is essential as the poor, minorities, and elderly share a disproportionate amount of preventable oral disease. The primary goal of oral health promotion is to reduce the prevalence of oral disease through education and other interventions.

Professionals abide by a rule or code of ethics that promotes health for the public. Current statistics clearly reveal that oral disease is one of the most prevalent health problems in society. As community members and as health care providers, we have a responsibility to be involved in health promotion to address this issue. The oral health professional can be involved in oral health promotion and help meet the objectives of Healthy People 2010 by resolving to influence social change, implement community programs, and work with existing effective programs.

RESOURCES

Healthy People 2010: Available at:
http://www.healthypeople.gov/
http://odphp.osophs.dhhs.gov/pubs/hp2000/
    consort.htm
Governmental Agencies: Available at:
http://www.nidr.nih.gov/
http://www.cdc.gov
http://www.health.gov
Fluoride/Fluoridation Web Sites:
http://www.fdiworldental.org/guidelines/
    index.htm
http://www.cdc.gov/oralhealth/topics/
    fluoridation.htm

http://www.who.int/environmental_information/
    Information_resources/htmdocs/Fluoride/
    fluoride.html#FLUORIDE%20OCCURENCE
http://www.health.gov/environment/
    ReviewofFluoride/default.htm
http://fluoride.oralhealth.org/
http://www.ada.org/public/topics/fluoride/
    facts-toc.html
http://www.who.int/water_sanitation_health/
    GDWQ/Chemicals/fluoridefull.htm
http://www.gov.on.ca/molt/english/pub/
    ministry/fluoridation/fluor.pdf
http://www.gov.on.ca/MOH/english/pub/
    ministry/fluoridation/fluor.pdf
http://www.dns.vic.gov.au/phd/fluoridation/
http://www.york.ac.uk/inst/crdl/fluoride.htm
http://www.bfsweb.org
**Nevada Healthy Smile, Happy Child
    Program:**
http//www.health2K.state.nv.us/index.htm

Review Questions

1. Most disparities in oral health fall along lines of:
    a. age, race/ethnicity, and socioeconomic level.
    b. age and socioeconomic level.
    c. age, race/ethnicity, educational level, and gender.
    d. age, race/ethnicity, gender, and socio-economic level.
    e. race/ethnicity, gender, and socioeconomic level.

2. Why is community water fluoridation considered a model for oral health promotion?
    a. It is safe, effective and socially equitable.
    b. It is easy to implement, effective, and inexpensive.
    c. The CDC recommends it.
    d. The public is uniformly supportive of fluoridation.
    e. It is safe, reaches everyone, and is expensive.

Learning Activities

1. Go the Centers for Disease Control and Prevention Web page (http://www.cdc.gov) to read about health disparities related to dental caries and water fluoridation.
   a. Which populations have the greatest proportion of dental caries?
   b. What does the Surgeon General say about community water fluoridation?
2. Interview an uninsured member of a population that is at greater risk of dental caries and who has experienced a toothache.
   a. Ask them about their frustration in accessing dental care when they were in pain.
   b. What steps did they have to go through to receive dental care?
3. Conduct an Internet search, using your favorite search engine, to read the opinions of those opposing community water fluoridation. Simply type in water fluoridation, you will find many sites.
   a. Create a list of reasons for opposing community water fluoridation
   b. Describe how you would respond to someone with those views.
4. Write a letter to the editor expressing your support for community water fluoridation. Use supporting evidence to convince the reading audience of your opinion.

5. Write a letter to the editor expressing your opposition to community water fluoridation. Use supporting evidence to convince the reading audience of your opinion.
6. Write a review of community water fluoridation after conducting a literature search to locate pertinent articles. This paper should be based on scientific research, therefore, it must cite at least 10 referenced works. It should include:
   a. Risks, benefits, and use
   b. Type of fluoride used
   c. Who benefits most from community water fluoridation
   d. Current dose
   e. Toxic level
   f. Signs and symptoms of acute and chronic toxicity
7. Choose a health promotion topic (e.g., tobacco cessation, community water fluoridation, early childhood caries). List the social factors at the micro, meso, and macro levels that would be barriers to success of the program.

3. The primary goal of any oral health program should be to:
   a. change individual habits.
   b. educate the public.
   c. empower people to attain equity in health.
   d. teach people oral hygiene care.
   e. provide clinical services.

4. Education should be included in which stages of a community water fluoridation program?

   a. Community assessment
   b. Early planning
   c. Implementation
   d. Evaluation
   e. All stages

5. What are three options to community water fluoridation that provide systemic fluoride?
   a. Professional application of fluoride, salt, and milk fluoridation

b. School water, salt, and milk fluoridation

c. Fluoride rinse, professional application, fluoride tablets

d. Fluoride varnish, school water fluoridation, and fluoride tablets

e. Fluoride varnish, salt fluoridation, and fluoride tablets

6. Who benefits from community water fluoridation?
   a. Small children younger than age 7
   b. All children younger than age 18
   c. Adults
   d. The elderly
   e. Everyone who has teeth

7. All of the following are examples of primary prevention EXCEPT:
   a. community water fluoridation.
   b. pit and fissure sealants.
   c. preventive education.
   d. professional fluoride applications.
   e. remineralization of dental caries.

8. A single educational program is not effective as a health promotion program because:
   a. individuals learn at different rates.
   b. health behavior is complex and includes many factors, such as psychosocial issues, health habits, and cultural influence.
   c. people are difficult to educate in groups.
   d. everyone has a different learning style.
   e. educators should be calibrated.

9. It is important for the oral health professional to understand risk factors for oral disease, health behaviors, determinants, and disparities in oral health so they can:
   a. identify a target audience and design a program specifically for that audience.
   b. demonstrate compassion for the populations.
   c. change the risk factors.
   d. change the health behaviors.
   e. explain it to their patients.

10. Social factors operating on a micro level include:
    a. social institutions.
    b. the family unit.
    c. age.
    d. cultural beliefs.
    e. government policies.

REFERENCES

1. American Dental Education Association. Competencies for entry into the profession of dental hygiene. exhibit 7 J Dent Educ 2003;67(7):1–5.
2. Duhl L. Guide to community preventive services: A commentary. Am J Prev Med 2002;23(1):10–11.
3. World Health Organization. WHO/HPR/HEP/98.1 Health Promotion Glossary, 1998. World Health Organization.
4. Peterson PE. The World Oral Health Report 2003. Oral Health Programme, Noncommunicable Disease Prevention and Health Promotion. Geneva, Switzerland: World Health Organization, 2003;1–45. Available at: http://www.who.int.
5. Green LW, Kreuter MW. Commentary on the emerging guide to community preventive services from a health promotion perspective. Am J Prev Med 2002;(23)1:7–9.
6. World Health Organization. Available at: http://www.wpro.who.int/hpr/docs/rf_intro.pdf. Accessed February 2004.
7. Ottawa Charter for Health Promotion (hpr). First International Conference on Health Promotion, Ottawa, Canada, 21 Nov, 1986. Available at: http://www.who.int/hpr/archive/docs/ottawa.html. Accessed February 2004.
8. U.S. Department of Health and Human Service. Healthy People 2010. Volume 2/21, Oral Health. Centers for Disease Control and Prevention. Available at: http://www.health.gov/healthypeople/state/toolkit. Accessed February 2004.
9. Healthy People 2010 Toolkit: A field guide to health planning. public health foundation. Available at: http://www.health.gov/healthypeople/state/toolkit. Accessed February 2004.
10. A New Perspective on the Health of Canadians. Available at: http://www.hc-sc.gc.ca/hppb/phdd/pube/perintrod.htm. Accessed February 2004.
11. Lawrence HP, Leake JL. The U.S. Surgeon General's Report on Oral Health in America: A Canadian Perspective. J Can Dent Assoc 2001;67:(10)587.
12. Beck JD, Offenbacher S. Oral health and systemic disease: periodontitis and cardiovascular disease. J Dent Educ 1998;62(10):859–870.
13. Oral Health in America. A Report of the Surgeon General. Executive Summary. Available at: http://www.nidr.gov/sgr/sgrohweb/chap4.htm. Accessed February 2004.

14. U.S. Department of Health and Human Service, Oral Health in America. A Report of the Surgeon General. Section 4, The Magnitude of the Problem. 2000. Available at: http://www.nidr.gov/sgr/sgrohweb/chap4.htm. Accessed February 2004.

15. Missing the Mark. Oral Health in America. The Oral Health in America National Grading Project. Oral Health Report Card. Fall 2000/United States.

16. Gift HC. Prevention of oral diseases and oral health promotion. Curr Opinion Dent 1991;1:337–347.

17. Blinkhorn A. Evaluation and planning of oral health promotion programmes. In: Schou L, Blinkhorn A, eds. Oral Health Promotion. Oxford: Oxford University Press, 1999, p 249–270.

18. Blaxter M. Health services as a defense against the consequences of poverty in industrialized societies. Soc Sci Med 1983;17:1139–1148.

19. Milbank Memorial Fund. Pediatric dental care in CHIP and Medicaid: Paying for what kids need getting value for state payments. July 1999 Available at: http://www.milbank.org/reports/990716mrpd.html. Accessed February 2004.

20. Loe H. Oral hygiene in the prevention of caries and periodontal disease. Int Dent J 2000;50:129–139.

21. Chu R, Craig B. Understanding the determinants of preventive oral health behaviours. Probe 1996;30(1):12–18.

22. Centers for Disease Control and Prevention. National Oral Health Surveillance System: Dental visits. 1999. Available at: http://www2.cdc.gov/nohss/ListV.asp?qkey=2. Accessed February 2004.

23. Mckenzie JF, Smeltzer JL. Planning, Implementing, and Evaluating Health Promotions Programs: A Primer. 3rd Ed. Needham Heights, MA: Ally and Bacon, 2001.

24. Edmunds M, Fulwood C. Strategic Communications in oral health: influencing public and professional opinions and actions. Amb Ped 2002;2:180–184.

25. Task Force on Community Preventive Medicine. Recommendations on selected interventions to prevent dental caries, oral and pharyngeal cancers, and sports-related craniofacial injuries. Am J Prev Med 2002; 23(1):16–20.

26. Truman BI, Gooch BF, Sulemana I, et al. The Task Force on Community Preventive Services. Reviews of evidence on interventions to prevent dental caries, oral and pharyngeal cancers, and sports-related craniofacial injuries. Am J Prev Med 2002;23(1):21–54.

27. Crall JJ. Reviews and recommendations to prevent dental caries, oral and pharyngeal cancers, and sports-related craniofacial injuries. Am J Prev Med 2002;23(1):81–82.

28. Gooch BF, Truman BI, Griffin SO, et al. A comparison of selected evidence reviews and recommendations on interventions to prevent dental caries, oral and pharyngeal cancers, and sports-related craniofacial injuries. Am J Prev Med 2002;23(1):55–80.

29. Oral Health Resource (Press Release). Community water fluoridation and school-based sealant programs. Centers for Disease Control and Prevention. Available at: http://www.cdc.gov/OralHeal/pressreleases/cwf-sealantshtm. Accessed February 2004.

30. Chronic Disease Prevention: Oral Health. Centers for Disease Control and Prevention, 2002. Available at: http://www.cdc.gov/nccdphp/exemplary/oral_health.htm. Accessed February 2004.

31. Stavisky J, Bailit H. The Robert Wood Johnson Foundation's response to improving the nation's oral health. Am J Prev Med 2002;23(1):13–15.

32. Treadwell H, Ro M. Community-based oral health prevention. Issues and opportunities. Am J Prevent Med 2002; 23(1):18–21.

33. What is Oral Health? America's NSTEP. Available at: http://www.nstep.org/whatis/whatis,htm. Accessed February 2004.

34. Centers for Disease Control and Prevention. Achievements in Public Health, 1900–1999: Fluoridation of drinking water to prevent dental caries. MMWR 1999;48(41): 933–940.

35. Easley MW. Celebrating 50 years of fluoridation: A public health success story. Brit Dent J 1995;21:72–725.

36. Featherstone JDB. The science and practice of caries prevention. J Am Dent Assoc 2000;131(7):87–89.

37. Horowitz HS. The effectiveness of community water fluoridation in the United States. J Public Health Dent 1996; 56:253–258.

38. Population receiving optimally fluoridated public drinking water—United States, 2000. MMWR 2002;57(7):144–147. Available at: http://www.cdc.gov/mmwr/preview/mmwrhtml/mm5107a2.htm. Accessed February 2004.

39. The impact of fluoride on health. J Am Diet Assoc 2000; 100:1208–1213. Available at: http://www.eatright.org/adap1000.html. Accessed February 2004.

40. Dietary reference intakes of calcium, phosphorus, magnesium, vitamin D, and fluoride. Institute of Medicine; National Academy of Science, Food and Nutrition Board Washington DC: Nation Academy Press, 1997.

41. Brunelle JA, Carlos JP. Recent trends in dental caries in U.S. children and the effect of water fluoridation. J Dent Res 1990;47:89–92.

42. Newbrun E. Effectiveness of water fluoridation. J Public Health Dent 1989;49(special issue):17–44.

43. Griffin SO, Gooch BF, Lockwood SA, Tomar SL. Quantifying the diffused benefit from water fluoridation in the United States. Comm Dent Oral Epidemiol 2001; 29:120.

44. American Dental Hygienists' Association. ADHA Code of Ethics for Dental Hygienists. Available at: http://www.adha.org/aboutadha/codeofethics.htm. Accessed February 2004.

45. Cappella JN, Turow J, Jamieson KH. Call-in talk radio: background, content, audiences, and portrayal in mainstream media. Annenburg Public Policy Center's Series. Aug 7,1996;1–68.

46. The British Fluoridation Society for Evidence-Based Information. The Ethics of Fluoridation. Harris J. Center for Social Ethics & Policy, University of Manchester, November 1989. Available at: http://www.liv.ac.uk/bfsethicsharris.html. Accessed February 2004.

47. Forum on Fluoride, Section 7. Fluoridation status worldwide: the international context. Available at: http//www.doh.ie/publications/fluoridation/section7.html. Accessed February 2004.

48. New FDI statements. Fluoride and dental caries. FDI World Mar 2001; 24–26. Available at: http://www.fdiworldental.org/. Accessed February 2004.

49. The National Alliance for Equity in Dental Health: 2001 Annual Symposium on Inequalities in Dental Health. Report of the 6th Annual Symposium of Inequalities in Dental Health. Available at: htpp://wwliv.ac.uk/bfs/alliance01report.htm. Accessed February 2004.

50. The British Fluoridation Society for Evidence-Based Information. Available at: http://www.liv.ac.uk/bfs/support.html. Accessed February 2004.

51. World Health Organization. Environmental health criteria 36: Fluorine and fluoride. Geneva, Switzerland: World Health Organization, 1984.

52. U.S. Department of Health and Human Services, Centers for Disease Control and Prevention. Recommendations for using fluoride to prevent and control dental caries in the united states. MMWR 2001;1–42.

53. Klein SP, Bohannan HM, Bell RM, et al. The cost and effectiveness of school-based preventive dental care. Am J Public Health 1985;75:382–391.

54. American Dental Hygienists' Association. Symposium on Fluoride Varnish. National Oral Health Conference, April 2003.

55. Clarkson JJ, McLoughlin J. Role of fluoride in oral health promotion. Int Dent J 2000;50:119–128.

56. Preventing and controlling oral and pharyngeal cancer recommendations from a National Strategic Planning Conference. Centers of Disease Control and Prevention. MMWR August 8, 1998/(RR14). Available at: http://www.cdc.gov/mmwrhtml/00054567.htm. Accessed February 2004.

57. U.S. Department of Health and Human Services. Centers for Disease Control and Prevention. A framework for assessing the effectiveness of disease and injury prevention. MMWR 1992;41:1–7.

58. Capilouto E. Partnering to unlock the mysteries of oral diseases and injuries. Am J Prev Med 2002;23(1):6–7.

59. Horowitz AM, Goodman HS, Yellowitz JA, Nourjah PA. The need for health promotion in oral cancer prevention and early detection. J Public Health Dent 1996;56(6):319–330.

60. Kleinman DV. The guide to community preventive services and oral health. Am J Prev Med 2002;23(1):1–2.

61. Weintraub JA, Millstein SG. Community preventive services and oral health: Wishes for the future. Am J Prev Med 2002;23(1):3–5.

62. McGinnis JM, Foege W. Guide to community preventive services: harnessing the science. Am J Prev Med 2002;23(1):1–2.

63. Watt AG, Fuller S, Harnett R, Treasure ET, Stillman-Lowe C. Oral health promotion evaluation—time for development. Comm Dent Oral Epidemiol 2001;29:161–166.

64. Centers for Disease Control and Prevention. Oral Health Promotion and Disease Prevention Activities. Critical role of prevention research: Focus on oral health prevention research and practice. Available at: http://www.cdc.gov/nccdphp/aag/aag_prc.htm. Accessed February 2004.

Community Oral Health Education

9

Objectives

After studying this chapter and completing the study questions and activities, the learner will be able to:

- Define health education.
- Describe the goal of health education.
- Describe the traditional, cognitive approach to health education.
- Discuss why the traditional model is not always effective.
- Discuss the evolution of health education.
- Give examples of health education in individual and group education settings.
- Describe health behavior theories.
- Discuss components of common theories of health behavior.
- Explain Maslow's Hierarchy of Needs.
- Describe the components of the Learning Ladder Continuum.
- Apply appropriate health behavior theory, motivational and learning concepts, and teaching methods to guide an education effort.

KEY TERMS

Community focus
Community Organization Theory
Compliance
Consumer Information Processing Model
Diffusion of Innovations Theory
Enabling factors
Focus groups

Health Belief Model
Health education
Interpersonal focus
Intrapersonal focus
Learning Ladder
Learning styles
Maslow's Hierarchy of Needs
Oral health education

Organizational Change Theory
Predisposing factors
Reinforcing factors
Social Cognitive Theory
Social Learning Theory
Social Marketing Theory
Stages of Change Model

The American Dental Education Association competencies addressed in the chapter include[1]:

C.8:   Communicate effectively with individuals and groups from diverse populations, both verbally and in writing.

HP.1:   Promote the values of oral and general health and wellness to the public and organizations within and outside the profession.

HP.4:   Identify individual and population risk factors and develop strategies that promote health and quality of life.

HP.5:   Evaluate factors that can be used to promote patient adherence to disease prevention and health maintenance strategies.

CM.3:   Provide community oral health services in various settings.

Introduction

Dental hygienists play a vital role in the health of individuals and groups. As oral health educators, they design, develop, and implement oral health education efforts for diverse populations. Theoretic guidance for this aspect of dental hygiene has been borrowed from educational theory, communication, and social and behavioral psychology. This chapter introduces some basic concepts for guiding oral health education efforts.

HEALTH EDUCATION

Health education provides the decision-making foundations needed for attaining and maintaining health. Defined as learning opportunities or educational interventions designed to help individuals or groups learn new health information and develop new health behaviors, it is a process of communicating information about evidence-based methods of disease prevention and encouraging responsibility for self-care.[2,3] Health education services are developed in various formats and are presented in various settings. They can be directed toward either individuals or groups. To be considered successful, health education must result in behavioral change.

The terms *health education* and *health promotion* are sometimes used interchangeably. Both are important in modifying detrimental behaviors and promoting self-wellness concepts. Although the concepts are similar, the differences are significant. The goal of health education is to have a positive impact on health through accurate knowledge of health behaviors and lifestyles. Health promotion, which may include health education, is a broad concept that addresses the general process of advocating health, increasing awareness of health issues, and identifying appropriate strategies to address health issues and prevent disease.[4] (For a full discussion of health promotion, refer to Chapter 8.)

Many different types of health care providers offer health education; it is not restricted to any one profession or field. Dentists and dental hygienists, as well as physicians and nurses, have a key role in health education delivery because the care they provide often includes educational information. Whether working with individual patients in the clinical setting or with groups in a community setting, the dental hygienist is an educator. In the American Dental Hygienists' Association (ADHA) role of Health Educator/Wellness Promoter, they are vital to oral health.

ORAL HEALTH EDUCATION

Oral health education is a planned package of information, learning activities, or experiences that are intended to produce improved oral health. With the primary goal of disease prevention, its purpose is to facilitate decision-making for oral health practices and to encourage appropriate choices for these behaviors. Oral health education has evolved from the traditional approach of simply providing information to incorporating various models of sociology, psychology, learning styles, and methods to better facilitate learning and behavior change.

Historically, many health recommendations have centered on avoidance behaviors, such as "Brush this way . . . to avoid periodontal disease" or "Don't eat sweets . . . to avoid dental caries." Contemporary health education strategies emphasize the positive aspects of health and often encourage health achievement through a wellness approach.[5]

Not all oral health education activities produce positive changes in oral health behaviors. The traditional method of merely dispensing information on ways to improve oral health has been shown ineffective in producing changes in oral health behaviors.[2] To be successful, an oral health education plan must assess and accommodate the knowledge levels, cultural norms, values, beliefs, attitudes, opinions, and environment of the intended audience. When identified, indicated adjustments and modifications must be incorporated into the educational plan.

LEVELS OF FOCUS

Health education may be designed to address the needs of individuals, groups, or entire communities. A framework has been described with three different levels of focus for designing components of health education programs.[6] These levels include **intrapersonal focus** (individualistic), **interpersonal focus** (microsocial), and **community focus** (macrosocial).[4-6]

An intrapersonal approach to health education focuses on the individual as the target of change. It uses behavior modification techniques to effect changes in knowledge, attitudes, or beliefs.[4] One example is one-to-one chairside instruction on the relationship between plaque and dental diseases. In a health education program with individual focus, the program recipients have the ability and resources to start and maintain the desired behavior change on their own.

In contrast, the interpersonal approach focuses on groups as targets of change. This has been referred to as a "people helping people" approach to health education in which small group strategies between families, neighbors, peers, or work groups try to achieve behavioral change. A health education program that focuses on the group as the target of change is based on the belief that interpersonal interactions and characteristics are the forces that initiate and reinforce behavioral changes in group members. Group dynamics are a factor in the effectiveness of these educational programs.[4] An example of this type of program is a chemical dependency support group in which group members give each other reinforcement.

A community approach to health education focuses on the impact of economy, politics, or other factors within the community on behavior. Health education efforts that include decision-makers in regulatory or legislative bodies illustrate this level of focus. Community-focused education programs take advantage of community strength for problems that cannot be effectively addressed by the individual or small group.[4] Community organizing and social marketing are examples of change strategies at the community level of focus. Table 9-1 further describes these levels of focus and gives examples.

HEALTH BEHAVIOR THEORIES

Theories from sociology, education, and psychology that describe learning and behavioral change can help the health educator design and develop educational efforts. Some basic theories and principles are presented here.

Theories With Intrapersonal Focus (Individualistic Approach)

HEALTH BELIEF MODEL

The **Health Belief Model** is useful in predicting the likelihood of an individual's **compliance** with professional recommendations for preventive

TABLE 9-1 LEVELS OF FOCUS IN HEALTH EDUCATION

APPROACH	TARGETS OF CHANGE	EXPLANATION	EXAMPLE
Intrapersonal (Within the individual/Individualistic)	Knowledge; attitudes; skills; behavior; self-concept; self-esteem; developmental processes	Focuses on the person Uses behavior modification to effect change Strategies used: • information dissemination • skill development and repetitive learning experiences • increased cognitive awareness	Chairside, one-to-one instruction on the plaque-dental disease relationship
Interpersonal (People helping people/Microsocial)	Families; work groups; peers; neighbors; social networks; social support	Focuses on interactions between people Uses: • individual and small group strategies • peer group influences • counseling in the oral health care setting	Town Hall meetings on community water fluoridation Oral health education workshop for caregivers to special needs patients
Community (Creating public policy/Macrosocial)	Regulatory agencies; legislation; governmental structures; formal and informal leadership; social and health services	Focuses on the impact of economy, politics, social, cultural, and environmental factors on oral health behavior	Letter writing campaign to legislators regarding supervision
		Broad efforts to include decision-makers, governmental bodies, and public interest groups	Regulations that put limits on access to care for some populations

Sources: Locker D. Preventive Dental Services. 2nd Ed. Canada: Health and Welfare, 1988; Darby ML, Walsh MM. Dental Hygiene Theory and Practice. Philadelphia, PA: WB Saunders, 1995; and Dignan MB, Carr PA. Program Planning for Health Education and Promotion. 2nd Ed. Philadelphia, PA: Lea & Febiger, 1992.

health behaviors. Based on experiences with public participation in a screening program for tuberculosis, this model was first introduced in the 1950s by I.M. Rosenstock[7] and other psychologists working with the U.S. Public Health Service. It remains a major construct that is still consulted for understanding behaviors.

This model is based on the theory that behaviors are directed by perceptions and beliefs and suggests that whether or not a person engages in preventive health actions depends on these beliefs. In short, it provides an outline of the essential factors involved in behavioral change. The belief components of this model are:

- Susceptibility: The individual must believe that they are susceptible to a given disease or condition.
- Severity: The individual must believe that the disease will have an impact of at least moderate severity or seriousness on their life.

- Beneficial: The individual must believe that there are effective actions that can be taken to reduce the risk of, or control, the disease.
- Benefits outweigh barriers to action: The individual must believe that the benefits of taking the recommended action exceed any difficulties that might be encountered.[2,5,8,9]

The stronger the beliefs, the higher the probability that an appropriate health action will be taken. If dental diseases are not perceived as a serious health threat, it is unlikely that an individual will participate in daily preventive dental behaviors, proceed with professional interventions, or accept professional recommendations.

Cues to action, that activate readiness to change and stimulate overt behavior change, are a concept that has been added since the model was first described. The concept of self-efficacy, or confidence in one's ability to successfully perform an action, was added by Rosenstock and others in 1988 to help this model better fit the challenges of changing unhealthy habitual behaviors, such as overeating, smoking, or sedentary lifestyles.[10]

Observations and questioning during assessment can provide clues to existing health beliefs. Age, gender, race, ethnicity, peer or reference group pressure, and prior knowledge about health problems are all factors that play a role in modifying beliefs and potential compliance with recommendations for health behaviors.

The Health Belief Model can help identify leverage points for change and can be a useful tool for designing change strategies, as well. Developing persuasive health messages that can guide individuals toward making healthy decisions is one promising application. Box 9-1 illustrates the Health Belief Model.

STAGES OF CHANGE MODEL

The **Stages of Change Model,** introduced by James O. Prochaska and Carlo C. DiClemente in 1979, grew from their work with smoking cessation and drug and alcohol addiction. It has recently been applied to various other health behaviors. This theory is concerned with an individual's readiness to adopt a behavioral change for a healthier life. It views behavior change as a process rather than an event, with people at varying levels of motivation or readiness to change.[11]

The primary concept of this theory is that people cycle through different stages of readiness and that an individual can be in any stage at any given time. This is a circular, not a linear model. People can enter or exit the circular cycle at any point and may often recycle through the stages. The oral health educator can use this theory to assess the

---

BOX 9-1 Illustrating the Health Belief Model

Susceptibility	"I could develop periodontitis."
Severity	"Periodontitis is a serious disease and can lead to bleeding gums, halitosis, and loss of teeth, which will affect my life."
Beneficial	"There are specific things I can do, such as using the recommended brushing method and following the prescribed home care regimens, which will prevent the disease."
Benefits Outweigh Barriers	"It is worth the extra time I spend to clean my teeth and mouth to be free of the threat of periodontitis."

individual's readiness for behavioral change and match health education efforts accordingly. The major stages of this model and their explanations are:

- Precontemplation: unaware of the health problem, without any thought of need for change
- Contemplation: aware of problem and thinking about possibility of making change
- Decision/Determination: making a plan for change
- Action: putting a plan for change into action
- Maintenance: continuing desired health action.[11]

Observations and responses to questions asked during assessment can provide indications to the readiness stage. Educational efforts that match readiness to change are more likely to effect behavioral change. Box 9-2 describes using the Stages of Change Model.

The main point to remember here is that people can be at different places in the process of change. They can benefit from different interventions that are matched to the stage they are in at the time.

CONSUMER INFORMATION PROCESSING MODEL

The **Consumer Information Processing Model,** which evolved out of the study of human problem solving and information processing, addresses the ways consumers take in and use information in their decision-making. The consumer information processing theory makes two key assumptions: (1) people are limited in how much information they can acquire, use, and remember, and (2) people combine bits of information into useable summaries and create decision rules to enable faster and easier choices.

James R. Bettman, a marketing theorist, developed one of the best-known models of consumer information processing. In it, he describes a cyclical process of information search, choice, use and learning, and feedback for future decisions.[12] The model has been extended to address the information environment and the way it affects how people obtain, process, and use information. The ap-

BOX 9-2 Using the Stages of Change Model

For the individual who is unaware of a given health problem, begin by providing and personalizing information on the risks for the health problem and the need for behaviors that decrease the risks. In sequence, provide information that encourages making a specific change and offer activities that foster the development of goals and firm action plans.

When a change has been implemented, provide feedback, support, and reinforcement. Offer ongoing and continuing support to assist the individual in coping with the acquired differences that occur because of the behavior change and to minimize relapsing behaviors.

plication for health education is that, before people will use health information, it must be available, it must be thought of as useful and new, and it must be user friendly. Box 9-3 gives an example of the Consumer Information Processing Model.

The concept to note here is that the oral health educator should evaluate the information environment to ensure the target audience finds the information materials convenient, attractive, and easy-to-use.

Theories With Interpersonal Focus (Microsocial Approach)

SOCIAL LEARNING THEORY

The **Social Learning Theory** assumes that people and their environments are continuously interacting. The basic premise of this theory is that people learn through their own experiences, as well as by observing the actions of others and the results of those actions.[10]

The **Social Cognitive Theory,** developed by Albert Bandura in the 1970s, is the dominant version of social learning theory.[13] It proposes that

BOX 9-3 Consumer Information Processing Model

In point-of-purchase (POP) nutrition information programs in grocery stores, information is given in summary form and only carefully chosen, useful points are provided (e.g., information processing capacity, decision rules). Labels or stickers with symbols or catch-phrases, such as "low fat" or "low calorie," are conveniently shown on shelf tags or the food items themselves so that it is easy to locate (information search). The most successful POP programs offer information that is new and helpful in choosing items with nutritional value and by not providing information consumers already know, such as labeling all fresh vegetables as "healthy."

behaviors are learned socially, through direct or vicarious experiences, and through observations of others' actions and their results. Reactions to a behavior, such as testimonies or judgments or advocacy by experts, provide negative or positive reinforcements to perpetuate or terminate a behavioral change.

Self-efficacy, or the confidence in one's ability to successfully perform an action and persist in it, is the single most important aspect of the sense of self that determines one's effort to change behavior. Greater self-efficacy promotes higher motivation when confronting obstacles and increases the chances of a behavior persisting over time in the absence of formal supervision.

Two other relevant concepts are observational learning, or modeling, and behavior reinforcement. Modeling allows people to observe others for an understanding of the consequences of an action. It is most powerful when the person being observed is powerful, respected, or like the observer. Reinforcement is a response to a behavior that affects the likelihood of it being repeated.

Positive reinforcements increase the chances that a behavior will be repeated. Tangible rewards, or praise and encouragement for self-reward, encourage people to establish positive health habits. Extrinsic rewards are often useful as motivators for continued participation, but they do not sustain long-term change. These should be used with caution to avoid developing dependence. Negative reinforcements include punishments or absence of response. Box 9-4 describes using the Social Learning Theory.

Theories With Community Focus (Macrosocial Approach)

COMMUNITY ORGANIZATION THEORY

Identifying common problems, activating resources, and developing and implementing methods for reaching goals that have been collectively set are the constructs upon which the **Community Organization Theory** is based.[14] It emphasizes active participation and the development of communities to evaluate and solve health and social problems. In contrast to professionally designed and implemented activities, this is a

BOX 9-4 Using the Social Learning Theory

Involve significant others or relevant others together with the individual. Give accurate information and skill development training about proposed behaviors. Include advance information about probable results of behavior change. Approach behavioral change in small steps and give encouragement. Use persuasion and emphasize strengths and capabilities. Identify role models; point out the experiences of others. Provide praise, rewards, and incentives. Minimize negative responses that decrease the probability of positive change.

process of self-led improvement within the group. The community (or group) is the medium for change. In this theory, group members:

- participate in, and have ownership of, the change process.
- believe that they have control (empowerment) over their lives and the lives of their group.
- assume responsibility for, and take leadership roles in, change.
- effectively collaborate to identify problems, achieve consensus on goals and priorities, and implement actions.[14]

Box 9-5 illustrates the Community Organization Theory.

DIFFUSION OF INNOVATIONS THEORY

Before new ideas, behaviors, products, or services become part of society, they must be communicated, accepted, and adopted. The **Diffusion of Innovations Theory,** which describes how new ideas, social practices, or products spread through a society or from one society to another, helps assess how this happens. This theory, pioneered by Everett M. Rogers in 1962 to describe the acceptance of a hardier corn variety by Midwest farmers in a depression-era rural society, is still general enough to be applicable to contemporary public health challenges for disseminating new prevention, early detection and treatment methods, and to increase the use of beneficial programs.[15]

How well an innovation is received, or how quickly it is accepted and adopted, is determined by several factors. Inclusion of the target population in innovation development is critical. Their values, needs, experiences, and habits are important considerations. This theory also suggests that it is important to identify opinion leaders within a community and to gain their support for new experiences, ideas, or proposed behavior changes. Community leaders who reiterate information that has been provided through mass media channels increase the chances that people will decide to accept an idea or practice.

Another important component of this theory is the view of communication as a two-way process. Instead of merely persuading an audience to accept or adopt an idea, communication flows reciprocally in two directions. Both formal and informal communication channels and social systems for disseminating new knowledge should be identified and used. Box 9-6 describes using the Diffusion of Innovations Theory.

Not all community members will adopt or even accept new ideas. For those that do, adoption occurs at varying rates and within the category descriptions shown in Table 9-2. Determining where group members are on the *adopter curve* allows health educators to better select the intervention

BOX 9-5 Illustrating the Community Organization Theory

A group of mothers who use the same local day care facility for their young children meet regularly to discuss parenting and child care. They have all noticed the recent occurrence of brown cavity spots on many of their toddlers' upper front teeth. They ask an acquaintance who is a dental hygienist to meet with them to discuss pediatric oral health.

After learning about Early Childhood Caries, the mothers inquire about naptime routines at the facility and learn that the children receive bottles at naptime. The mothers explain the oral problems associated with this routine to the day care staff and then work with them to change naptime behaviors to eliminate nursing bottle sugar exposures. At subsequent meetings, the oral hygiene procedures that are being used at home are described. Successes and challenges are discussed, with the group offering support and suggestions for further improvement.

BOX 9-6 Using the Diffusion of Innovations Theory

Identify the values, needs, habits, and experiences of the target population and adapt the innovation so that it is consistent with them. Involve the group in developing and providing feedback on the new idea. Identify opinion leadership and solicit their support. Ask yourself: Who are the influential community members that are likely to be early adopters of the innovation? Use media (e.g., public service announcements, press releases, and community announcements at social, recreational, or church events) to expose the group to the innovation. Design the innovation so that the group will find it easy to use or understand. Give opportunities for trial experiences (e.g., free samples) with the innovation. Identify possible causes for dissatisfaction with the innovation and develop ways to overcome them. Ensure tangible, visible results through feedback and publicity.

strategies to use for individuals within a particular category.[2]

Some important characteristics of innovations that can improve the chances that they will be adopted include relative advantage (Is it superior to a past idea?), compatibility (Is it consistent with the adopter's experiences and values?), complexity (ease of use), trialability (Can it be experimented with or tried on a limited basis?), and observability (the visibility of successful tangible results). These factors enhance acceptance and adoption of a new idea, behavior, product, or service innovation.[10]

TABLE 9-2 RATE OF ACCEPTANCE OF CHANGE

Innovators	2.5% of population	May be viewed as *mavericks;* eager risk-takers; alert to the national media; more educated; usually not a part of the prevailing social structure
Early Adopters	13.5% of population	Respected, knowledgeable opinion leaders within the community; active in the community; alert to the national media; use innovations successfully; can be consulted before a potential adopter will accept a new idea
Early Majority	34% of population	Accept change, though not the first; are followers rather than leaders; more educated; more influenced by interpersonal interactions than media; more alert to local and regional media than national; above average age
Late Majority	34% of population	Skeptical members of the community; cautious but can be convinced by peer persuasion; not willing to take many risks; older, less educated and lower in socioeconomic status
Laggards	16% of population	Suspicious of innovations; very slow to change; often oriented toward past; usually have little influence on prevailing social structure; lower socioeconomic status and often feel alienated from society; use media primarily for entertainment; * This group is a likely potential target for government-sponsored oral health programs.

NOTE: There is a small segment of the community that will not accept innovation.

Source: DeBiase CB. Dental Hygiene in Review. Baltimore, MD: Lippincott Williams & Wilkins, 2001.[2]

ORGANIZATIONAL CHANGE THEORY

The **Organizational Change Theory** is applied to improve the problem-solving and renewal processes of large organizations or entire communities. Its premise is that organizations move through stages, or a series of steps, as they initiate and adopt changes.[16] By recognizing the stages, strategies to promote change can be developed to match various points in the process of change. These four stages are:

- Defining the problem: recognize and analyze problems; seek and evaluate solutions
- Initiating action: formulate policies and directives; allocate resources
- Implementing change: put the change into action
- Institutionalizing change: the new policy of change becomes integrated into the organization.[16]

For organizational change to be complete, new policy must become entrenched within the organization as the new goals and values are internalized. Box 9-7 illustrates the organizational change model.

Table 9-3 summarizes the theories and key concepts that have been presented thus far.

SOCIAL MARKETING THEORY

Kotler and Andreasen define **social marketing** as the adaptation of commercial marketing principles to the development of programs in order to influence the behavior of target audiences to improve physical and mental well-being and/or the society of which they are a part.[17] Social marketing focuses on tailoring products or programs to match a defined target audience. It is a planning model that is used to design, implement, evaluate, and manage large-scale, broad-based behavior change programs.

A marketing mix of the "four *P*s" summarizes the formula for marketing success: product, promotion, place, and price. The formula advocates promoting a product and making it available at the right place and at the right cost. In health education, the product is an educational program that has been developed for the needs and interests of the target population. Promotion refers to the strategies used to make it familiar, acceptable, and desirable. Place refers to the logistics of accessing the product, its availability and distribution. Price refers to the time, money, and energy costs of participating in the program.[5]

Focus groups, a marketing technique for understanding consumer behavior, can be a useful

---

BOX 9-7 Illustrating the Organizational Change Theory

The oral health educator for a military installation notice that the majority of manual toothbrushes offered for sale at the post exchange (PX) store were poorly-designed, low quality brushes with design features that can be damaging to oral structures.

The educator asked the manager of the PX to include brushes of recognized quality in addition to those already offered for sale. To initiate the change, specific brands of brushes had to be identified, priced, and advertised for sale. Once stocked and offered, shoppers began to make choices from the new stock, purchasing better brushes.

Eventually, shoppers began to request automated brushes and a larger selection of oral health items and self-care devices. The oral health educator and the PX manager collaborated to identify and stock these and other items of recognized quality and efficacy, accomplishing institutional change.

TABLE 9-3 SUMMARY OF THEORIES: FOCUS AND KEY CONCEPTS

	THEORY	FOCUS	KEY CONCEPTS
Intrapersonal Level (Individualistic)	Health Belief Model	Person's perception of threat of a health problem and their appraisal of recommended behaviors for preventing or managing the problem	Perceived susceptibility Perceived severity Perceived benefits of action Perceived barriers to action Cues to action Self-efficacy
	Stages of Change Model	Readiness to change or try to change toward healthy behaviors	Precontemplation Contemplation Decision/Determination Action Maintenance
	Consumer Information Processing Model	Processing by which consumers acquire and use information in decision-making	Information processing Information search Decision rules Information environment
Interpersonal Level (Microsocial)	Social Learning Theory	Behavior is explained as a three-way, dynamic reciprocal theory in which personal factors, environmental influences, and behavior continually interact	Behavioral capability Reciprocal determinism Expectations of self-efficacy Observational learning Reinforcement
Community Level (Macrosocial)	Community Organization Theory	Active participation and development of communities to better evaluate and solve health and social problems	Empowerment Community competence Participation and relevance Issue selection Critical consciousness
	Diffusion of Innovations Theory	Addresses how new ideas, products, and social practices spread within a society or from one society to another	Relative advantage Compatibility Complexity Trialability Observability
	Organizational Change Theory	Concerns processes and strategies for increasing the chances that healthy policies and programs will be adopted and maintained in formal organizations	Problem definition (awareness) Initiation of action (adoption) Implementation of change Institutionalization of change

Adapted from: Glanz K, Lewis FM, Rimer BK: Theory at a Glance: A Guide for Health Promotion Practice. National Institutes of Health, Bethesda, 1997.[16]

tool for collecting information on community needs, attitudes, norms, and other issues. A focus group usually consists of 6 to 12 people with similar backgrounds who meet over approximately 1 to 2 hours for guided discussion. A moderator leads the discussion, asking a series of questions to elicit group reactions to various issues. The session may be audiotaped or videotaped for later review and analysis. Generalizations can be inferred to the larger group from which the focus group is drawn. The information collected can be helpful in developing new educational programs.[4]

Campaigns against social behaviors or practices that are not conducive to health, such as substance abuse, drinking and driving, or abusive behavior toward others, are examples of programs grounded in social marketing theory. Credible organizations with a public image of integrity and accountability are successful social marketers. Box 9-8 gives an example of Social Marketing Theory.

PRECEDE—PROCEED MODEL

Lawrence Green and Marshall Kreuter developed the PRECEDE—PROCEED planning model for health education and health promotion programs.[18] (See Fig 5-4) It is useful because it provides a format for identifying factors related to health problems, behaviors, and program implementation.

PRECEDE refers to **p**redisposing, **r**einforcing, and **e**nabling **c**onstructs in **e**cosystem **d**iagnosis and **e**valuation (Box 9-9). This portion of the model considers the behavioral factors relevant to the emergence and occurrence of a health problem.

Three categories of factors—predisposing, enabling, and reinforcing—make it possible to sort behaviors into segments for program planning. **Predisposing factors** provide the reason behind, or motivation for, a behavior. They include knowledge, beliefs, attitudes, values, cultural mores and folkways, and existing skills. **Enabling factors** include the personal skills and available resources needed to perform a behavior. They enable, or make it possible for, actions to occur. The extent to which their absence will prevent an action from

---

BOX 9-8 Social Marketing Theory

Product: Tobacco Cessation Campaign

Promotion: Posters, radio, and television public service announcements; free oral cancer screenings by dental professionals

Place: Public schools and libraries; screening booths at local malls

Price: Anxieties and emotional stressors associated with "quitting"; transportation to screening location; time lost from work to attend screening

---

occurring is the key to identifying enabling factors. **Reinforcing factors** provide incentives for the repetition or persistence of health behaviors once they have begun. Praise, reassurance, symptom relief, and social support are examples of reinforcing factors.[4]

Program planning is facilitated by the ability to classify health behaviors in terms of the factors that predispose their occurrence, provide reinforcement for repetition, and enable their expression. Once categorized, priorities must be identified. Priority is assigned to factors on the basis of their significance in effecting the behavior in question, the degree to which the factor can be changed, and the resources available to contend with the causative factor(s). Priority factors provide the basis for developing the objectives that direct the future action of the program.

The PROCEED portion of this planning model involves the administrative and policy components of the model. It represents the **p**olitical, **r**egulatory, and **o**rganizational **c**onstructs that affect **e**ducational and **e**nvironmental **d**evelopment (Box 9-9).

MOTIVATION AND LEARNING

Motivation, which can be explained as *the will to act*, is an important factor in learning. Human motivation theory offers several models for under-

BOX 9-9 PRECEDE—PROCEED Acronym

P	**P**redisposing
R	**R**einforcing and
E	**E**nabling
C	**C**onstructs in
E	**E**cosystem
D	**D**iagnosis and
E	**E**valuation
P	**P**olitical
R	**R**egulatory and
O	**O**rganizational
C	**C**onstructs that affect
E	**E**ducational and
E	**E**nvironmental
D	**D**evelopment

standing the internal and external forces that can move an individual to action. Some useful models are included here.

Maslow's Hierarchy of Needs

Psychologist Abraham H. Maslow (1908–1970) attempted to synthesize a large body of research related to human motivation in his conceptualization of a hierarchical arrangement of needs as motivating factors. His work, first published in 1954, has become one of the most popular and most cited theories of human motivation. It may be helpful to oral health educators in identifying motivational factors that can be targeted for facilitating behavioral changes.

Maslow's Hierarchy of Needs suggests that inner forces (needs) drive a person into action and that some needs take precedence over others.[2,8] It provides a framework for identifying, classifying, and assigning priorities to these human needs and values. In this concept, needs are classified into a pyramid arrangement, according to their importance to the individual and the importance attached to their satisfaction. Based on their

power and strength, the most imperative needs are positioned at the base of the pyramid and the least imperative needs are at the top. The relative importance of each level to the other needs in the hierarchy is represented by its size within the pyramid. According to Maslow's theory, the individual can become concerned about higher level needs only when lower level needs are met; once needs for a level are satisfied, they are no longer motivators. If a situation arises that causes deficits in lower level needs, the drive to satisfy those needs reverts back into the predominant motivator. Figure 9-1 illustrates Maslow's pyramid.

The hierarchical arrangement used by Maslow, in ascending order, is as follows:

1. Physiologic Needs: These are basic survival needs and include oxygen, food, water, and rest. This is the dominant and most powerful need level; these needs must be satisfied before any others can become relevant. If not reasonably satisfied, all other categories become irrelevant or are relegated to low priority.

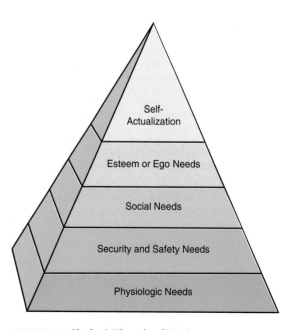

FIGURE 9-1 Maslow's Hierarchy of Needs.

2. Security and Safety Needs: This level represents human requirements to be safe from harm, for protection against physical or psychologic injury. It includes needs for the stability of a well-organized environment (shelter), economic self-sufficiency (job), protection, and freedom from fear and anxiety. These needs become paramount in times of danger; everything else loses importance. Examples of threats to safety include war, parental protection loss, new tasks, strangers, and illness.

3. Social Needs: These are love and social belonging needs (to love and belong). They include needs for affectionate relationships and a place in one's culture, group, or family; they are expressed in a desire for face-to-face contacts, intimacy, and a desire to overcome feelings of alienation or aloneness.

4. Esteem or Ego Needs: This level refers to feelings of self-worth (competence, achievement, mastery, or independence), as well as to the need to gain the respect (status, esteem) of others. Deprivation leads to feelings of inferiority, helplessness, and discouragement; fulfillment leads to feelings of capability and a willingness to contribute to society.

5. Self-Actualization or Self-Realization: This level represents the state of fully achieving one's potential, being able to control one's needs rather than being controlled by them. It is achieved as driving needs to reach the top of one's chosen areas of interests are satisfied.[2,8]

Since it was originally described, gains have been made toward the abundance of commodities and a decrease in personal concerns for basic survival and safety needs. Subsequent generations have been able to devote more and more energy to esteem and self-fulfillment needs. To correspond to these changes in needs systems, the pyramid configuration morphs. An inverted pyramid shape, as in Figure 9-2, emerges as greater emphasis is placed on fulfillment of higher order needs.[19]

To apply Maslow's hierarchy of needs, the oral health educator must assess where oral health fits into this arrangement of the individual's needs. Certain people may value oral health because it is perceived as related to the need for loving human relationships. Dental appearance may be important in making friends, getting a job, dating, and sex appeal. For others, a desire for white teeth may be tied in with a need for status within one's culture.[8]

The main point is that identifying and targeting operative need levels of the intended audience may be one avenue through which behavioral changes can be achieved through an educational plan.

The Learning Ladder

The **Learning Ladder,** also known as the Decision-Making Continuum, is based on the concept that people learn in a linear series of sequential steps. It illustrates the progression away from ignorance to the acquisition of information and

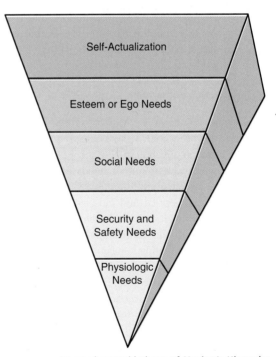

FIGURE 9-2 Inverted pyramid shape of Maslow's Hierarchy of Needs. Greater emphasis is placed on higher order needs by emerging generations.

through to adoption of a new behavior.[2,9] The learning ladder steps, in sequence from lowest to highest (shown in Fig. 9-3 and explained in Table 9-4), are:

- Unawareness
- Awareness
- Self-Interest
- Involvement
- Action
- Habit

In this theory, the learner must move through each step on the continuum to acquire and make a commitment to a new behavior. If a step is omitted, long-term behavior change (habit) will not take place. To apply the theory, the educator determines the learner's entry level on the continuum and develops a plan for movement up the steps in sequence. An example is given in Box 9-10.

Assessing location on the Decision-Making Learning Ladder enables the development of an

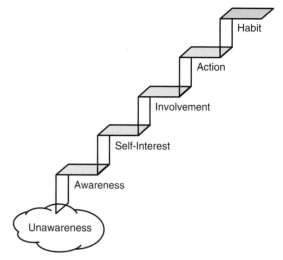

FIGURE 9-3 Learning Ladder Continuum.

educational plan that addresses the learner with messages specifically designed for their particular stage of educational readiness.

TABLE 9-4 LEARNING LADDER DECISION-MAKING CONTINUUM

STEP	EXPLANATION
Unawareness	Ignorance; no information or misinformation
	The learner lacks information or has incorrect information about the problem.
Awareness	Receives correct information but has no real sense of personal meaning or desire to act at that time
	The learner knows problem can or does exist, but does not act on the knowledge.
Self-Interest	New information becomes meaningful; intrinsic drive … realizes that the information is relevant to self
	The learner recognizes problem and shows a tentative inclination to act.
Involvement	Desire for action: realizes that values are inconsistent with actions; value is strong, but behavior is missing; develops an urge to act
	The learner's attitudes and feelings are affected and the desire for knowledge increases
Action	Moves to act to test the new concepts and practices
	The learner institutes new behaviors aimed at solving the problem.
Habit	Balances values and behaviors by making permanent changes that produce a lifelong habit
	The learner practices new behaviors over time that become part of the lifestyle.

Sources: Harris NO, Christen AG. Primary Preventive Dentistry. 4th Ed. Stanford, Appleton and Lange, 1995; DeBiase CB. Dental Hygiene in Review. Baltimore, MD: Lippincott Williams & Wilkins, 2001.[2,19]

Learning Styles

Not all people learn in the same way. Individuals have their own **learning styles** or characteristic ways of processing information, feeling, and behaving in learning situations.[20] Understanding the various ways people learn can help the oral health educator coordinate compatible teaching strategies with different learning styles. Ideally, health education programs should use educational strategies that match the individual's learning style or the predominant learning style of the target audience.

Certain people are self-learners who learn best through solitary study methods, such as reading. These learners like to be able to work on their own, reading instructions, texts, or other written information to increase their understanding. Others may learn better in group learning situations. These peer-learners benefit from group activities or pairings with another person whenever possible.

Certain people are auditory learners and learn best through listening activities. These people do well with lectures and discussions, but may also be more sensitive to extraneous noises. Others are visual learners who learn best when they receive various visual stimuli. For example, color is a powerful visual stimulus, and these learners often find it helpful to use different color highlighters or pens as they are reading and taking notes. Visual learners do well through observational experiences, such as demonstrations, but they may also be more sensitive to visual distractions. Still others learn best when they have an opportunity to actively participate in hands-on activities, or other types of movement-related experiences. Potential for learning is maximized when these kinetic learners to have the opportunity to do something for themselves.

Learning styles determine how much, and how fast, learning occurs. People typically remember 10% of what they read, 20% of what they hear, 30% of what they see, 70% of what they see and hear, and 90% of what they see, hear, and do. These percentages demonstrate that the more effective formats for retaining knowledge appear to be hands-on, interactive, multimedia formats as compared with simple reading or listening to a message.[3]

BOX 9-10 Learning Ladder Example

- Expectant parents have no knowledge of Early Childhood Caries.
- They receive information on Early Childhood Caries at prenatal class.
- During predelivery discussions and imagery, they realize the implications of using a bottle with formula or sugary liquid when putting a baby to bed.
- Before delivery, expectant parents role-play desirable bedtime behaviors.
- At their new baby's bedtime, parents clean the infant's mouth with a damp cloth and offer water at bedtime.
- Gratification derived from providing appropriate infant oral care over time produces lifelong habit.

Most groups have a diversity of learning styles within them. To reach all members of diverse target audiences, oral health educators are encouraged to use various methods. This increases the likelihood that most learners will have the opportunity to learn in at least one way that matches their learning style.

Learning Principles

Although numerous theories that describe how people learn have been developed, several principles are found repeatedly. Educational programs built around these principles are more likely to result in positive outcomes. Some highlights are:

- Without readiness, learning may be inefficient, or even harmful.
- Without motivation, there will be no learning. Identify and exploit motives for learning, such as desire for recognition, security, new experiences, and satisfaction of basic needs or wants.
- There is greater involvement in learning if learners have participated in selection and planning of the project.

- Learning is faster and is retained longer when content has meaning, organization, and structure.
- People learn by doing; learners should be actively involved.
- Repetition, review, and reinforcement enhance learning.
- Learning is most effective when many channels of information, or senses, are stimulated.
- Learner responses must be immediately reinforced.
- For best transfer of learning, behaviors should be learned in the way they will be used.
- Learners progress only as far as they need to achieve their purposes.[9]

Teaching Methods

Educators have options; there are various methods to choose from when deciding on an instructional strategy for oral health content. Lecture is an expert-centered method, distilling important points and presenting factual material to large audiences in a short time. Although lecture is one of the more common methods, it may not be the most appropriate choice. Discussion, which involves the audience and encourages pooling of ideas and experiences from the group, is a frequent method for delivery of health education. The demonstration method of instruction is especially beneficial for use with procedures and manipulative tasks. It is often used as a follow-up strategy to complement an earlier lecture or discussion. Instructional methods that may have particular application in oral health education are discussed in Chapter 10.

SUMMARY

Understanding and accepting information necessary for achieving and maintaining health is essential to the adoption of a preventive oral health behavior. This is the oral health educator's challenge. Other disciplines offer useful health behavior theories that can provide some insight into why human beings behave as they do. Needs, motivations, readiness to learn, and diverse learning styles are among the factors that influence willingness to engage in preventive health behaviors. Familiarity with the theories and models in this chapter prepares the oral health educator to better meet the challenges associated with oral health education for individuals and groups.

 Learning Activities

1. Obtain examples of available oral health education programs or lessons from your local county or state dental health department.
   a. Evaluate each to assess its health behavior theory basis.
   b. What motivational and learning strategies does it use?
   c. Identify the teaching method(s) it uses.
2. Check out copies of the texts and other books that contain the oral health education content used in your local elementary, middle, and high school curricula.
   a. Identify the learning principles that are demonstrated.
   b. Which of these materials are, in your opinion, most likely to create behavioral changes toward preventive health behavior, and why?
3. Collect several examples of free brochures and pamphlets from commercial companies that produce oral health products. Review each of these for suitability.
4. Look through a recent issue of the ADA Publications Catalog; select several pamphlets for review. Request the one free review copy of your selections that the ADA will send at no charge.
   a. Review each of these for suitability.
   b. Compare and contrast the free commercial materials from number 3, with those from the ADA.

RESOURCES

Glanz K, Rimer BK. Theory at a glance: A guide for health promotion practice. National Institutes of Health. Available at: http://cancer.gov/aboutnci/os/theory-at-a-glance/.

Review Questions

1. An individual who has successfully completed a health education experience:
   a. will not get any new cavities for the next 18-month period.
   b. can correctly describe flossing techniques.
   c. answers 5 of 7 oral health questions correctly.
   d. practices new oral health behaviors regularly.

2. Factors that play a role in modifying potential compliance with recommendations for preventive health behaviors include all of the following EXCEPT:
   a. age.
   b. gender.
   c. marketing techniques.
   d. cultural norms.
   e. health attitudes.

3. Precontemplation, contemplation, decision/determination, action, and maintenance are components of which of the following theories, or models?
   a. Health Belief Model
   b. Stages of Change Theory
   c. Diffusion of Innovations Theory
   d. Community Organization Theory

4. Which of the following does NOT affect the likelihood that a new idea, product, or practice will be accepted and adopted?
   a. It is advocated by health professionals.
   b. It is superior to a past idea, product, or practice.
   c. Tangible results can be observed.
   d. It can be tried out on a limited basis.

5. For a health education program, the oral health educator chose brochures that were clear and concise, sturdy, and easy to handle and manipulate. These educational materials demonstrate principles from:
   a. the Health Belief Model.
   b. Social Marketing Theory.
   c. Consumer Information Processing Model.
   d. the Social Learning Theory.

6. Which of the following is/are correct about a focus group?
   a. 6 to 12 people with similar backgrounds
   b. Moderator-led guided discussion
   c. Useful tool for collecting information on community needs, attitudes, and norms
   d. Inferences can be made for the larger group
   e. All of the above

7. According to Maslow, a well-organized environment, economic self-sufficiency, familiar surroundings, tasks, and activities are:
   a. physiologic needs.
   b. ego or esteem needs.
   c. social needs.
   d. security and safety needs.
   e. self-fulfillment needs.

8. Learning occurs as a series of sequential, liner steps from unawareness to commitment. This describes:
   a. Stages of Change Model.
   b. Learning Ladder.
   c. learning styles.
   d. learning principles.

9. For which of the following is observational learning an important tool?
   a. Group empowerment
   b. Social Cognitive Theory
   c. Health Belief Model
   d. Learning Ladder

10. Learning is most effective when many channels of information or senses are stimulated. Learners should be actively involved.
    a. Both statements are correct.

b. The first statement is correct, but the second statement is incorrect.

c. The first statement is incorrect, but the second statement is correct.

d. Neither statement is correct.

REFERENCES

1. American Dental Education Association. Competencies for entry into the profession of dental hygiene, exhibit 7. J Dent Ed 2003; July;67(7):1–5. Available at: http://www.adea.org/cepr. Accessed January 2004.

2. DeBiase CB. Dental Hygiene in Review. Baltimore, MD: Lippincott Williams & Wilkins, 2001.

3. Geurink KV. Community Oral Health Practice for the Dental Hygienist. Philadelphia, PA: WB Saunders, 2002.

4. Dignan MB, Carr PA. Program Planning for Health Education and Promotion. 2nd Ed. Philadelphia, PA: Lea and Febiger, 1992.

5. Darby ML, Walsh MM. Dental Hygiene Theory and Practice. Philadelphia, PA: WB Saunders, 1995.

6. Locker D. Preventive Dental Services. 2nd Ed. Canada: Health and Welfare, 1988.

7. Rosenstock IM. Historical origins of the health belief model. In: The Health Belief Model and Personal Health Behavior. Becker MH, ed. Thorofare, NJ: Charles B. Slack, 1974.

8. Cormier PP, Levy JI. Community Oral Health. New York: Appleton-Century-Crofts Prentice-Hall, 1981.

9. Darby ML. Mosby's Comprehensive Review of Dental Hygiene. 5th Ed. St. Louis, MO: Mosby Elsevier Science, 2002.

10. Glanz K, Lewis FM, Rimer BK. Theory at a glance: A guide for health promotion practice. Publication No. 95-3896. Bethesda, MD: National Institutes of Health, 1997.

11. Prochaska JA, Norcross JC, DiClemente CC. Changing for good: A revolutionary six-stage program for overcoming bad habits and moving your life positively forward. New York: Avon Books, 1994.

12. Bettman JR. An Information Processing Theory of Consumer Choice. Reading, MA: Addison-Wesley, 1979.

13. Bandura A. Social Foundations of Thought and Action. Englewood Cliffs, NJ: Prenctice-Hall, 1986.

14. Bracht N. Health Promotion at the Community Level. Newbury Park, CA: Sage Publications, 1990.

15. Rogers EM. Diffusion of Innovations. 3rd Ed. New York: The Free Press, 1983.

16. Glanz K, Lewis FM, Rimer BK. Health Behavior and Health Education: Theory, Research, and Practice. San Francisco, CA: Jossey-Bass, 1990.

17. Kotler P, Andreasen A. Strategic Marketing for Nonprofit Organizations. 4th Ed. Englewood Cliffs, NJ: Prentice-Hall, 1991.

18. Green LW, Kreuter MW. Health Promotion Planning: An Educational and Environmental Approach. 2nd Ed. Mountain View: Mayfield, 1991. Mountain View, CA: Mayfield Publ.

19. Harris NO, Christen AG. Primary Preventive Dentistry. 4th Ed. Stamford,CT: Appleton and Lange, 1995.

20. Smith RM. Learning How to Learn: Applied Theory for Adults. Englewood Cliffs, NJ: Cambridge, 1982.

Developing Educational Materials

10

Objectives

After studying this chapter and completing the study questions and activities, the learner should be able to:

- Design health educational materials for a target audience.
- Evaluate the utility of existing health educational material and methods.
- Develop a lesson plan.
- Discuss options for teaching methods and evaluate each for learning principles.
- Create culturally sensitive educational materials.

KEY TERMS

Body	Instructional set	Target audience
Closure	Layout	Type font
Educational goal	Lesson plan	Type size
Instructional objectives	Reading level	Visuals
Instructional planning	Subject content	

The American Dental Education Association competencies addressed in this chapter include[1]:

C.8: Communicate effectively with individuals and groups from diverse populations, both verbally and in writing.

HP.1: Promote the values of oral and general health and wellness to the public and organizations within and outside the profession.

HP.4: Identify individual and population risk factors and develop strategies that promote health and quality of life.

HP.5: Evaluate factors that can be used to promote patient adherence to disease prevention and health maintenance strategies.

CM.3: Provide community oral health services in various settings.

Introduction

Techniques for creating experiences that lead to learning have been used and refined by generations of educators. An understanding of the processes involved can help dental hygienists make effective contributions to the planning and development of successful oral health education interventions. This chapter introduces the instructional process. Educational materials for oral health education are discussed and described. Applying the information in this chapter can assist in the development of new educational materials, as well as the critique of existing materials.

INSTRUCTIONAL PLANNING

A meaningful learning experience is the carefully crafted result of a deliberate process known as **instructional planning.** In addition to subject matter expertise, instructional planning requires an understanding of learning principles and teaching techniques, as well as information about the background and learning levels of the intended audience. The purpose of oral health education is to produce an appropriately tailored oral health educational plan for specific learners.

Instructional planning is a systematic series of equally important events in the design and development of an educational plan. It is a purposeful, learner-centered activity that includes:

- Analysis of the **target audience** and their unique learning needs
- Identification of learning objectives that define the quality and extent of the learning to be achieved
- Identification of specific subject content to meet those needs
- Selection of methods to deliver that content
- Selection of materials and learning activities to support the learning experience.

Target Audience

Chapter 6, Planning for Community Programs, discussed the significance and function of the community profile in the planning and development of successful community health programs. This information, which is collected as part of community assessment, has instructional planning applications, as well. Population demographics are core considerations when planning learning experiences. Age, gender, ethnicity, cultural background, socioeconomic status, and educational levels all exert an influence on attitudes, values, and readiness to learn. It is necessary to adapt learning experiences to accommodate these characteristics to make them meaningful and motivating for those who receive them. Ignoring the significance of cultural influences on values, beliefs, and attitudes can result in a failed experience. Some general guidelines for communicating effectively across cultures are discussed at the end of this chapter.

Learning Needs

The types and kinds of learning to be effected should be identified early in the planning process. Instructional methods and materials are chosen by how well they support the learning experience. Do the learners need to know something that they did not know before (i.e., facts, or *cognitive* information)? Lecture might be an appropriate method for delivering a lesson that puts heavy emphasis on facts and the delivery of factual content.

Do the learners need to be able to do something that they could not do before (i.e., skills, or *psychomotor* abilities)? A demonstration showing the skills being performed correctly by someone who already possesses the skills may be the most appropriate method in this situation.

Do the learners need to be able to think differently about something than they could before (i.e., develop or modify attitudes, or *affective* conditions)? Discussion, which has been shown to be an effective strategy for dealing with attitudes, might be the method chosen. Instructional methods are covered in more detail later in the chapter

THE EDUCATIONAL PLAN

An educational plan, known to educators as a **lesson plan,** is a well-organized, written guide for presenting a specific block of instruction. In addition to an outline of the content to be presented, it specifies the procedures to follow when presenting. Lesson plans ensure that all information and materials required to meet specific learning goals are presented in the most effective order and supported effectively by carefully chosen instructional materials.

Stability and standardization are two benefits from using lesson plans. When an educator follows the same lesson plan each time they deliver the same presentation, it is reasonable to expect consistency of results across time. Additionally, instructional interventions can be standardized when different individuals using the same lesson plan are able to present the same topic and accomplish the same learning goals. To illustrate the need for this kind of standardization, consider a sealant program in which different teams of oral health educators present background lessons to different groups of first- and second-grade children before their sealants are applied. Because all program participants need the same information and values regarding sealants, the educators must achieve the same learning objectives. A standard lesson plan contributes to this result.

Components

Lesson plans begin with a broad general statement that describes the overall purpose of the block of instruction. This **educational goal** is a nonspecific statement that serves as the foundation on which to develop all subsequent plans.[2] For example, if the target audience is a group of expectant parents at a prenatal class, the goal statement might be: "To increase prospective parents' awareness of the need for oral hygiene care and good oral health for their children."

Instructional objectives, in contrast, are specific statements that describe what the learner is expected to be able to do, know, or think differently about when the lesson's content has been provided and successfully completed. These objectives clearly define the goals of the learning experience by describing a pattern of behavior (or performance) that the learner should be able to demonstrate when the learning experience has been completed successfully.

Meaningful instructional objectives that are written in behavioral terms have several components. They are constructed according to the performance–conditions–criteria format.[2]

1. Identify the behavior (that will be accepted as evidence of learning) by name; use action verbs to describe what the learner will do (*performance*). Action verbs that are useful in describing behaviors are shown in Box 10-1.
2. Include specific conditions under which the behavior will occur (*condition*); describe any important or relevant circumstances that accompany the action.

BOX 10-1 Action Verbs for Behavioral Objectives

KNOWLEDGE (COGNITIVE)	SKILLS (PSYCHOMOTOR)	ATTITUDES (AFFECTIVE)
analyze	act	accept
choose	assemble	adopt
compare	brush	advocate
complete	carry	ask
copy	catch	evaluate
define	climb	promote
describe	demonstrate	question
find	draw	recommend
identify	fit	share
label	floss	volunteer
list	form	
match	manipulate	
name	operate	
place	paint	
plan	perform	
point	prepare	
predict	press	
recall	roll	
select	show	
sort	wipe	
state	wrap	

3. Specify a measurable standard that must be met to be considered acceptable (*criteria*); describe how well the behavior must be performed to provide evidence that learning has occurred.

The following examples contain each of the performance–condition–criteria components. They describe exactly what the learner is expected to be able to do and how well the learner is expected to be able to do it after successfully completing the educational experience. For example: (1) Using a mirror, adequate lighting, and 2×2 gauze, the learner should be able to perform an oral self-exam that exposes all specified oral structures for observation; and (2) Using a food diary form, the learner should be able to develop a personal 1-week food intake plan that is 90% consistent with healthful dietary concepts. Box 10-2 identifies the performance–condition–criteria components of each example.

Objectives for health education interventions often follow a more general approach, specifying the behavior with the expectation that required conditions are met and satisfactory competency is achieved. For example: "The learner will demonstrate disease control in his own mouth through proper daily brushing and flossing for plaque control" may be more appropriate for a health education plan than "Given a quality toothbrush and floss, the learner will demonstrate disease control in his own mouth through daily brushing and flossing to achieve a score of 100% plaque-free surfaces."

Well-stated instructional objectives guide the selection of lesson content and the relevant presentation strategies. Guesswork is eliminated and random coverage of irrelevant material is minimized. Instructional objectives also serve as guides for evaluation of learning and the evaluative process. The degree to which learners do or do

BOX 10-2 Examples of Instructional Objectives and Their Components

INSTRUCTIONAL OBJECTIVE	P–C–C COMPONENTS	
Using a mirror, adequate lighting, and 2x2 gauze, the learner should be able to perform an oral self-care exam that exposes all specified oral structures for observation.	Performance	• perform an oral self-exam
	Conditions	• using a mirror, adequate lighting, and 2x2 gauze
	Criteria	• all specified oral structures observed
Using a food diary form, the learner should be able to develop a personal 1-week food intake plan that is 90% consistent with healthful dietary concepts.	Performance	• develop a personal food intake plan
		• using a food diary form
	Conditions	• 90% consistent
	Criteria	

not achieve expected learning outcomes can serve as a basis for drawing inferences about the effectiveness of the educational intervention.[3]

Subject content is the main focus of the lesson plan. This is the portion of the lesson plan that addresses the new facts, attitudes, or skills that the learner needs to know. It consists of information that has been collected about the topic, researched, and selected for presentation. When deficiencies in previously learned health information or practices are identified during the needs assessment segment of community program planning, adjustments and corrections are incorporated in the subject content portion of the educational interventions lesson plan.

Subject content information should be organized effectively to fit the time and facilities available. Chronologic order is a simple organization and well suited to explanation of processes, procedures, or historic information. Logical order arranges information according to some plan, such as from cause to effect, general statements to particulars, or least important to most important.

PRESENTATION STRATEGIES[2-5]

Teaching strategies are methods for relating content to the learners. They are typically identified during content development and selected on the characteristics of the learners, the learning objectives, and the type of content being delivered. A

number of methods are available. Some types of content are better served by specific methods of presentation.

Lecture is a classroom-style presentation that presents factual material in a direct, logical manner. It is a one-way communication that is developed almost entirely by the lecturer. The lecture audience passively sits and takes notes. Discussion is problem-solving or seminar-style instruction, during which group members pool ideas to derive information and reach conclusions. It is an active process that allows everyone to participate, but can be dominated by a few people or sidetracked without a competent group facilitator.

Demonstrations involve the presentation of a technique, procedure, or sequence of steps in a process by a person who already possesses the skills being shown. Table 10-1 describes and compares some common instructional methods.

LEARNING ACTIVITIES AND MATERIALS

Instructional materials and learning activities support the educational plan. They enliven a presentation and help learners form concepts and internalize information. Only activities and materials that make a contribution toward the desired learning should be used. They can be used to motivate and increase interest, to reinforce content, to supplement verbal information, or to provide opportunities for learner reinforcements and

TABLE 10-1 TEACHING METHODS

Lecture	**Formal informative talk, prepared and organized in advance**
	• Leader-centered • Easy to use; economical • Good for creating awareness of new ideas • Can present many facts in short time • Most effective in large groups when time is limited • Learners are not actively involved; communication is one-way • Poor presentation skills detract from learning • Best when complemented with other methods
Discussion	**Leader and learners define a problem and interact to find its solution**
	• Group activity, learner-centered • Often used in health education • Leader uses questions to stimulate participation and interaction • Two-way communication between participants and leader • Useful for problem-solving; fosters reasoning and critical thinking • Strong personalities can dominate the discussion • Requires competent facilitator to keep interactions on topic
Problem-Based Learning aka: **Inquiry**	**Learners research narratives of real problems to learn new information and solve problems**
	• Learner-centered; Leader gives guidelines on the process and serves as facilitator • Uses all levels of learning (recall through analysis and synthesis) • Produces cognitive and affective outcomes • Fosters motivation • Can be superficial and unorganized if not complemented with other methods and capable facilitator • Limited gains in immediate new knowledge • Requires time and committed involvement
Collaborative (or Cooperative) Learning aka: **Interactive Learning**	**People work in small groups to develop learning projects**
	• Learner-centered; leader facilitates team development and gives feedback • Small group peer interaction enhances learning and increased retention • Possible conflicts among team members can decrease efficiency or produce poor project outcomes
Demonstration	**Shows steps in a procedure to allow learner to see actions to be performed**
	• Illustrates and reinforces theory content • Can be used to complement lecture or discussion • Leader needs the skills to perform the task to be demonstrated • If more than one demonstrator, should be calibrated for consistency • Can be difficult for larger groups to see • Requires careful preparation, appropriate equipment and facilities
Simulation	**Opportunities for learners to practice actions or behaviors in safety of a classroom setting**
	• Fosters skill development without fear of irreversible outcomes • Leader provides constructive feedback • Can be used with a wide range of abilities • Experience and outcome can have unsatisfactory outcome if learner has high level of anxiety

(continued)

TABLE 10-1 TEACHING METHODS *(continued)*

Dramatizations, Role-Playing, and Storytelling	**Dramatizations:** Learner plays a part in scripted play, skit, or puppet show • Effective for elementary and middle school aged children • Requires preparation and focus on learning concepts **Role-Playing:** Learner receives written information on, assumes, and acts out a role in front of learning group • Leader guides follow-up discussion on the topic being role-played • Effective for middle school age through adult • Useful in problem analysis and solution development • Poor learning experience if learner is not an effective role-player **Storytelling:** Leader tells or reads a story that illustrates the learning concepts • Effective for preschool to early elementary school age • Helpful in increasing awareness of ideas, attitudes, and behaviors

repetitions. Using multiple activities and learning assessments facilitates more effective evaluations of learning. "Alerts" that cue the initiation of an activity or introduction of a particular material at the appropriate time should be written into the content outline.

Activities

Learning activities are experiences that lead to learning. Problem solving, experimenting, discussing, observing, demonstrating, collecting, interviewing, writing, and composing are some examples. Games and puzzles add fun to educational experiences and are useful ways to review lesson content. Educators often develop their own topic-specific games. The Grocery Bag Game, described in Box 10-3 is an example. Software programs for developing subject-related crossword puzzles are widely available and easy to use.

Materials

No longer called "aids," media materials for learning experiences are basic essentials for effective instruction. Examples of these **visuals** include chalkboards, bulletin boards, flannel boards, posters, charts, audio and video recordings, models, and samples of authentic real-world objects.

Professionally prepared materials are often free or available at low cost from many sources, such as the American Dental Association, the National Dairy Council, and commercial manufacturers. Many oral health product companies offer educational materials. Brochures, pamphlets, activity books, and fact sheets are some common examples. Any item used should have an obvious relationship to the topic being studied. General guidelines for choosing and using free and inexpensive materials are included in Box 10-4.

All visuals should meet some basic requirements. They should be colorful; however, color should be used wisely. Yellow, for example, is typically a poor choice for lettering. Visuals should be large enough to be seen easily from a distance. **Type font** should be easy to read and **type size** should be large enough to be seen easily. Box 10-5 shows examples of several fonts and type sizes. Layout designs that draw the viewer's eye from one point to the next assist the visual in quickly making its learning point. These basics are discussed in detail in the following section as they relate to some common types of visuals.

"NO-TECH" MEDIA MATERIALS

The Chalkboard/Whiteboard.[6,7] Chalkboards and whiteboards are inexpensive teaching tools, one of which is usually available in most classroom

BOX 10-3 Examples of Simple Games

Grocery Bag Game	Collect pictures or empty cartons, packages and cans of various foods. Choose common inclusions in culturally acceptable diets of the target audience. Put one half in one grocery bag and one half in another. Label pieces of felt or construction paper with the names of a food group category and place on the floor in a clear area. Place the grocery bags at one end of the area at some distance from each other. Divide the audience into two groups, or teams. Assign a bag to each team. Have each team send one group member at a time to place one of the foods from their bag onto the correct food group category. The first team to finish is the winner. Follow with a discussion of the foods and the category to which the teams have assigned them.
Riddles:	I'm thinking of something that . . .
I'm Thinking Of . . .	• we should do after we eat and before we go to bed. (*brush*)
	• is a long string and is used to clean between teeth. (*floss*)
	• sticks to our teeth, is invisible, and causes decay. (*plaque*)
	• bacteria and sugar make this to dissolve tooth enamel. (*acid*)
	• is in toothpaste and drinking water to make teeth strong. (*fluoride*)

settings. They are useful for spontaneously producing graphic information and as a means for giving instructions or for following special procedures. Certain skills are necessary to use these boards to maximum advantage, however. Common sense suggestions for effective chalkboard and whiteboard use are:

1. Write clearly:
   - Make chalk or marker lines bold enough to be seen in the back of the room.
   - Print everything for children in third grade or below.
   - Block letters are easier to read from the back of the room.
   - Make letters large enough to be read from the back of the room, between 2 and 4 inches high.
   - If using colored chalk or markers, choose colors vivid enough to stand out against the background of the board.
   - Use soft chalks, which are most easily erased.
   - Use plain rubbing alcohol for marker inks that are difficult to remove.
2. Stand to one side as you write. Do not turn your back toward the audience.
3. To help those with vision problems, repeat aloud what you have written.
4. Talk to the audience; do not talk into the board.
   - A good pattern to use is: state the topic first when facing the audience; turn and write on the board; then, turn back to the audience and discuss the topic.
5. Make sure nothing obstructs anyone's full view of the board.
6. Organize information rather than scatter it all over the board.
   - Avoid writing near the bottom of the board.
7. Erase the board before you leave.

A well-known trick that is useful for drawing illustrations on a large board is to use a template. This is particularly useful for frequently redrawn illustrations (e.g., a tooth). First, draw the object

BOX 10-4 Choosing and Using Free and Inexpensive Materials

Choose materials that:

- do not present false claims or mislead with half-truths or incomplete information.
- do not contain exaggerated claims for a product or situation.
- are accurate and consistent with the latest scientific information.
- are appropriate to the learning levels of the intended population in vocabulary, difficulty of concepts, and sentence structure.
- present both sides of controversial issues.
- include illustrations pertinent to the reading content, not merely "attention-getters" with little or no relationship to the subject.

Use materials that:

- reinforce information already given verbally.
- make a constructive contribution to the educational program of the patient, school, or group.
- match the educational and reading levels of the target audience.
- are adequately and effectively colorful.
- have durable physical and mechanical features.

BOX 10-5 Type Font and Type Size

Serif Fonts	Times New Roman
	Courier
	Century Schoolbook
Sans Serif Fonts	Arial
	Tahoma
	Century Gothic
Elaborate Fonts	*Brush Script*

Lu

onto heavy cardboard. Cut the object out and use it against the board as a pattern for quick and accurate tracing. If available, lightweight plywood or masonite materials and power cutting tools can be used to make more permanent patterns.

Bulletin Boards.[3,6] Oral health educators often prepare bulletin board displays to deliver a dental message. Bulletin boards are devices used to graphically display materials relevant to the attainment of instructional objectives. They are used to motivate and arouse interest, to establish conducive learning environments, and to provide focal points for more intensive research and study. A good display is the result of advance thought and careful planning. Four points to be considered are caption, color, illustrations or illustrative materials, and layout.

Caption.[6] A good caption will gain attention and make the intended audience want to see and learn more. The caption might ask a question (What does fluoride do?) or it might make a positive statement (Spit tobacco stinks!). Direct the words to the viewer. To be readable from any area of the room, captions should be in print style, using 2-inch block letters. Figure 10-1 shows a quick and simple way to make a guide for placing letters in a straight line by taping or pinning a taut string or dental floss to the borders of the board where the caption is to be placed.

Lettering can be time consuming—stencils, precut letters, and pressure-sensitive letters from art or office supply stores can be used. Precut letters can be spray painted in advance with enamel paint of any color. Words can be printed from a computer program onto colored paper and pinned on the board. Letters made with the flat side of a crayon are interesting. Letters can be drawn with a heavy glue, then yarn, string, or twine can be quickly applied to the wet glue. Yarn can be dipped in heavy starch and formed into words or letters; pin them to the board when dried.

Color.[8,9] Color is one of the first things viewers notice about a bulletin board. It can be used to attract attention, create moods, and emphasize impor-

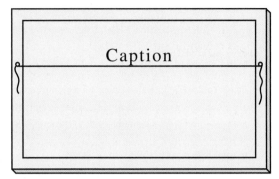

FIGURE 10-1 String Guide for Lettering in Straight Lines. A taut string taped or pinned across the board makes a quick guide for positioning letters in a straight line.

tant areas. A good general rule for color use is to keep it simple by minimizing the number of colors on any one display. Limit the color scheme to two or three major colors to avoid an overuse of color. Contrasting colors, such as dark on light and vice versa, are effective for emphasizing important areas.

There are two families of colors: hot and cool. Cool colors are blues, greens, and purples. These are considered calming colors and are thought to evoke a relaxed, yet sufficiently serious mood. They have been associated with decreased circulation and body temperatures. Cool colors are good for background and foreground elements, such as shapes and designs. Hot colors are reds, oranges, and yellows. These are considered stimulating, energizing, and exciting colors. They have been associated with increased circulation and body temperatures. Hot colors may be useful for calling attention to or marking the most important elements of the design. A background of hot colors might be too intense for the audience.

Color symbolism and emotional connotations vary with culture. For example, in American culture, red means danger, green means go, yellow alerts to caution, and red, white, and blue suggest national patriotism. Seasons and holidays suggest particular color schemes. Autumn suggests a combination of browns, yellows, greens, and reds.

Spring suggests bright greens and pastel colors. Halloween uses orange and black, and Valentine's Day uses red and white.

Illustrations or Illustrative Materials.[6] The illustrations that communicate the idea(s) of the bulletin board may be pictures, photographs, drawings, cartoons, or actual objects. The attention a display demands might be attributable to the contrast and various shapes and materials used or to their dramatic or unusual arrangement.

Many materials can be used to create interest in what the board has to say. Styrofoam, burlap, and ribbons are just a few examples. Box 10-6 gives a minimum listing of interesting materials. Everything must be fixed securely to the surface of the background covering. Straight pins, staples, glue, double-sided adhesive tape, and double-sided foam mounting tape can be used to attach materials to the bulletin board.

Layout.[6] **Layout** refers to the basic compositional form of a display. Balance is a major compositional aspect of layout; arranging the materials to avoid them from being top-heavy or lopsided. The three basic balance designs, radial balance, symmetrical (or formal) balance, and asymmetrical (or informal) balance, are illustrated in Box 10-7.

Radial balance has lines or shapes growing from a central point or spot. In symmetrically (formal) balanced designs, elements are more or less evenly distributed from the center. Both sides of an imaginary line through the center of the design are weighted the same. Asymmetrically (informal) balanced designs have elements that appear to balance even though each side of the arrangement is different. Each side of an imaginary line is different, but equal.

Other fundamental characteristics in a good layout are emphasis, harmony, and contrast.

- Emphasis: The central idea is brought out by effective use of lettering techniques, and dominant colors, for example.
- Harmony: All visual elements (eg, lettering, color, materials) appear to "go together" and create a feeling of unity.
- Contrast: Techniques that draw attention to the main parts of the display are used (eg, contrasting areas of light and dark, using dark papers for mounting light pictures).

Like any display, bulletin boards can become distracting if topics and materials are not changed periodically or confusing if materials are too

BOX 10-6   Materials for Bulletin Board Displays

VARIOUS MATERIALS CAN BE USED TO CREATE INTEREST IN THE BULLETIN BOARD'S MESSAGE

Toothbrushes	Floss	Brochures
Newsprint	Enlarged photographs	Magazine pictures
Posters	Burlap	Raffia
Wallpaper	Mirrors	Sandpaper
Ribbons	Thread	Pipe cleaners
Wire screening	Fabric patches	Corrugated cardboard
Scrapbooking materials	Quilt batting	Artificial flowers
Styrofoam cutouts	Aluminum foil	Party decorations
Yarn	Cardboard arrows	Rotating turntables
Pennants	Self-check sheets	Wooden tongue blades

BOX 10-7 Basic Balance Designs

A. Radial Balance

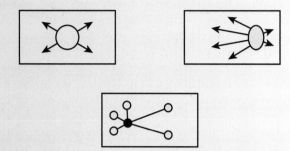

B. Symmetrical Balance

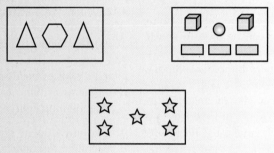

C. Asymmetrical Balance

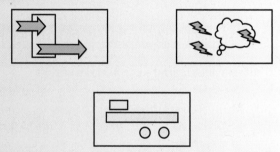

A. Radial Balance: design units grow from a central point. **B.** Symmetrical Balance: both sides of an imaginary line are the same. **C.** Asymmetrical Balance: each side of an imaginary line is different, but equal.

Adapted from: Dearth F. Construction and Utilization of Visual Aids in Dental Health Education. Thoroughfare: Charles B. Slack, 1974.

cluttered. Box 10-8 highlights four main considerations for a graphic display.

Storyboards.[3,6] Flannel and felt boards, hook and loop boards, and magnetic boards are inexpensive, easy-to-use teaching tools that can be used to help communicate abstract ideas and guide organized thinking about oral health through storytelling. They are particularly applicable for putting concepts, principles, generalizations, and facts into visual form. A good example of an oral health concept for the storyboard is the classic equation:

$$plaque + sugar = acid$$

$$acid + tooth = decay$$

Effective and successful use depends on the storyteller knowing the story well enough that manipulation of characters and pieces is free and easy. Children enjoy placing the items on the board and retelling the story, so durability is important.

Making a Flannel or Felt Board.

1. Choose lightweight plywood board or reasonably heavy foam core board.
2. Cut it to size. It should be large enough for children in the back of the room to see the visuals placed on it, but not so large that it is unwieldy.
3. Choose a good grade flannel or felt material to use as board covering. Popular colors are green and beige. Avoid red because it is difficult to look at for long periods.
4. Cut the covering material to size and fold it over the edge of the board. Tack, or staple it on the back every six inches.
5. For a smoother look, tape around the edges of the flannel and over the loose edges with wide tape.

Making Display Materials.
Many materials cling to a flannel surface with no special preparation. Colored felt is one example and can be easily cut into many shapes, designs, and symbols. Patterns for characters, shapes, or designs can be found in children's coloring books. Two or more pieces of material may be adhered together with white glue to increase stiffness and durability. Smooth cardboard, small three-dimensional objects, and other flat surfaces can be backed with a rough textured material to give them holding capabilities. Coarse sandpaper or Velcro pieces are easy options. Adhere magazine pictures, or other pictures that require some lightweight backing, directly to the sandpaper or Velcro with a light application of rubber cement.

Hook and Loop Board.
A hook and loop board is similar to the felt/flannel board, but offers some advantages. Various odd-shaped and heavier objects (up to several pounds) can be put onto the board. Attachment is firm, yet objects can be instantly removed and reattached. A sturdy board is prepared according to Steps 1 and 2 of the directions for a flannel board. Then, the board is covered with loop fabric yardage from the fabric

---

BOX 10-8 Considerations for a Graphic Display

Caption	Color	Illustrations	Layout
• Gains attention for and stimulates interest in the display	• Emphasizes important areas, creates moods, and focuses attention	• Conveys the content and communicates the ideas of the display	• Provides compositional form for the display
• Use print style with block lettering	• Limit to 2 or 3 major colors	• Use pictures, cartoons, photographs, drawings, or real objects	• Direct the eye with a balanced design format

section of a department or variety store. (The loop portion of the Velcro system is the softer, fuzzy-sided portion. The hook portion is the rougher, stiffer side and is surfaced with minute nylon hooks.) Back display materials with small patches or strips of hook material.

Magnetic Board. This board, like the others, allows items to be temporarily displayed and easily manipulated while speaking. Magnetic chalk-boards, with surfaces that have been prepared with a magnetic coating or paint, are available in many classrooms. Portable magnetic boards can be easily made. Purchase a piece of flat metal from a home supply store and have it cut to size. Carefully wash the surface with white vinegar, rinse thoroughly and dry carefully. Cover sharp edges with duct tape. Paint the surface with flat black paint or use several coats of chalkboard paint, sanding in between coats. Attach magnets to the backs of the display items. Small magnets or thin strips of adhesive-backed magnet material, available at office supply stores, can be used.

Samples, Specimens, and Real Objects.[4] Opportunities to interact with authentic objects, samples, or specimens from the real world make a learning experience personal and give meaning to subject content. Interactions with these three-dimensional objects can be tactile and auditory, as well as visual. Some real-world materials are readily available and inexpensive, while others are difficult or impossible to acquire. Disadvantages for the use of real objects include handling and distribution difficulties and storage space requirements.

Radiographic film packets and radiographs, or digital printouts, dental mirrors or other nonsharp instruments, soft disposable saliva ejectors, individual units of polishing paste, and disposable cotton and paper products used in the clinical setting are examples of real objects that might find applications in an oral health presentation.

"LOW-TECH" MEDIA MATERIALS

Posters and Charts. Even in a high-tech world of computer-generated presentations, posters and charts are effective and easy to use **visuals.**

They have several advantages:

- They do not require electricity or specialized, elaborate equipment.
- They are easy to use and inexpensive to make and update.
- They are portable and transportable.
- They can remain in view of the audience while important points are being discussed.
- They provide good opportunities for interaction with the audience.

One major disadvantage is that posters and charts are not suitable for use with large groups. Because of their relatively small size, it is difficult for groups of more than 35 persons to see them well enough during a presentation.

Posters are pictorial designs that convey a message visually within a few seconds and quickly make a point. They can be effective with all age-groups. Their purpose is to draw attention to an idea or topic, which makes them useful in creating or increasing levels of awareness. To be effective, a poster should focus on only one main idea.

Many oral health product companies offer free, commercially-prepared posters that may be suitable for selected topics. Student-made posters can be a useful activity for building learner interest and developing positive attitudes and values for oral health. When incorporated into a carefully designed lesson, they can be educational for those who make them and those who view them. Health professionals are cautioned, however, about using these projects as competition in "poster contests." Producing an artful poster to win a prize does not necessarily translate into an ability, or commitment, to practice oral health behaviors.[10]

Charts are used to highlight important points that are covered in a presentation. They are particularly useful for complementing the verbal commentary in a small group presentation. Charts can be used to outline information or to present a mixture of pictures, drawings, diagrams, or graphs.

Flip charts can be prepared in advance or developed spontaneously during a presentation. A large, commercial flip chart pad, an easel or flip chart stand, and markers are the required materials for typical flip charts. Pages are turned or removed as sequential points are developed and discussed. Some suggestions to simplify preparation of a flip chart in advance are offered here[11]:

- Lightly write your text in pencil first before using markers. This allows adjustments to be made in spacing and in any figures you will be drawing. Pads with grid lines make it easier to keep lines of text straight.
- Use print lettering that is large enough for easy legibility. One-inch letters can usually be seen from a distance of 32 feet; 2-inch letters from a distance of 64 feet.
- Do NOT use all capital letters. Upper case and lower case lettering is easier to read.
- Follow the "6 × 6 rule." Use no more than six words on each line and no more than six lines on a sheet.
- Avoid writing with too many colors; one dark color and one accent color works best. Avoid yellow, pink, or orange for lettering. These are extremely difficult for the audience to see.
- Write any notes you may want lightly in pencil where needed. The audience won't be able to see them, and they can help you remember key points. You may also want to make a note at the bottom of the page to help you lead into or introduce the next sheet.

A simple, tabletop, mini-flip chart for use with individuals or small groups can be made using a notebook and clear document protectors. Figure 10-2 shows tabletop flip charts.

A strip chart, shown in Figure 10-3, is another chart design that presents information in sequence. It is a single chart with various sequential parts covered, or masked, by strips of paper. The paper strips are attached to the chart with a lightly adhesive tape. Important points are exposed gradually, one at a time. Each strip is removed at the appropriate time when the point is being discussed. The sequenced parts remain in view, showing the *building* relationship of each part to

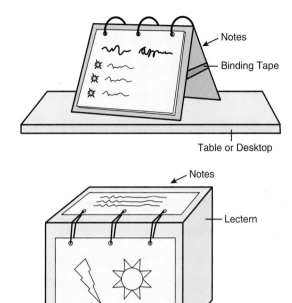

FIGURE 10-2 Table Top Mini-Flip Chart. A simple, portable, tabletop flip chart can be made from a 3-ring notebook and clear document protectors. Visuals are positioned toward the side facing the audience, while speaking notes are directed toward the speaker.

the next. Strip charts are especially effective with primary grade learners.

Overhead Transparencies.[6,12] In spite of predictions otherwise, overhead transparencies remain a popular and commonly used teaching visual. Most classrooms and most facilities have an overhead projector, which is a simple box containing a light source, a lens, and a glass presentation stage. When the light source is turned on, a transparency is placed on the glass stage and the image from the transparency is projected onto the screen. Overhead projectors require minimal operational skills and are relatively damage-proof.

Materials for projection are easy to prepare and update. Simple drawings or notes can be prepared spontaneously during a lesson by marking directly onto clear acetate sheets with a grease pencil or special water-based marking pen for transparency sheets. More permanent transparencies can be

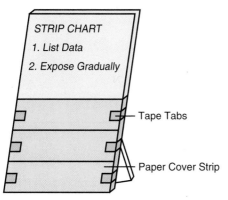

FIGURE 10-3 Strip Chart. A strip chart is used to progressively reveal masked points during a presentation.

prepared in advance. One quick method is to print directly from a computer program onto a transparency sheet adapted for printers. Another method uses a regular copier machine to make a copy of a prepared drawing or picture onto a transparency sheet adapted for copiers. Transparency sheets and marking pens are available at office supply stores.

Because they project large images in a lighted room, overheads offer several advantages to instructional situations. The images are big enough to be a practical choice for use with large groups. The projector is positioned in front of the group, which allows eye contact between the group leader and learners. Being able to observe reactions encourages interaction with the audience and enables adjustments in the presentation when needed. The room remains fully lighted, which reduces drowsiness and inattention. Content is easy to update or change because new transparencies can be produced quickly and easily.

Some suggestions for effective use of overhead transparencies follow:

- Stand to one side of the projector, facing the audience. If the screen is not raised or set at a diagonal, standing between the projector and screen will cast a shadow of your body onto the screen.

- If writing by hand onto the transparency, make your letters at least $\frac{1}{2}''$ high.
- Control the rate of presenting information by masking (covering) part of the transparency and exposing subsequent information when you are ready to discuss a point. Use an opaque piece of paper or cardboard; by placing the cover sheet on the glass stage first with the transparency over it, you will still be able to see all of the transparency yourself.
- Face the audience, not the screen. Too often, speakers face, and end up talking to, the screen.
- Whenever information needs to be pointed out, point to the transparency with a pen to cast a pointing shadow on the screen.
- Do not crowd too much information onto one transparency. To illustrate complex ideas, use overlays of additional transparencies to superimpose elements progressively onto a base transparency (e.g., progression of decay).
- Enlarge graphs, charts, or tables from books before reproducing them onto a transparency sheet.
- Leave the material on the projector long enough for the audience to see and absorb.
- Store overhead transparencies in a sturdy box so they will stay clean and protected for future use.

"HIGH-TECH" MEDIA MATERIALS

Slides and Videos. Professionally prepared videos or slides are available from commercial sources. Commercial production lends a professional appearance to a presentation. The American Dental Association (ADA), the American Dental Hygienists' Association (ADHA), certain professional product companies, and companies that manufacture dental devices and materials are some examples of resources.

Both slides and videos are suitable for use with large groups. Although both require special equipment for projection, the equipment is often a common feature in many classrooms and facilities, and is easy to operate. Slides can be arranged into any desired sequence and can be projected onto the screen for any length of time. Slides have two major disadvantages: (1) they require a darkened environment for optimum viewing, and (2) they cannot effectively portray motion. Slides can be expensive to purchase and cannot be updated unless replaced.[3]

Videos are particularly useful for presenting concepts that involve motion. They can be viewed by individuals or small groups, as determined by screen size. Due to production costs, videos are usually more expensive than other types of visuals. Not conducive to discussion and audience interaction, they can be effective if the audience is "set up" to receive them. Prior to showing, give your audience a task to do as they watch. Otherwise, they may decide to just doze instead. Say something like, "As you look at how the brush is moved, see how it compares with your current brushing method." Immediately after the video is finished, follow up on your question by asking something like, "So, how does your brushing method compare with the one you saw in the video?"[13]

Computer-Generated Electronic Presentations.[4,13,14] Electronic presentations are rapidly becoming the medium of choice in the business world and increasingly popular in educational situations, as well. This type of media has several advantages:

- They lend a professional appearance to a presentation.
- They are suitable for use with large and small groups.
- They are easy to integrate into audience discussions.
- They offer opportunities to bring a message to life with color, sound, pictures, and various effects.
- They are easy to change and update.
- The technology is up-to-date.

Significant skill with the particular software program is required to generate/create the electronic presentation. Time to learn how to use the software application is necessary if not already a part of your skill set. Each electronic presentation requires considerable development time to compose content and create graphics, as well. The computer equipment that runs the electronic presentation and the special equipment needed to project it for viewing are expensive and not commonly available in classrooms or other facilities. Arrangements to ensure its availability must be made in advance.

Basic guidelines for creating electronic presentations include the following points:

- Use clear, standard type fonts.
  - Sans serif fonts do not have "side arms" and "curlicues." Arial or Helvetica are examples of standard sans serif fonts.
  - Times New Roman and Courier are examples of standard serif fonts. Box 10-5 shows examples of standard serif and sans serif fonts.
  - Use a type size that is large enough to be read from the back of the room. Recommendations for type size are 32–40 point for headings and 24–28 point for main text. Consider using boldface lettering to make text thicker. Box 10-5 shows examples of various type sizes.
- Do not use all capital letters for the main text. Use upper case and lower case lettering.
- Avoid putting too much text in italics, which can slow down reading.
- Limit the text to a few phrases on a screen. A good rule of thumb is six words across and six lines down.
- Write phrases, not sentences. When you use sentences, you have little or nothing to add and the tendency is to just read the words on the slides. Reading visuals aloud conveys the perception of lack of subject matter expertise and poor preparation.
- Use parallel grammar structure on each screen slide. Begin each point on a slide with the same part of speech, all verbs or all nouns. The

continuity in such structuring links smoothly from point to point.

- Assume your audience will want to write down everything you present on the screen. Keep information clear, simple, and minimal.
- Use color consistently, but avoid overuse. Keep the number to a maximum of four colors per slide. Choose colors that convey your message appropriately.
- Use contrasting colors. For example, put dark lettering against a light background and vice versa.
- Keep the background simple. It should show off the information, not overwhelm it.
- Curb the urge to go overboard with technology! Just because you can animate graphics and add sound does not mean you should. Visuals should make a point, not compete for Oscars in special effects!

OTHER MEDIA AND MATERIALS

"Mass media" communication tools reach large numbers of people with a common message (e.g., magazines, newspapers, pamphlets, advertisements, radio, and television). Oral health educators can take advantage of these readily available materials. Some applications for oral health education include:

- To communicate current, accurate scientific information to the public at-large
- To publicize special events and bring special projects to the public's attention
- To periodically present information, which keeps oral health in the public's attention.

Many newspapers and magazines find their way into school classrooms. When written at the **reading level** of the intended students, these items can contribute to improved learning in a number of ways. They can provide:

- new information that may not yet be available in textbooks
- opportunities for extra or specialized reading for students who want, and can manage, more detailed information

- material for classroom teaching displays, bulletin boards, and scrapbook collections
- topics for panel discussions of controversial issues
- materials for career guidance.

The reading level of written material is based on readability scores, such as the Flesch Reading Ease Score and the Flesch-Kincaid Grade Level Score. Some commercial word processing and desktop publishing software programs have the ability to calculate readability statistics based on these scores.

The Flesch Reading Ease Score rates written text on a 100-point scale; the higher the score, the easier the material is to read and understand. The Flesch-Kincaid Grade Level Score rates text on a United States grade-school level. A score of 6.0 indicates that the material is written on a sixth grade level, 8.0 on an eighth grade level, and 12.0 on a twelfth grade level. The Flesh-Kincaid Grade Level Score for this chapter, for example, is 11.2.

Both scoring systems consider the average sentence length (ASL: the number of words divided by the number of sentences) and the average number of syllables per word (ASW: the number of syllables divided by the number of words). The formula for the Flesch Reading Ease Score is: $206.835 - (1.015 \times ASL) - (84.6 \times ASW)$. The formula for the Flesch-Kincaid Grade Level Score is: $(0.39 \times ASL) + (11.8 \times ASW) - 15.59$.[15]

Radio and television can be potent forces in health education learning. Much of the world's population does not read or write, but they can listen and observe effectively. Health education promotions and health advertising aired over these mediums can stimulate thought about new ideas. They can take advantage of the motivational impact of the human voice to convey feelings and attitudes. Certain broadcasting companies voluntarily provide time occasionally for health education programs, such as during National Dental Health Month.

All articles published, radio or television stories aired, or advertisements campaigned may not necessarily be favorable or accurate. The oral health educator must be prepared to respond appropriately to misinformation. Several questions should be considered when evaluating statements about health practices or products. First, "Who said it?" Are they a recognized authority or reliable expert in the subject? Second, "Does the statement present verifiable facts or is it merely an emotional appeal?" In other words, is the product or practice necessary for attaining and maintaining health and is absolute success promised? Finally, "What is the reason for making the statement?" Profit-driven motives can be, but are not always, a cause for skepticism. Considerations for evaluating media sources are given in Box 10-9.

Table 10-2 gives an overview of common media and materials.

Presentation Structure[16]

Good presentation structure is similar to this well-known guideline for public speakers: Tell them what you are going to tell them—Tell them—Then, tell them what you told them. There are three basic components for this aspect of the lesson plan: the **instructional set,** content **body,** and **closure.**

The instructional set establishes the climate for the presentation. Its purpose is to make learners aware of what it is they are to learn and to cause them to want to learn it. Comments that arouse interest or indicate the use or value of the upcoming information are made to motivate learners and make it real for them. Instructional objectives and procedural aspects for the upcoming presentation are given here.

The content body is the bulk of the lesson information. All of the major learning points are presented here. Be sure you have done sufficient research and preparation in this area. No amount of drama or theatrics can make up for content inadequacies or poor sequencing. The closure summarizes the presented material. Main points are reviewed here to give a sense of unity to the lesson as a whole. If time permits, questions should be taken from the learners. A closing statement of concluding comments formally closes the block of

---

> ### BOX 10-9 Considerations for Evaluating Media Sources
>
> - Who said it? Are they a recognized authority or reliable expert in the subject?
> - Are verifiable facts presented or is this statement merely an emotional appeal?
> - What is the motive, or reason, for making the statement?

instruction. Examples of set, body, and closure are shown in the sample educational plans in Box 10-10 and Box 10-11.

Communicating Across Cultures[17]

Expectations for health-related interactions, including oral health education, can be strongly influenced by culture. An awareness of, and respect for, cultural influences can help in the creation of culturally acceptable educational plans. Recognizing the many ways in which people are different, as well as the many ways in which they are the same, assists communications between oral health educator and recipient. Of paramount importance, however, is to understand and accept that we are all people with health needs and concerns.

The following guidelines are suggested for increasing communication and building trusting relationships across cultures.

1. Behave formally in interactions with people who were born in another culture.
   - Using first names to show equality within exchanges is a uniquely American behavior. People from many cultures offer, and expect to receive, respect throughout the health care relationship. Address adults with deference to their age and status by using their title and last name (e.g., Mr./Señor X; Mrs. Señora X; Miss/ Señorita X). This is especially important for Hispanic, Middle-Eastern, former Soviet bloc, and some Asian

TABLE 10-2 EXAMPLES OF MATERIALS AND MEDIA FOR LEARNING EXPERIENCES

MATERIAL	ADVANTAGES	DISADVANTAGES
Audio: tape, disc, or CD	• Useful in groups and with individuals • Easy to make original recordings and duplicate tapes • Commercial software is widely available • Equipment is inexpensive, easy to use, and portable	• Information is presented at a fixed rate and sequence • Existing recordings are difficult to revise or update
Video: video recordings, videodiscs	• Useful in groups and with individuals • Deliver information through multiple senses • Show actions and illustrate relationships • Are reusable • Typical equipment is widely available and easy to use	• Information is presented at a fixed rate and sequence • Existing recordings are difficult to revise, and updating can be expensive • Equipment is moderately costly
Print Media: books and magazines, newspapers, brochures, pamphlets, flyers and fact sheets, posters, charts	• Easy to use • Useful in many locations • Simple forms can be easily prepared • Some are commercially available at no, or low, costs	• Reading skills are needed • Best with small groups • Advanced forms may require costly preparation
Technology-Based: Overheads	• Useful with large groups • Simple preparation; Easily updated • Used in a lighted room, facing audience • Equipment is common	• Overcrowded or cluttered transparencies can be distracting • Can get out of sequence easily
Technology-Based: 35 mm Slides	• Useful with individuals and large groups • Compact and easy to use • May be used singularly or in sequence; can be rearranged for various situations • Equipment is common and simple to use	• Requires a darkened room • Do not convey motion • Difficult to update
Technology-Based: Videos	• Useful with individuals and medium groups • Combines motion and sound with visuals • Can be used to illustrate motion relationships and special effects • Instant replays are possible	• Fixed rate and sequence • Expensive to update or revise
Technology-Based: Electronic Presentations	• Useful with all group sizes • Presentation pace can be controlled by presenter • Can combine visuals with sound and motion • Easily revised	• Preparation is extensive and requires special skills • Too many elaborate animations and/or sounds can be distracting • Requires expensive equipment that is not always available at program sites

Adapted from: DeBiase CB. Dental Hygiene in Review. Baltimore, MD: Lippincott Williams & Wilkins, 2001.[2]

BOX 10-10 Sample Educational Plan: A

Title: Being a Good Dental Parent   **Target Group:** Prenatal class for expectant parents

Estimated Length: 50 minutes, evening   **Instructional Method:** Discussion

Educational Goal: To increase prospective parents' awareness of the need for dental care and good dental health for their children.

Instructional Objectives:
1. State the number of teeth in the primary dentition and in the permanent dentition.
2. Identify the ages when formation of the primary teeth begins, eruption and exfoliation of primary teeth typically occur, and eruption of permanent teeth typically occurs.
3. Discuss methods for cleaning the gums of infants.
4. Describe a technique for effective brushing and flossing.
5. Discuss nutrients needed during pregnancy for proper tooth development.
6. Rebut the myth "You lose a tooth for every baby you have."

Instructional Materials: Eruption and Exfoliation Chart, brochures illustrating brushing and flossing techniques, handouts: "Dental Myths" and "Being a Good Dental Parent" quiz

Learning Activity: Quiz: "Being a Good Dental Parent," with multiple choice questions about timing of tooth development in utero, eruption and exfoliation, fluoride, etiology of tooth and oral hygiene techniques

Instructional Set: We are all excited about the anticipated arrival of the soon-to-be new members of our families and have come to this class tonight to discover ways to help them have a healthy life!

Body:
1. Distribute quiz and "Dental Myths" handout, 1 each per couple. Allow ~ 8 minutes for participants to complete quiz and review myths.
2. Read questions aloud and allow spontaneous responses from the audience. Discuss to highlight and explain:
   a. Basic dental embryology
   b. Basic eruption and exfoliation   → Point out on Chart
   c. Oral Hygiene for infants
   d. Plaque: Sugar: Acid: Tooth Decay relationships
   e. Basic brushing and flossing techniques   → Distribute OH brochures

Closure: In the past hour, we have talked a lot about things as tiny as "baby teeth" and how to safeguard them . . . to the importance of our children's teeth to their dental health and overall well-being. We have seen that many dental myths we may have grown up believing actually have no basis in fact. If you have further questions that I might be able to help you with, please feel free to contact me at my office!

BOX 10-11 Sample Educational Plan: B

Title: Sugar Q and A

Target Group: 4th Grade Elementary

Estimated Length: 45 minutes

Instructional Method: Discussion

Educational Goal: To increase students' awareness of the damaging effects of a high sugar diet on teeth and encourage food choices that promote good dental health.

Instructional Objectives:
1. Explain the plaque-sugar-acid-tooth decay chain of events.
2. Identify food package labeling as a source of consumer information on ingredients and nutrient content.
3. Differentiate between "tooth healthy" foods and foods that promote tooth decay.

Instructional Materials: "Plaque Chain" Chart; Samples of food labels from food cartons, packages and cans; Clean food wrappers, bags, and packages; Pictures of high sugar foods from magazines.

Learning Activity: "OK Snacks" Game (variation of Grocery Bag Game)

Instructional Set: Think for a minute about all of the things you ate yesterday. Did any of those things contain sugar? Today we are going to take a close look at sugary foods and the effects they can have on your teeth.

Body:
1. Explain food labeling regulations and listing by volume and discuss examples.
   NOTE: Break students into small groups of four. Give each group three food labels (one showing sugar ingredient near top of list, one without sugar or near end of list, and one somewhere in between).
2. Explain plaque and its etiological role in tooth decay using "plaque chain" concept.
   NOTE: Use Plaque Chain chart; begin with each link masked and reveal as each is discussed.
3. Review and reinforce with "OK Snacks" game.

Closure: Now that we have taken a close look at some of the foods we eat every day, it is apparent that we eat more sugary foods than we realize. It is important to break the "plaque chain."

cultures. Handshakes at the beginning of each meeting are important in Hispanic and Polish cultures.
2. Pay careful attention to nonverbal communication and communication styles.
   - Body language, eye contact, and communication patterns are important communicators.

- Make eye contact, without necessarily expecting it in return. Certain cultures consider it disrespectful to look authority figures in the eye, while in others, avoiding eye contact is a way of showing respect for authority.
- Conversational distance space for Westerners is about five feet. For people from the Middle East, an appropriate distance is

Learning Activities

1. A sample file of available materials that can be obtained at low or no cost allows the oral health educator to identify and select those that are appropriate as supplemental materials for specific target audiences when developing an educational plan.
   a. Compile a file of examples of various free or inexpensive oral health brochures, pamphlets, and posters from commercial companies or other sources.
   b. Evaluate the materials based on the criteria in Box 10-4.
   c. Organize the file to facilitate retrieval (e.g., by topic, category, or other logical system).

2. Collect examples of newspaper or magazine articles about oral health.
   a. Share the articles with a group of your classmates.
   b. Discuss the accuracy, source, and motivation behind each article.

3. Write a short feature about an oral health topic of your choice that would be suitable for publication in a small, locally operated newspaper. Calculate its readability statistics (Flesch Reading Ease Score and Flesch-Kincaid Grade Level Score).

4. Assume that you and a classmate have been asked to present a 30-minute oral health program for a group of 15 Girl Scouts, ranging from 11 to 14 years in age.
   a. Brainstorm ideas for age-appropriate topics.
   b. Write an educational goal and three specific instructional objectives for the chosen topic.

5. Do a Web search for companies that make oral health products. Visit their Web sites
   a. Examine and evaluate any educational programs they have developed and posted at the site.
   b. Determine whether the company offers any free or inexpensive learning materials or activities.

6. Do a Web search for translation services in your area and in the nearest major cities. Find out what is available and how services can be obtained.

7. Develop at least one learning activity to support a tobacco cessation educational plan.

8. Develop an idea for an appropriate media/material for a tobacco cessation educational plan. Sketch out your idea and write a brief page describing it and how you envision its use. (This is brain work; you do not have to produce the item.)

2. "To introduce age-appropriate oral health concepts to second grade teachers attending the Teacher Training Workshop at the beginning of the school year." This statement best exemplifies which of the following?
   a. Lesson plan
   b. Educational goal
   c. Instructional objective
   d. Condition criteria

3. Complete this instructional objective. "On completion of the learning experience, the learner should be able to:
   a. appreciate the value of good oral hygiene."
   b. know four brushing methods."
   c. demonstrate the Bass brushing technique."
   d. understand why brushing and flossing are important."

4. Presentation structure for the content of a lesson plan includes:
   a. set, body, and closure.
   b. staging, action, and ending.

c. objectives, goal, and closure.

d. content, body, and summary.

5. Develop an argument for student-made posters but against a poster contest.

6. A middle school teacher has never used newspapers or magazines in the classroom. Describe to this teacher at least three ways these materials can be used to support learning experiences.

7. A person from a Middle Eastern culture may convey the importance they attach to what they are saying by:

a. repeating it several times.

b. saying it loudly.

c. pointing their fingers at the person to whom they are speaking.

d. speaking in a high-pitched voice.

8. Identify the central focus for all instructional planning events.

a. The teaching strategy that will be used

b. The instructional materials that are available

c. The content that must be presented

d. The target audience of intended learners

9. What is the purpose for covering parts of the information on a strip chart?

10. The typical conversational distance between people in Western cultures is about ___ feet; the typical distance for Middle Eastern cultures is ___.

a. 5; 5

b. 5; 2

c. 3; 1

d. 6; 3

REFERENCES

1. American Dental Education Association. Competencies for entry into the profession of dental hygiene, Exhibit 7. J Dent Educ 2003 July;67(7):1–5. Available at: http://www.adea.org/cepr. Accessed January 2004.

2. DeBiase CB. Dental Hygiene in Review. Baltimore, MD: Lippincott Williams & Wilkins, 2001.

3. Foder JT, Dalis GT. Health Instruction: Theory and Application. 4th Ed. Philadelphia, PA: Lea and Febiger, 1989.

4. Faculty Development Guidebook: Teaching tips. Honolulu Community College. Available at: http://www.hcc.hawaii.edu/intranet/committees/FacDevCom/guidebk/teachtip/teachtip.htm. Accessed April 2003.

5. Darby ML. Mosby's Comprehensive Review of Dental Hygiene. 5th Ed. St. Louis, MO: Elsevier Science, 2002.

6. Dearth F. Construction and Utilization of Visual Aids in Dental Health Education. Thoroughfare: Charles B. Slack, 1974.

7. Instructional Aids. Available at: http://www.isd.uga.edu/teaching_assistant/ta-handbook/instaids.html. Accessed April 2003.

8. Study Art. Available at: http://www.sanford-artedventures.com/study/g_color.html. Accessed April 2003.

9. Wilder C. Some basics on color. Available at: http://www.presentersuniversity.com/courses/show_vadesigning.cfm?RecordID=246 Accessed April 2003.

10. Stoll FA. Dental Health Education. 5th Ed. Philadelphia, PA: Lea and Febiger, 1977.

11. Laskowski L. 11 Tips for using flip charts successfully. Available at: http://www.powerpointers.com/showarticle.asp?articleid=246. Accessed April 2003.

12. Designing Effective Visual Aids. Available at: http://www.presentersuniversity.com/courses/cs_visualaids.cfm. Accessed April 2003.

13. Miller A. Visual aid virtuosity. Available at: http://www.presentersuniversity.com/courses/show_vachoosing.cfm?Record=104. Accessed April 2003.

14. Wilder C. 8 basic guidelines for visuals. http://www.presentersuniversity.com/courses/show_vadesigning.cfm?RecordID=161. Accessed April 2003.

15. Flesch Reading Score/Flesch-Kincaid Grade Level Score. Available at: http://csep.psyc.memphis.edu/cohmetrix.

16. Nelson DM. Saunders Review of Dental Hygiene. Philadelphia, PA: W.B. Saunders, 2000.

17. Salimbene S. What Language Does Your Patient Hurt In? A Practical Guide to Culturally Competent Patient Care. EMC Paradigm, 2001.

EPIDEMIOLOGY AND RESEARCH

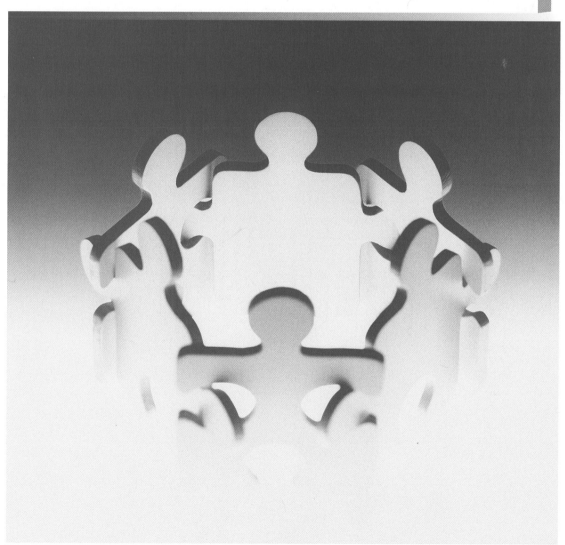

Concepts in Epidemiology

11

Objectives

After studying this chapter and completing the study questions and activities, the learner will be able to:
- Define epidemiology and oral epidemiology.
- Describe an epidemiologic triangle for dental caries.
- Describe the difference between morbidity and mortality.
- Describe the difference between incidence and prevalence.
- List the types of study designs commonly used in epidemiology.
- Explain the importance of sensitivity and specificity for a screening test.

KEY TERMS

Agent	Environmental factors	Oral epidemiology
Analytic	Epidemic	Pandemic
Associated	Epidemiology	Predictive value
Case-control	Experimental	Prevalence
Causative factors	Host factors	Proportion
Cohort	Incidence	Prospective
Confounding variables	Index	Retrospective
Count	Morbidity	Risk factor
Cross-sectional	Mortality	Sensitivity
Descriptive	Multiple causation	Specificity
Endemic	Observational	

The American Dental Education Association competencies addressed in this chapter include[1]:

HP.4:   Identify individual and population risk factors and develop strategies that promote a health-related quality of life.

CM.1:   Assess the oral health needs of the community and the quality and availability of resources and services.

CM.6:   Evaluate the outcomes of community-based programs and plan for future activities.

Introduction

By turning to basic medical terminology, we can learn the literal definition of the term **epidemiology.** The prefix, *epi,* means "on, upon, befall." The root, *demo,* means "people, population, man," and the suffix, *ology,* means "the study of." If taken literally, epidemiology is "the study of that which befalls man."

Epidemiology, often considered the core science of public health, can be more accurately defined as the study of the distribution and determinants of disease and injuries in human populations.[2] In other words, epidemiologists study how often disease occurs in different population groups and why. In epidemiology, the primary units of concern are groups of persons, not separate individuals. For this reason, thinking in epidemiologic terms often seems foreign to clinicians trained to think of the unique problems of each individual patient. By studying groups of individuals, epidemiologic information can be used to plan and evaluate strategies to prevent illness and as a guide in the management of patients in whom disease has already developed.

Public health has found the principles of epidemiology useful in assisting with its mission of protecting the health of populations and groups. General uses of epidemiology include, but are not limited to, the following:

- To study the history of disease
- To assess and evaluate public health and clinical health services

- To determine the cause and source of disease
- To determine what diseases, conditions, injuries, or disorders cause illness, health problems, or mortality in a community
- To complement and complete the clinical picture of disease.

An Historic Event: John Snow's Natural Experiment

One of the most famous events in the history of epidemiology was a natural experiment reported more than 150 years ago by John Snow, a British physician. In 1854, a cholera outbreak in London claimed thousands of lives. During this time, several water companies piped drinking water to community pumps throughout London (this was before indoor plumbing), and Snow found that many of the deaths were occurring around one particular water pump—the Broad Street pump in Soho. The company that provided water to this particular pump, the Southwark and Vauxhall Company, piped water from the Thames river within London's city limits, and Snow hypothesized that the cholera outbreak was due to water contaminated by sewage (although this was before the formulation of the germ theory). Snow compared the cholera mortality (death) rates for residents subscribing to the Southwark and Vauxhall Company and for residents subscribing to the Lambeth Company that obtained its water upstream of London (therefore, not contaminated by London's sewage). During 1854, there were 4,093 cholera deaths among the 266,516 customers of the Southwark and Vauxhall Company and 461 cholera

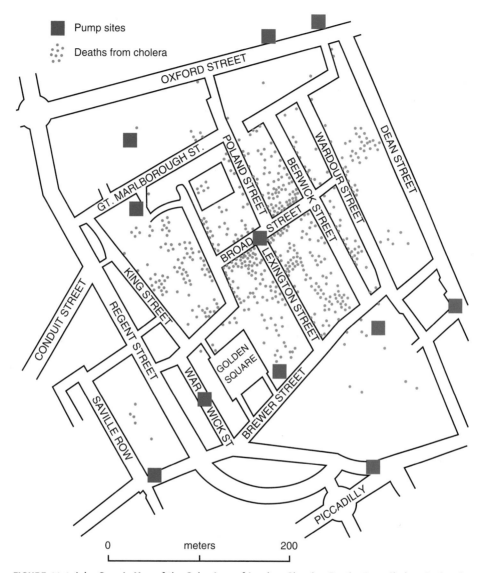

FIGURE 11-1 John Snow's Map of the Soho Area of London, Showing Deaths From Cholera During the Epidemic of 1854.[3]

deaths among the 173,748 customers of the Lambeth Company (Table 11-1 and Fig. 11-1).[3]

In September 1854, Snow convinced local authorities to remove the handle from the Southwark and Vauxhall water pump at Broad Street and the epidemic soon subsided.

Epidemiology and Oral Health

Although you may be aware of the role of epidemiology in the practice of medicine and public health, the science of epidemiology is also basic to the practice of dentistry, dental hygiene, and

TABLE 11-1 ATTACK RATE OF FATAL CHOLERA AMONG CUSTOMERS OF SOUTHWARK AND VAUXHALL (EXPOSED COHORT) AND LAMBETH (UNEXPOSED COHORT), LONDON, 1854[3]

	WATER COMPANY	
	SOUTHWARK AND VAUXHALL	LAMBETH
Cholera deaths:	4,093	461
Population served by water company:	255,516	173,748
Attack rate:	0.0154	0.0027

dental public health. When epidemiology is applied to oral health issues, it is often referred to as **oral epidemiology.** One classic example of the use of epidemiology in oral health was the discovery of the relationship between mottled teeth, dental caries, and fluoride. In 1916, Black and McKay[4] presented the first of a series of reports on what was then called "mottled enamel" in children in certain areas of Colorado. The search for the cause of mottled enamel culminated in a report by Smith et al.[5] in 1931 that implicated a relatively high amount of fluoride in the soil and water. Up to this time and for several years thereafter, mottled enamel was considered a pathologic condition, with fluoride as the undesirable causative agent. During the 1930s, however, several investigators began to notice a possible relationship between the high fluoride content of soil and water, mottled enamel, and an apparent resistance to dental caries. By the mid- to late 1930s, it became apparent that fluoride in drinking water was inversely related to dental caries experience; as fluoride level increased, caries rates decreased.

A more modern example of the use of epidemiological research in oral health relates to the association between smoking and periodontitis. Based on epidemiologic investigations, there is compelling evidence that cigarette smokers are more likely than nonsmokers to experience the onset and progression of periodontal destruction and that smokers have a poorer prognosis following periodontal therapy.[6,7,8] To estimate that proportion of adult periodontitis in the United States that could be attributed to cigarette smoking, Tomar and Asma[9] used data from the Third National Health and Nutrition Examination Survey (NHANES III)—a multipurpose health survey conducted from 1988 to 1994 by the National Center for Health Statistics of the Centers for Disease Control and Prevention.

The investigators found that current smokers were about four times as likely to have periodontitis as persons who had never smoked, former smokers were about two times as likely to have periodontitis as persons who had never smoked, and that among current smokers there was a dose-response relationship between cigarettes smoked per day and the odds of periodontitis. Using standard epidemiologic formulas, the investigators calculated that 41.9% of periodontitis cases in the U.S. adult population were attributable to current cigarette smoking and 10.9% to former smoking. Based on epidemiologic studies such as this, we now know that a large proportion of adult periodontitis may be preventable through prevention and cessation of cigarette smoking.

The Scope of Epidemiology

As previously stated, epidemiology is the study of the distribution and determinants of diseases. In the early history of epidemiology, the primary diseases of concern were generally infectious in nature (e.g., cholera, typhoid). Today, the science of epidemiology is applied to all diseases, conditions, and health-related events, including chronic disease, health services research, program planning, and program evaluation. It is concerned not only with epidemics but also with interepidemic periods and sporadic and endemic occurrences of disease.

Endemic is defined as the constant presence of a disease or infectious agent within a given geographic area; it may also refer to the usual prevalence of a given disease within an area. An **epidemic** is an unusually high occurrence of disease or the occurrence in a community or region of cases of an illness clearly in excess of expectancy.[10] The definition of unusually high or in excess of expectancy may differ depending on the circumstances, so there is no clear demarcation between an epidemic and a small fluctuation. Even a single case of smallpox would exceed expectancy anywhere in the world today, whereas, until recently, 100 cases in a single year might have been within the expected number in Ethiopia or India.

A disease that remains epidemic over many years may eventually be considered endemic and many chronic diseases or problems are endemic in nature. That is, they are widespread and do not exhibit great variability in frequency from year to year. For example, hypertension, one of the risk factors for cardiovascular and cerebrovascular disease, is one of the more prevalent conditions in the United States. Approximately 23% of all Americans 20 to 74 years of age have hypertension and more than 75% of women aged 75 and older have hypertension. In 2000, more than 23,700 deaths were attributed to hypertension, for a death rate of 8.6 per 100,000 population.[11] This illustrates the fact that both endemic and epidemic conditions are important to public health and the science of epidemiology.

Another term used to describe the occurrence and distribution of disease is **pandemic.** A pandemic is a disease or infection that has spread over an entire country or the world. Acquired Immune Deficiency Syndrome (AIDS) is an example of a pandemic.

With an infectious or communicable disease, a single factor, or agent, must be present for the disease to occur. The presence or absence of the agent alone, however, does not determine if an individual will get a disease. Other factors, including the immunity of the host, play a role in the onset of disease. The concept that more than one factor must be present for disease to develop is referred to as **multiple causation.** A single bacterium living in isolation is not sufficient to cause an outbreak of a disease and cannot by itself be responsible for the outbreak or labeled as the cause. The mode of transmission, ability of the organism to grow and propagate, communicability of the organism, level of immunity within the population, and the density of the population or the proximity of the cases to one another are other factors that contribute to the level or intensity of an outbreak. Therefore, an agent may be a necessary but not a sufficient cause of disease.

In epidemiology, it is customary to consider three primary factors when assessing the development of disease: (1) the agent, (2) host factors, and (3) factors in the environment. The **agent** is the cause of the disease (for infectious diseases), **host factors** affect an individual's susceptibility to a disease, and **environmental factors** influence exposure and may indirectly affect susceptibility as well. These three factors comprise what is often referred to as the epidemiologic triangle (Fig. 11-2). A fourth factor—time—is also a component of any disease process.

The epidemiologic triangle is basic and fundamental to all epidemiologic principles; however, it was based on communicable diseases, which are no longer the leading cause of illness or death in most industrialized nations. For this reason, the model is often modified when referring to chronic diseases such as dental caries and heart disease. For instance, the term agent is often replaced by a reference to **causative factors;** and host factors include important behavioral and lifestyle factors, such as smoking. Figure 11-3 depicts an epidemiologic triangle or epidemiologic model for dental caries.

MEASURES OF DISEASE OCCURRENCE

To study the distribution and determinants of disease, disease must be accurately measured.

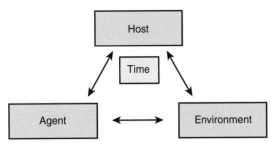

FIGURE 11-2 The Epidemiologic Triangle

Measures of disease range from simple counts to more complex measures, such as rates and indices.

Counts

The simplest measurement of disease is a **count** of the number of persons in a group who have a particular disease or characteristic. It may be noted that 50 children in an elementary school have dental caries or that 12 dental patients with advanced periodontitis smoke cigarettes.

Proportions and Rates

For a count to be descriptive of a group, it must be seen as a **proportion** (i.e., it must be divided by the total number in the group). The 50 dental caries cases mentioned earlier would have a different significance if the elementary school had an enrollment of 600 or if the school only had an enrollment of 100. In the first case, the proportion would be 50/600, 0.08, or 8% (percentage, or number per one hundred, is one of the most common ways of expressing proportions). In the second case, the proportion would be 50/100, 0.50, or 50%.

Certain kinds of proportions are frequently used in epidemiology. These are referred to as rates. The various types of rates involve or imply some time relationship. The numerator of a rate is the number of people with the disease being counted; the denominator is the population at risk of the disease or event (Box 11-1). Rates of disease are called **morbidity** rates, and rates of death are called **mortality** rates. Two commonly used rates that every dental professional should understand and remember are incidence and prevalence.

INCIDENCE

Incidence describes the rate of development of a disease in a group over time, which is included in the denominator; or, the rate at which new disease

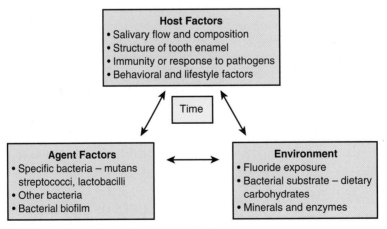

FIGURE 11-3 Epidemiologic Triangle for Dental Caries

BOX 11-1 Formula for Rate

$$\text{Rate} = \frac{\text{Number of events, cases, or deaths}}{\text{Population in same area}}$$
in a time period

cases occur in a population during a specified period (Box 11-2). Think of incidence as a video—it captures a series of events (cases of disease) during a period (usually a year). As an example, the age-adjusted incidence of cancer of the oral cavity and pharynx in the United States during 1998 was 15.7 new cases per 100,000 population in men and 6.4 new cases per 100,000 population in women.[12]

Occasionally, measurement of incidence is complicated by changes in the population at risk during the period when cases are ascertained, such as through birth or death. This problem is overcome by relating the numbers of new cases to the person years at risk, calculated by adding together the periods during which each individual member of the population is at risk during the measurement period. Therefore, incidence can also be defined as the number of persons developing a disease divided by the total time experienced for the subjects followed (Box 11-3).

PREVALENCE

Prevalence describes a group at a certain time. It is like a snapshot, rather than a video, of an existing condition or a measure of disease status. The

BOX 11-2 Formula for Incidence Rate

Incidence Rate =

$$\frac{\text{Number of persons developing a disease}}{\text{Total number at risk}}$$
per unit of time

BOX 11-3 Another Formula for Incidence Rate

Incidence Rate =

$$\frac{\text{Number of persons developing a disease}}{\text{Total time experienced for the subjects followed}}$$

simplest way of considering disease status is to consider disease either present or absent. Prevalence is the proportion of people in a population that have disease. For example, the prevalence of gingivitis in a middle school during a dental screening on November 10 was 54%; or, the prevalence of untreated decay in third grade children during Dental Health Month was 25%.

Several factors affect disease prevalence, including disease occurrence (incidence) and duration of disease. The greater the incidence of disease, the greater the number of people who will have it. The longer the duration of disease once it occurs, the higher the prevalence. Diseases with short duration may have a low prevalence even if the incidence rate is high. The prevalence of upper respiratory infection may be low despite a high incidence because, after a brief period, most people recover. Duration may also be short for a grave disease that leads to rapid death. Therefore, the prevalence of aortic hemorrhage would be low even if it had a high incidence because it generally leads to death within minutes. In contrast, a disease with low incidence could have a high prevalence if the duration of the disease is long or the effects not reversible. For example, the prevalence of gingival recession (≥ 1 mm) in adults between 55 to 64 years of age was 78% in 1988–1991.[13]

Because prevalence reflects both incidence rate and disease duration, it is not as useful as incidence for studying the causes of disease. It is extremely useful, however, for measuring the disease burden in a population.[14] Refer to Box 11-4 for the formula

BOX 11-4 Formula for Prevalence Rate

$$\text{Prevalence Rate} = \frac{\text{Number of persons with a disease}}{\text{Total number in group}}$$

for prevalence rate and to Box 11-5 for the difference between incidence and prevalence.

Indices

Dentistry uses another measure of disease referred to as an **index** (plural, indices or indexes). An index is a graduated, numeric scale with upper and lower limits. Indices allow for the measurement of disease severity, rather than just disease incidence or prevalence. For example, a teenager with dental caries on 4 of 28 teeth has a lower level of disease than a teenager with caries on 12 of 28 teeth; however, both would be considered to have disease in the calculation of caries prevalence. By using an index, we can quantify how much disease a person has. Common indices used in dentistry include the DMFT/DMFS index and the Plaque Index. Chapter 13 contains a detailed description of dental indices.

GENERAL TYPES OF EPIDEMIOLOGIC STUDIES

Descriptive, Analytic, Experimental, and Observational

Learning about causes of disease through epidemiologic studies is generally a gradual process that requires different types of study design, depending on the nature of the disease, possible etiologic agents, and the current state of knowledge about the disease. One overall way to classify epidemiologic studies is into two broad categories: (1) **descriptive** studies, which are usually undertaken when little is known of the epidemiology of a disease; and (2) **analytic** studies, which are carried out when leads about etiology are already available (Box 11-6). Descriptive studies study the amount and distribution of disease; analytic studies evaluate the determinants of or risk factors for disease. Descriptive studies tell you who is affected, where cases occur, and when cases occur; analytic studies tell you why disease rates are high in a particular group.

Descriptive studies are usually the first step in looking at a disease and often use existing data sources. A descriptive study usually looks at the prevalence of disease by person (e.g., age, gender, race, ethnicity, socioeconomic status, occupation), place, and time to describe groups at higher risk of developing a disease. The most common descriptive study is a **cross-sectional** or prevalence study. In a cross-sectional study, disease status and exposure to risk factors are measured at one point in time. An oral health status survey is an example of a cross-sectional study.

Information gathered during a descriptive study is used to build a model and develop a hypothesis for further research. An analytic study design is then used to test the causal hypotheses generated through descriptive studies. Traditionally, analytic studies have been classified as either experimental or observational, although these terms are used less frequently today. In an **experimental** study, an investigator studies the impact of a factor that he or she controls. If an investigator is interested in the health effects of secondhand cigarette smoke on a litter of rats, the investigator can

BOX 11-5 The Difference Between Incidence and Prevalence

To remember the difference between incidence and prevalence, think of incidence as a video and prevalence as a snapshot. Incidence measures the number of new disease cases during a period (like a video); prevalence measures the number of cases of disease at a given point (like a snapshot).

BOX 11-6 The Difference Between Descriptive and Analytic Studies

DESCRIPTIVE STUDY	ANALYTIC STUDY
Looks at amount and distribution of disease: Who gets the disease and where and when does disease occur?	Looks at determinants of disease: Why do people get the disease?
Used to *develop* hypotheses	Used to *test* hypotheses

expose one half of the litter to secondhand smoke and not expose the other half. Experimental studies on humans, however, are often not possible because of ethical considerations, with the exception of intervention trials or clinical trials testing a treatment for a disease. Examples of experimental studies in dental public health are the clinical trials testing chlorhexidine or fluoride varnish and gels for the prevention of dental caries in which one half of study participants receive the active agent and the other one half receive a placebo.[15]

Because experimental trials are not always possible or appropriate, investigators may select a study design in which they "observe" the impact or health effect of a factor in a population that is already segregated into groups on the basis of some experience, exposure, or disease (married versus single, smoker versus nonsmoker, periodontitis versus no periodontitis). This study design is called an **observational** study. To determine if smoking is associated with advanced periodontitis, an investigator could look at pocket depth and loss of attachment in smokers compared with nonsmokers. To determine if alveolar bone loss is associated with skeletal bone loss (osteoporosis), an investigator could follow adults for several years to determine if individuals with skeletal bone loss also have alveolar bone loss.

The primary difficulty with observational studies is that observed groups may differ, not only in the factor under study but also in other factors. In the previous example on advanced periodontitis and smoking, nonsmokers may differ from smokers in ways other than their smoking habit. They may differ in terms of oral hygiene, education, and

access to preventive dental care; factors that may influence periodontal health regardless of smoking status. These other factors—known as **confounding variables**—may make it more difficult to demonstrate the role of the specific factor under study (smoking).

A common sequence in the discovery of a causal association between an agent and a disease—using each of the previously described study designs—is as follows. First, clinical observations suggest a possible causal association between a factor and a disease. Second, descriptive epidemiologic studies establish the association on a population level. Third, analytic epidemiologic studies establish the association on an individual level. Fourth, experimental studies reproduce the disease when the risk factor is introduced and/or elucidate potential pathogenic mechanisms between the disease and the risk factor. Finally, observational studies find that removal of the risk factor alters the incidence of disease (Fig. 11-4).

Let us return to the previous example of mottled teeth, dental caries, and fluoride. Early in the 20th century, observations of mottled enamel and tooth decay prevalence in communities throughout the United States led to the discovery in analytic epidemiologic studies, and then in animal studies, that fluoride in drinking water was responsible for mottled enamel and also for protection against dental caries. Belief in the causal nature of the association was further strengthened by studies showing that the frequency of mottled enamel decreased and the frequency of dental caries increased when communities changed from drinking water sources high in fluoride to sources

Clinical Observations

> *Physicians who treat patients with Disease X report that the patients appear to consume less of a certain nutrient, referred to as Anti-X.*

↓

Descriptive Studies

> *Disease X is 20 times more common in countries where people get less Anti-X.*

↓

Analytic Studies

> *You contact people who already have Disease X (cases). Then you find a group of similar people who do not have Disease X (controls). You ask both groups about their eating habits over the last 10 years to find out if the cases and controls differed in their intake of Anti-X.*

↓

Experimental Studies

> *You randomly assign thousands of healthy people to get either Anti-X or placebo. After 5 years, you look and see if Disease X is less common in those who took Anti-X compared with those who took the placebo.*

FIGURE 11-4 Potential Sequence in the Discovery of a Causal Association

low in fluoride. Finally, experimental studies in which fluoride was added to the water of some communities but not others clearly established both the causal nature of the relationship and the efficacy of fluoridated drinking water in reducing the frequency of dental caries.

Retrospective, Prospective, Cohort, and Case-Control

As previously mentioned, the terms experimental study and observational study are being used less frequently to describe a general type of epidemiologic study design, mainly because experimental studies and observational studies often use similar epidemiologic techniques to study the relationship between disease and a potential risk factor. The more common terms now used to describe differ-

ent types of epidemiologic studies are **retrospective, prospective, cohort,** and **case-control.** Retrospective and prospective refer to the timing of the information and events of a study; cohort and case-control refer to the type of population being studied.

Let us start with a description of cohort study and case-control study. In epidemiology, a cohort is defined as any designated group of individuals who are followed or traced over time.[16] In a cohort study, new cases of disease are measured in a group of people who are or have been exposed to a factor believed to influence the occurrence of the disease. The cohort is followed over time, usually with the aim of comparing disease rates for two or more cohorts. Because most cohort studies look toward the future, they are occasionally referred to simply as prospective studies, although some cohort studies can be retrospective in nature. If you see a reference to a prospective study design, you can usually assume that the study is actually a prospective cohort study. Prospective studies are also referred to as longitudinal studies.

The following is an example of a prospective cohort study designed to assess potential risk factors for osteoporosis in women aged 65 years and older.[17] During the 1980s, four clinical sites recruited a cohort of almost 10,000 older women. Detailed information on potential risk factors for osteoporosis was obtained from each woman through a questionnaire, physical examination, bone mineral density test, and an interview. The women were then followed over time, with a contact every 4 months to determine if they had fractured a bone. If a woman reported a fracture, medical records were obtained to verify that a fracture actually occurred. In simplistic terms, women within the cohort were classified according to a specific risk factor. Fracture incidence in women with and without the risk factor was then compared.

Although most cohort studies are prospective in nature (e.g., they follow a cohort forward in time), a cohort study may also be retrospective. In a retrospective cohort study, occasionally referred to as an historic cohort study, the cohorts are identified from recorded information, with the time during which they were at risk for disease occurring before the beginning of the study.

Although a cohort study provides a vast amount of information on risk factors for disease, following a large cohort over time can be expensive. The case-control study design aims at achieving the same goals as a cohort study, but more efficiently. In a case-control study, persons with a given disease (the cases) and persons without the given disease (the controls) are selected; the proportion of cases and controls who have a certain background characteristic or who have been exposed to possible risk factors are then determined and compared. Because a case-control study often looks to the past for exposure, it is often referred to as a retrospective study.

Case-control studies are one of the most frequently undertaken types of epidemiologic study. They can generally be carried out in a much shorter period than cohort studies, do not require nearly so large a sample size, and, consequently, are less expensive.

The following is an example of a case-control study designed to evaluate the association between fluoride exposure and hip fractures.[18] The county of Cleveland in northeast England has one area with water naturally high in fluoride (>1.0 ppm); the rest of the county has water with a low fluoride concentration. In this case-control study, the cases were adults who were admitted to the county's three hospitals with newly diagnosed fractures of the femoral neck (hip fractures). The controls were adults randomly selected from those registered with the National Health Service, matched to the cases by age and sex.

Both the cases and controls were interviewed to obtain information on demographic variables, height, weight, lifetime residential history, usual physical activities, age at menopause, alcohol consumption, smoking history, recent medication use, and dietary sources of calcium and fluoride. As presented in Table 11-2, the investigators found no evidence of any increase in the risk of hip fracture from fluoride in drinking water at concentrations of about 1 ppm.

THE CONCEPTS OF CAUSALITY AND RISK

At the beginning of this chapter, "determining the causes and sources of disease" was listed as one of the general uses of epidemiology. Unfortunately, determining the "cause" of a particular disease is not an easy task, especially given the multiple causation or multifactorial etiology of chronic diseases. What epidemiologic studies provide us with is information on which host and environmental factors are **associated** with an either increased or decreased risk of developing disease in a population, together with the strength of the association. In fact, many statistical measures obtained from epidemiologic studies are referred to as measures of association or measures of risk.

The concept of risk for disease is widely used in public health and is measured on the same scale and interpreted in the same way as a probability. In other words, risk is the probability that a specified event will occur. A **risk factor** is an attribute or exposure that increases the probability or risk of

TABLE 11-2 ASSOCIATION OF HIP FRACTURE WITH EXPOSURE TO FLUORIDE IN DRINKING WATER[18]

LIFETIME EXPOSURE TO WATER CONTAINING:	CASES	CONTROLS	ODDS RATIO (ADJUSTED)
< 0.9 ppm fluoride	380	346	1.0*
≥ 0.9 ppm fluoride	80	77	1.0 (0.7–1.5)

* reference category

BOX 11-7 Formula for Sensitivity and Specificity		
	ACTUAL DISEASE STATE	
TEST RESULTS	**DISEASE**	**NO DISEASE**
Positive	A	B
Negative	C	D
	A+C	B+D

Sensitivity = A/(A+C)
Specificity = D/(B+D)

BOX 11-8 Sensitivity and Specificity for Pap Tests[18]		
	CERVICAL CANCER	
PAP TEST	**YES**	**NO**
Positive	109	488
Negative	31	7,926
	140	8,414

Sensitivity = 109/140 = 78%
Specificity = 7926/8414 = 94%

disease occurrence. For example, smoking is a risk factor for periodontitis and xerostomia is a risk factor for root caries.

SCREENING FOR DISEASE AND DISEASE RISK

Over the years, various diagnostic and screening tests have been developed to determine if an individual has oral disease or is at increased risk of developing either dental caries or periodontal disease. Unfortunately, clinical diagnosis is not necessarily a perfect process and two different diagnostic approaches to the same disease may not lead to the same classification for every patient. To obtain something more than an impression of the quality of a diagnostic or screening test, it is useful to calculate quantitative indices of the accuracy of a test. For a diagnosis that is dichotomous (disease or no disease), there are two separate aspects of the accuracy of diagnosis. One is **sensitivity,** defined as the proportion of those who truly have the disease that are correctly classified as having it. The other is **specificity,** defined as the proportion of those who truly do not have the disease that are correctly classified as not having it (Box 11-7). The goal of any diagnostic or screening test is to have a sensitivity and specificity as close to 100% as possible. In addition, an ideal test should also be simple, inexpensive, acceptable to the patient, and reliable.

The easiest way to conceptualize sensitivity and specificity is through an example from medicine. The Papanicolaou (Pap) test is the mainstay of cervical cancer screening. The Pap test, however, is not perfect—it results in both false positives and false negatives. Box 11-8 includes data from a study evaluating cervical cancer screening tests.[19] Of the 8,554 women in the study, 31 had a false negative (they had cervical cancer, but the Pap test was negative) and 488 had a false positive (they did not have cervical cancer, but the Pap test was positive). Using the formula in Box 11-7, the specificity and sensitivity of the Pap test in this study were 78% and 94%, respectively.

Although sensitivity and specificity describe the characteristics of a test by correctly classifying those who have or do not have a disease, **predictive value** is a measure of the usefulness of a test in classifying people with disease. It can be calculated from the same basic data used to calculate sensitivity and specificity. More information on sensitivity, specificity, and predictive value can be obtained from most epidemiology and biostatistics textbooks.

SUMMARY

This chapter defined the science of epidemiology and gave examples of how epidemiology is used in dentistry. Concepts and terms for measuring disease were introduced, as were study design models commonly used in epidemiology and oral epidemiology. The chapter also introduced the concepts of causality, risk, and risk factor. Now that you have a basic understanding of epidemiology, the next three chapters will focus on the application of epidemiology in the practice of dentistry, dental hygiene, and dental public health.

 Learning Activities

1. Read the following three articles about the relationship between fluoridation and hip fractures and briefly describe the study design. Was it a descriptive study, an analytic study, a cohort study, or a case-control study? Which study provides the "best" data regarding the potential association?
   a. Phipps KR, Orwoll ES, Mason JD, Cauley JA. Community water fluoridation, bone mineral density, and fractures: prospective study of effects in older women. BMJ 2000; 321:860–864.
   b. Li Y, Liang C, Slemenda CW, et al. Effect of long-term exposure to fluoride in drinking water on risks of bone fractures. J Bone Miner Res 2001; 16:932–939.
   c. Hillier S, Cooper C, Killingray S, Russell G, Hughes H, Coggon D. Fluoride in drinking water and risk of hip fracture in the UK: A case-control study. Lancet 2000; 355:265–269.
2. Go to the *American Journal of Epidemiology* Web site (http://aje.oupjournals.org/) and search for articles that contain "oral cancer" in the title or abstract. Read one article relating to risk factors for oral cancer. What risk factors were studied? What type of study design was used? What was the association between the risk factor and oral cancer?
3. The Cochrane Collaboration maintains a research glossary for consumers. Go to this glossary on the Web (http://www.cochrane.org/ cochrane/cngloss.htm) and look up the terms *epidemiology, case-control,* and *cohort.* Look up three other terms not included in this chapter. Define the three additional terms and briefly describe how they relate to dental public health.
4. Oral epidemiology is a viable career for dental hygienists. Go to the University of North Carolina's Oral Epidemiology PhD Program Web site and look at career options for oral epidemiologists (http://www.dent.unc.edu/ academic/programs/ade/epid/).

Review Questions

1. When a disease is constantly and consistently present in a population it is referred to as:
   a. pandemic.
   b. prevalent.
   c. epidemic.
   d. incident.
   e. endemic.
2. When the incidence of a disease is unusually high for a population it is referred to as:
   a. pandemic.
   b. prevalent.

c. epidemic.

d. incident.

e. endemic.

3. Although a triangle has three sides, the epidemiologic triangle actually consists of four parts. Which of the following is not part of the epidemiologic triangle?

a. Time

b. Confounding variable

c. Environment

d. Agent

e. Host

4. Rates of death are called:

a. Morton rates.

b. mortuary rates.

c. mortality rates.

d. morbidity rates.

e. proportion rates.

5. Which of the following describes the number of new disease cases that have occurred during a specific period?

a. Incidence

b. Mortality

c. Proportion

d. Analytic

e. Prevalence

6. Incidence rates are generally used to describe the amount of dental caries in the United States. True or False?

7. Which study design is usually the first step in looking at a disease?

a. Experimental

b. Longitudinal

c. Prospective

d. Descriptive

e. Cohort

8. Which study design follows a group of individuals forward in time?

a. Retrospective cohort

b. Prospective cohort

c. Cross-sectional

d. Retrospective case-control

e. Horizontal cohort

9. The goal of any diagnostic or screening test is to have:

a. Sensitivity, 0%; Specificity, 0%

b. Sensitivity, 100%; Specificity, 0%

c. Sensitivity, 0%; Specificity, 100%

d. Sensitivity and Specificity, 100%

e. Sensitivity and Specificity, 50%

REFERENCES

1. American Dental Education Association. Competencies for entry into the profession of dental hygiene, exhibit 7. J Dent Ed 2003; July;67(7):1–5. Available at: http://www.adea.org/cepr. Accessed January 2004.

2. Mausner JS, Kramer S. Epidemiology—An Introductory Text. Philadelphia, PA: W.B. Saunders, 1985.

3. Snow J. On the Mode of Communication of Cholera. 2nd ed. London, England: John Churchill, 1860. (Facsimile of 1936 reprinted edition by Hafner, New York, 1965.)

4. Black GV, McKay FS. Mottled teeth: an endemic development imperfection of the enamel of the teeth heretofore unknown in the literature of dentistry. Dent Cosmos 1916; 58:129–156.

5. Smith MC, Lantz E, Smith HV. The cause of mottled enamel. J Dent Res 1932;12:149-159.

6. Salvi GE, Lawrence HP, Offenbacher S, Beck JD. Influence of risk factors on the pathogenesis of periodontitis. Periodont 2000 1997;14:173–201.

7. Tonette MS. Cigarette smoking and periodontal diseases: etiology and management of disease. Ann Periodontol 1998;3:88–101.

8. Gelskey SC. Cigarette smoking and periodontitis: methodology to assess the strength of evidence in support of a causal association. Community Dent Oral Epidemiol 1999; 27:16–24.

9. Tomar SL, Asma S. Smoking-attributable periodontitis in the United States: finding from NHANES III. J Periodont 2000;71:743–751.

10. Beneson AS, ed. Control of Communicable Diseases In Man. 14th Ed. Washington, DC: The American Public Health Association, 1985.

11. National Center for Health Statistics. FastStats AtoZ: Hypertension. Available at: http://www.cdc.gov/nchs/fastats/hyprtens.htm. Accessed November 2003.

12. National Center for Health Statistics. FastStats AtoZ: Cancer. Available at: http://www.cdc.gov/nchs/fastats/cancer.htm. Accessed November 2003.

13. Brown LJ, Brunelle JA, Kingman A. Periodontal status in the United States, 1988-91: prevalence, extent, and demographic variation. J Dent Res 1996;75(Spec Iss):672–683.
14. Rothman KJ. Epidemiology: An Introduction. New York: Oxford University Press, 2002.
15. Brailsford SR, Fiske J, Gilbert S, Clark D, Beighton D. The effects of the combination of chlorhexidine/thymol- and fluoride-containing varnishes on the severity of root caries lesions in frail institutionalised elderly people. J Dent 2002; 30:319–324.
16. Last JM. A Dictionary of Epidemiology. 4th Ed. New York, NY: Oxford University Press, 2001.
17. Seeley DG, Browner WS, Nevitt MC, et al. Which fractures are associated with low appendicular bone mass in elderly women? The Study of Osteoporotic Fractures Research Group. Ann Intern Med 1991; 115:837–842.
18. Hillier S, Cooper C, Kellingray S, et al. Fluoride in drinking water and risk of hip fracture in the UK: A case-control study. Lancet 2000;355:265–269.
19. Schiffman M, Herrero R, Hildesheim A, et al. HPV DNA testing in cervical cancer screening: results from women in a high risk province of Costa Rica. JAMA 2000;283:87–93.

Oral Disease Patterns in the United States

12

Objectives

After studying this chapter and completing the study questions and activities, the learner will be able to:

- Describe trends in overall oral health during the last 20 years.
- Describe the prevalence of dental caries and dental fluorosis in U.S. children.
- Describe the prevalence of dental caries, periodontitis, and tooth loss in U.S. adults.
- Describe the prevalence of oral and pharyngeal cancer in the United States.
- Outline the disparities in oral health status in the United States.
- Discuss the determinants of oral disease in humans.

KEY TERMS

Behavioral Risk Factor
   Surveillance System (BRFSS)
Cleft lip
Cleft palate
Dental caries
Dental fluorosis

Federal poverty level
Gingivitis
National Health and Nutrition
   Examination Survey (NHANES)
Oral and pharyngeal cancer
Orofacial pain

Periodontitis
Tooth loss
Total tooth loss
Trends
U.S. National Fluorosis Survey

The American Dental Education Association competencies addressed in this chapter include[1]:

HP.4:   Identify individual and population risk factors and develop strategies that promote a health-related quality of life.

CM.1:   Assess the oral health needs of the community and the quality and availability of resources and services.

Introduction

Between 1971 and 1974, the National Center for Health Statistics of the Centers for Disease Control and Prevention conducted the first **National Health and Nutrition Examination Survey** (NHANES I)—a nationwide survey designed to measure and monitor indicators of nutrition and health among U.S. citizens. Data from the third NHANES survey—NHANES III—were collected between 1988 and 1994. Because both of these surveys included a comprehensive dental component, the information obtained can be used to evaluate the current oral health status of the U.S. population, in addition to evaluating changes in oral health status over time (**trends**). Using data from NHANES and other sources, this chapter focuses on the current oral health status of the U.S. population, together with trends in oral health status over time. In addition, this chapter highlights those population subgroups identified as having oral health disparities. The reader should note that the oral health data from NHANES IV (collected between 1999 and 2003) is scheduled for release in 2004.

DENTAL CARIES

Dental Caries in Children

During the 15 or so years between NHANES I and NHANES III, there was a significant decrease in the total amount of **dental caries** experienced by U.S. school children (≥ 6 years) along with an increase in the proportion of caries-free children. As presented in Figure 12-1, the number of decayed, missing, and filled permanent teeth (DMFT) in children aged 6 to 18 years decreased by approximately 59%—from 4.44 in 1971–1974 to 1.90 in 1988–1994. A similar, although less dramatic, decrease of about 45% was seen in the number of decayed and filled primary teeth (dft)

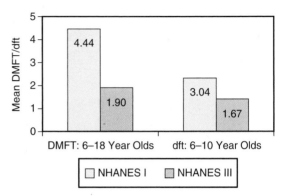

FIGURE 12-1 Mean DMFT and dft for Children Aged 6–18 and Aged 2–10. NHANES I (1971–1974) and NHANES III (1988–1994).[2]

among children aged 6 to 10 years (3.04 in 1971–1974 to 1.67 in 1988–1994). Although caries rates declined in U.S. school children age 6 and older, preschool children aged 2 to 5 years did not experience the same substantial decline. In fact, low-income preschool children saw a slight increase in caries rates.[2]

In addition to a decline in total decay experience, the amount of untreated decay in U.S. children also decreased. Overall, the number of decayed permanent teeth among children aged 6 to 18 years decreased by 77%—from 1.43 in 1971–1974 to 0.33 in 1988–1994.[3] For younger children, aged 2 to 10 years, the number of decayed primary teeth decreased by 56%—from 1.42 to 0.63.

Although there has been a reduction in overall caries rates, the reduction has not occurred evenly across all tooth surfaces. The reduction has been proportionately greater in interproximal and smooth surfaces than in pit and fissure surfaces. For all age, sex, race, and ethnic groups, the occlusal surface is the most commonly filled or decayed tooth surface.

Although national surveys have demonstrated a decline in the overall level of clinically detectable dental caries in U.S. children, caries is still one of the most common childhood diseases—five times as common as asthma and seven times as common as hay fever in 5 to 17 year olds.[4] Dental caries, however, is not evenly distributed among U.S. children. About 80% of permanent teeth affected by caries are found in about 25% of children aged 5 to 17 years.[5] In the United States, dental caries in both the primary and permanent dentition is disproportionately concentrated in children from low-income households and ethnic minority groups. This is especially true for untreated decay. This disproportional concentration of caries in low-income and minority populations is referred to as an oral health disparity.

Figure 12-2 presents the proportion of children with untreated decay in their primary and permanent teeth stratified by income level, using 200% of the **Federal Poverty Level** (FPL) as the income cut point. Compared with higher income children (income above 200% FPL), a higher proportion of lower income children (income at or below 200% FPL) have untreated decay. For children aged 2 to 5 years, 27% of lower income children have untreated decay in their primary dentition compared with 9% of higher income children. A similar difference can be seen in the permanent teeth of adolescents aged 15 to 18 years— 32% of the lower income children have untreated decay compared with 17% of the higher income children.[6]

Differences in the proportion of children with decay experience and untreated decay, stratified by race and ethnicity, is presented in Table 12-1. Compared with non-Hispanic White children, Hispanic, African American, and American Indian or Alaska Native children are more likely to have both decay experience and untreated decay.

Dental Sealants

As previously stated, the decline in childhood caries has been disproportionately higher in smooth surfaces compared with pit and fissure surfaces. For this reason, dental sealants continue to play an important role in the prevention of caries. Until recently, the prevalence of dental sealants in U.S. children has been relatively low.

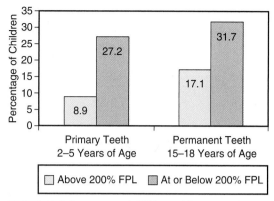

FIGURE 12-2 Percentage of Children With Untreated Decay by Income Level, NHANES III (1988–1994).[6]

In 1988–1994, 23% of children age 8 and 15% of children age 14 had at least one dental sealant on a permanent molar.[7] Although current national data are not available, data from state oral health surveys suggest that the prevalence of sealants has increased during the last 10 to 15 years. The Washington State Department of Health conducted a statewide oral health survey in both 1994 and 2000. In 1994, 19% of Washington's second grade children had a dental sealant compared with 41% in 2000.[8] Other state surveys have found the prevalence of sealants in third grade children ranges from 14–66%, with the majority of states reporting a prevalence of between 40–50%.[9]

Similar to dental caries, there are disparities in access to and prevalence of preventive dental sealants. On a national level, a significantly higher percentage of non-Hispanic Whites have sealants in comparison with their non-Hispanic Black and Mexican American counterparts.[10]

Dental Caries in Adults

When considering the distribution of dental caries in adults, a distinction must be made between coronal and root caries. In terms of coronal caries, most dentate adults have some evidence of treated or untreated decay. Of the dentate adults (≥18 years) examined in NHANES III (1988–1994),

TABLE 12-1 PERCENTAGE OF CHILDREN WITH DECAY EXPERIENCE AND UNTREATED DECAY STRATIFIED BY RACE AND ETHNICITY

	PERCENTAGE WITH DECAY EXPERIENCE			PERCENTAGE WITH UNTREATED DECAY		
	2–4 YEARS	6–8 YEARS	15 YEARS	2–4 YEARS	6–8 YEARS	15 YEARS
TOTAL	18	52	61	16	29	20
White non-Hispanic+	13	49	61	11	22	18
African American+	24	49	69	22	35	28
Mexican American+	27	68	57	24	43	27
American Indian or Alaska Native++	76	91	88	68	72	69

Source: Healthy People 2010 Database. Available at: http://wonder.cdc.gov/data2010. Accessed November 2003.[7]

+ NHANES III, 1988–1994

++ Oral Health Survey of Native American Dental Patients, 1999

94% had experienced coronal caries. Figure 12-3 presents the mean number of decayed and filled surfaces (DFS) for dentate adults, stratified by age and sex. As age increases, mean DFS also increases, until age 70 and older when it decreases slightly. In persons aged 20 to 29 years, mean DFS was 11.8; DFS was 30.7 in those aged 60 to 69 years. For each age-group between 20 to 59 years, females had a higher mean DFS than males, although males were more likely to have a higher percentage of untreated coronal surfaces.

Unlike children, differences in overall caries rates between adults of different racial/ethnic groups were not found in NHANES III. There were, however, racial and ethnic disparities in the number of surfaces with untreated decay. Non-Hispanic Whites had significantly fewer decayed surfaces (1.5) compared with non-Hispanic Blacks (3.4) or Mexican Americans (2.8).[11]

As would be expected, root caries prevalence increases significantly with age. Overall, 23% of dentate adults had root caries; with a low of 7% in persons aged 18 to 24 years and a high of 56% in those aged 75 years or older. As with coronal caries, non-Hispanic Whites had significantly fewer decayed root surfaces (0.6) compared with non-Hispanic Blacks (1.5) or Mexican Americans

(1.2).[11] Unlike coronal caries, however, more men (27.1%) than women (23.3%) had evidence of root caries.

As with decay rates in children, the amount of coronal caries in younger adults decreased during the last several decades. Among adults aged 18 to 45 years, the mean DMFS decreased from 38.3 in 1971–1974 to 27.9 in 1988–1994; a decline of

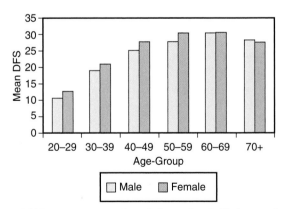

FIGURE 12-3 Mean number of decayed and filled coronal surfaces (DFS) by age and sex (U.S. population aged 20 years and older, 1988–1994). (Source: NIDCR/CDC Dental, Oral and Craniofacial Data Resource Center. NHANES III. Available at: http://drc.nidcr.nih.gov. Accessed February 2004.)

27.3%.[12] When stratified by age, the youngest age cohort had the most improvement, with a 44% decline in persons aged 18 to 24 years, a 39% decline in those aged 36 to 35 years, and a 21% decrease for adults aged 36 to 45 years. A decline in caries was noted in all racial and income subgroups.

Although total caries declined among people aged 45 years and younger, declines in caries experience among adults aged 46 to 65 years were not observed. In fact, there was a slight increase in mean DMFS between the early 1970s and the early 1990s. The small increase in mean DMFS from NHANES I to NHANES III consisted of a decreased number of decayed and missing surfaces and an increased number of filled surfaces.

Risk Factors

As previously stated, children from low-income and minority populations have a higher prevalence of dental caries and the prevalence and severity of caries in adults tends to increase with age and vary by gender. Dental caries is a complex, multifactorial disease and several other factors have been associated with the prevalence of dental caries in both children and adults. Salivary flow and composition play an important role in dental caries,[13] as does an individual's diet and intake of fermentable carbohydrates in foods and beverages.[14] Because caries is the result of a bacterial infection, the types and amounts of oral bacteria influence caries rates,[15] and limited data suggest that there may also be familial tendencies or genetic influences.[16] Last, but not least, is the important role of fluoride in the prevention of dental caries.[17]

DENTAL FLUOROSIS

With the substantial decline in the prevalence and severity of dental caries among U.S. children and young adults, there has been a corresponding increase in the prevalence of **dental fluorosis.** The **U.S. National Fluorosis Survey,** conducted by the National Institute of Dental Research in 1986–1987, found that 22% of children aged 7 years and older had some degree of dental fluoro-

sis, with the majority of the cases (76%) classified as very mild.[18] Approximately 16% of children in fluoride-deficient communities had fluorosis compared with 29% in fluoridated communities.

An in-depth review of all published studies of the prevalence and severity of enamel fluorosis in North American children, found a clear increase in fluorosis among populations with drinking water containing less than 0.3 ppm fluoride.[19] This same review also found that an increase in the prevalence of fluorosis in those drinking optimally fluoridated water likely has occurred as well; although the evidence for such a trend is not as clear as for fluoride-deficient communities.

Risk Factors

It is well documented that the prevalence of fluorosis is a direct result of the amount of fluoride ingested during tooth development, although some animal studies suggest the possibility of a genetic predisposition to dental fluorosis.[20] Excess fluoride ingestion may come from various sources, including fluoridated toothpaste, fluoride supplements, fluoridated water, or a combination of sources.

PERIODONTAL DISEASE

When the epidemiology of periodontal diseases is considered, a distinction must be made between **gingivitis** and **periodontitis.** Gingivitis is a reversible inflammation of the gingival tissue, which is generally assessed in community-based studies by the presence or absence of gingival bleeding. In populations, gingivitis is found in early childhood and becomes more prevalent and severe in adolescence, with the prevalence leveling off somewhat after adolescence.[21] The NHANES III survey found that 73% of adolescents aged 13 to 17 years had at least one site with gingival bleeding. The prevalence of gingival bleeding decreased to 66% of young adults aged 18 to 24 years and then stayed at about 60–63% in adults aged 25 years and older.[22] It is generally believed that the prevalence of gingivitis has declined over recent years in the United States, mainly because of greater attention to oral hygiene.[23]

The prevalence and severity of periodontitis in the United States is assessed in national surveys by evaluating clinical loss of attachment (LOA) and pocket depth (PD) at the mesiobuccal and mid-buccal sites of one mandibular and one maxillary quadrant. NHANES III found that approximately 26% of persons aged 20 years or older had destructive periodontal disease, defined as having a loss of attachment at one or more sites of at least 4 mm. The prevalence of more advanced attachment loss (≥5mm) increased with age, ranging from 1% of young adults aged 20 to 24 years to 40% of seniors aged 70 years and older (Fig. 12-4).

In regard to periodontal pocketing, 29% of persons aged 13 years or older had periodontal pockets of ≥4 mm, while 4% had pockets of ≥6 mm. Unlike clinical loss of attachment, there was not a clear increase in the prevalence of periodontal pockets with age (Fig. 12-5), although persons older than 45 had a slightly higher percentage of sites with deep pockets.[22]

For all ages, females tended to have better periodontal health. Forty-two percent of males compared with 37% of females had loss of attachment

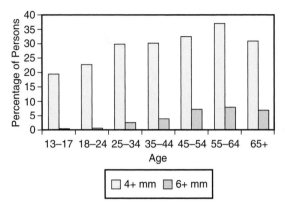

FIGURE 12-5 Prevalence of Pocket Depth of ≥4 mm and ≥6 mm by Age (U.S. population, aged 13 years and older, 1988–1991.[22]

of ≥3 mm, while 33% of males compared with 25% of females had periodontal pockets of ≥4 mm. With regard to race and ethnicity, non-Hispanic Whites exhibited better periodontal health than either non-Hispanic Blacks or Mexican Americans. Twenty-seven percent of non-Hispanic Whites compared with 44% of non-Hispanic Blacks and 34% of Mexican Americans had periodontal pockets of ≥4 mm.[22]

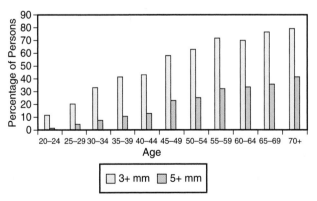

FIGURE 12-4 Prevalence of Clinical Loss of Attachment of ≥3 mm and ≥5 mm by Age (U.S. population, aged 20 years and older, 1988–1994). (Source: NIDCR/CDC Dental, Oral and Craniofacial Data Resource Center, NHANES III. Available at: http://drc.nidcr.nih.gov. Accessed February 2004)

Risk Factors

Smoking is a major risk factor in the United States for periodontitis, and a report suggests that smoking may be responsible for more than one half of all periodontitis cases among adults.[24] Other known risk factors include several systemic diseases, including Chediak-Higashi syndrome, Down syndrome, Ehlers- Danlos syndrome, and Papillon-Lefevre syndrome. In addition, insulin dependent diabetes and acquired immunodeficiency syndrome (AIDS) may exacerbate the effects of existing disease.[23]

TOOTH LOSS IN ADULTS

During the past several decades, there has been a steady decline in the prevalence of **tooth loss** and **total tooth loss** (edentulism) in the United States.[25] In the 30-year period from 1958–1988, the prevalence of total tooth loss in adults aged 75 years and older declined by 34% from 67% in 1957–1958[26] to 44% in 1988–1991.[11] The most current information on total tooth loss in the United States is from the **Behavioral Risk Factor Surveillance System (BRFSS).**[27] The 1999 BRFSS survey found that 24% of adults aged 65 years and older were edentulous, with the prevalence varying by education, sex, income, and race (Table 12-2). In general, older adults who have less than 12 years of education or have an annual income of less than $15,000 have a higher prevalence of total tooth loss.

In terms of tooth retention, NHANES III found that 90% of adults aged 18 years and older were dentate, while 30% had retained all 28 teeth. As would be expected, age is strongly related to both tooth retention and tooth loss. Adults between ages 18 to 24 years have an average of 27.1 teeth; persons aged 50 to 54 years average 18.7 teeth; and those 75 years or older average 9.0 teeth. The prevalence of total tooth loss increases from 12% in persons aged 50 to 54 years to 44% in those 75 years or older.[28]

TABLE 12-2 PERCENTAGE OF PEOPLE (AGE 65 AND OLDER) WHO HAVE LOST ALL NATURAL PERMANENT TEETH (UNITED STATES, 1999)

	HAVE LOST ALL NATURAL PERMANENT TEETH (EDENTULOUS)	HAVE NOT LOST ALL NATURAL PERMANENT TEETH (NOT EDENTULOUS)
United States, Total	24.4	75.6
<12 Years of Education	41.7	58.3
12 Years of Education	25.4	74.6
>12 Years of Education	13.8	86.2
Male	21.6	78.4
Female	26.4	73.6
<$15,000 Annual Income	40.4	59.6
≥$15,000 Annual Income	19.7	80.3
White, non-Hispanic	24.2	75.8
Black, non-Hispanic	32.7	67.3
Hispanic	19.2	80.8

Source: Complete Tooth Loss. National Oral Health Surveillance System, Centers for Disease Control and Prevention. Available at: http://www.cdc.gov/nohss. Accessed February 2004.[27]

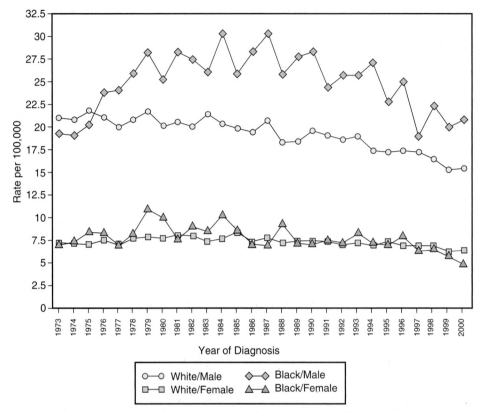

FIGURE 12-6 Trends in Incidence of Cancer of the Oral Cavity and Pharynx. (Source: SEER*Stat Database: Incidence. SEER 9 Regs Public-Use, Nov. 2002, Sub [1973–2000]. National Cancer Institute, DCCPS, Surveillance Research Program, Cancer Statistics Branch; released April 2003, based on November 2002 submission.)[32]

ORAL AND PHARYNGEAL CANCER

Cancer of the oral cavity and pharynx, which represents 3–4% of all cancers in the United States, includes tumors of the lip, tongue, gingival tissue, floor of the mouth, soft and hard palate, tonsils, salivary glands, oropharynx, nasopharynx, hypopharynx, and other less frequent sites.[29] In 2001, it was estimated that **oral and pharyngeal cancer** would account for 30,100 new cases and 7,800 deaths in the United States.[30] Except for salivary gland tumors, which are rare, almost all oral cancers are squamous cell carcinomas. The overall 5-year relative survival for oral cancer has remained stable at 40–50% for several decades.[31]

In Americans, oral cancer is two to three times more common among males than females, and more than 90% of cases occur in persons older than age 45.[31] Like most epithelial tumors, risk of oral cancer increases with age. This cancer occurs more frequently in Blacks than Whites. During 1992–2000, the average annual age-adjusted incidence rate for oral cancer in the United States was 17.0 cases per 100,000 persons/year among White men; 6.8 among White women; 22.8 among Black men; and 6.5 among Black women (Fig. 12-6).[32] In this country, differences in alcohol and tobacco use account for most of the racial differences in oral cancer.[33] As with incidence rates, mortality

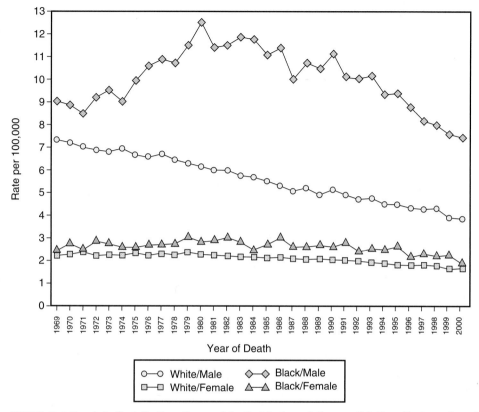

FIGURE 12-7 Trends in Mortality From Cancer of the Oral Cavity and Pharynx: U.S. Mortality Age-Adjusted Rates, Total United States (1969–2000). (Source: SEER*Stat Database: Mortality. All COD, Public-Use with State, Total U.S. [1969–2000]. National Cancer Institute, DCCPS, Surveillance Research Program, Cancer Statistics Branch, released April 2003. Underlying mortality data provided by NCHS [www.cdc.gov/nchs].)[32]

rates for oral and pharyngeal cancer are highest among Black males, followed by White males (Fig. 12-7).

Risk Factors

Tobacco and alcohol account for approximately three fourths of all oral cancers in the United States, and recent epidemiologic evidence indicates that smoking and drinking are independent risk factors for oral cancer that produce a synergistic effect when combined.[34] In some parts of the country, smokeless tobacco use contributes to the high rate of gum and buccal cancers.[35]

In addition to tobacco and alcohol, other potential risk factors for oral cancer include exposure to certain viruses (e.g., human papilloma, herpes simplex, Epstein-Barr),[36] exposure to sun for lip cancer,[37] and use of marijuana.[38] Nutritional factors, particularly the consumption of fresh fruits and vegetables, appear to be associated with decreased risk for these cancers.[39]

OTHER ORAL CONDITIONS

In 2000, approximately 3,259 babies were born with **cleft lip** and/or **cleft palate,** for a rate of 82.1 per 100,000 live births.[40] The rate for White mothers was 89.2 per 100,000, while the rate for Black mothers was 46.0 per 100,000 live births. The causes of cleft lip/palate are not well understood. Studies suggest that several genes and environmental factors, such as drugs, infection, maternal illness, maternal smoking and alcohol use and, possibly, vitamin B (folic acid) deficiency may be involved.[41]

In 1989, the National Health Interview Survey included a series of questions regarding **orofacial pain.** About 14% of the dentate adults reported having tooth pain during the past 6 months. As with other oral conditions, the prevalence of pain is higher in minority, low-income, and low-education groups. Thirteen percent of non-Hispanic Whites reported tooth pain compared with 16% of non-Hispanic Blacks and Hispanics. With regard to income, 21% of those below the FPL reported tooth pain compared with 13% of those above the FPL. Of adults with less than a high school education, 16% reported pain compared with 14% of those with a high school educa-

tion and 12% of those with higher than a high school education.[42,43]

SUMMARY

During the last 40 years, significant improvements have been made in the oral health of U.S. citizens— for both children and adults. Caries rates have declined, the prevalence of gingivitis is lower, more adults are keeping their teeth longer, and mortality rates from oral cancer are becoming lower. Despite these improvements, certain segments of the population continue to experience oral health disparities. Low-income and minority children carry the burden of dental caries, low-income and minority adults are more likely to have untreated decay, and African American men have a higher incidence of oral and pharyngeal cancer. To see continued improvements in the oral health of Americans, efforts must be made to address and resolve the oral health disparities outlined in this chapter.

 Learning Activities

1. This chapter presents data from NHANES I and NHANES III. In 2004, the NHANES IV oral health component will be released. Go to the NHANES Web site (http://www.cdc.gov/nchs/nhanes.htm) and look up the most current oral health data. Have dental decay rates in children continued to decline?

2. The Centers for Disease Control and Prevention maintains a Web site that tracks data related to the Healthy People 2010 objectives. Go to this Web site and select the oral health focus area (http://wonder.cdc.gov/data 2010/). Compare the baseline data and target data for

untreated decay in children aged 2 to 4, 6 to 8, and 15.

3. Look closely at Figures 12-6 and 12-7. Describe trends in oral cancer incidence and mortality rates over the last 30 years for Black males and White males.

4. Smoking is a significant risk factor for both periodontitis and oral cancer. For your next five adult patients who smoke, calculate the amount of time you talked with them about oral hygiene and smoking cessation. What did you spend more time talking about and why?

Review Questions

1. There has been a substantial decrease in the total amount of dental caries experienced by U.S. children aged 6 to 18 years; however, the amount of untreated decay has not changed. True or False?

2. Eighty percent of permanent teeth affected by caries can be found in what percentage of children aged 5 to 17 years?
   a. 45%
   b. 35%
   c. 25%
   d. 15%
   e. 5%

3. About twice as many low-income children have untreated decay compared with high-income children.
   a. True
   b. False

4. Which of the following groups of adults tend to have higher levels of coronal caries experience?
   a. Males
   b. Females
   c. Non-Hispanic Blacks
   d. Mexican Americans
   e. Hispanic Blacks

5. There has been a substantial decline in caries experience in all age-groups in the United States.
   a. True
   b. False

6. Which of the following describes trends in dental fluorosis?
   a. The prevalence has decreased.
   b. The prevalence has remained stable.
   c. The majority of dental fluorosis cases can be classified as very mild.
   d. The prevalence of fluorosis is lower in fluoridated communities compared with fluoride-deficient communities.
   e. Most dental fluorosis cases can be classified as moderate.

7. Which of the following groups has the highest prevalence and severity of gingivitis?
   a. Preschool children
   b. Elementary school children
   c. Adolescents
   d. Young adults
   e. Older adults

8. The prevalence of periodontal pocketing increases substantially with age.
   a. True
   b. False

9. Which of the following groups of adults tend to have lower levels of periodontal disease?
   a. Males
   b. Females
   c. Non-Hispanic Blacks
   d. Mexican Americans
   e. Hispanic Blacks

REFERENCES

1. American Dental Education Association. Competencies for entry into the profession of dental hygiene, exhibit 7. J Dent Ed 2003;July;67(7):1–5. Available at: http://www.adea.org/cepr. Accessed January 2004.
2. Brown LJ, Wall TP, Lazar V. Trends in total caries experience: permanent and primary teeth. J Amer Dent Assoc 2000;131:223–231.
3. Brown LJ, Wall TP, Lazar V. Trends in untreated caries in permanent teeth of children 6 to 18 years old. J Amer Dent Assoc 1999;130:1637–1644.
4. Oral Health in America: A Report of the Surgeon General. Rockville, MD: U.S. Department of Health and Human Services, National Institute of Dental and Craniofacial Research, National Institutes of Health, 2000.
5. Kaste LM, Selwitz RH, Oldakowski JA, et al. Coronal caries in the primary and permanent dentition of children and adolescents 1–17 years of age: United States, 1988–1991. J Dent Res 1996;75(Special Issue):631–641.
6. Vargas CM, Crall JJ, Schneider DA. Sociodemographic distribution of pediatric dental caries: NHANES III, 1988–1994. J Amer Dent Assoc 1998;129:1229–1238.
7. Data 2010 . . . The Healthy People 2010 Database. Centers for Disease Control and Prevention. Available at: http://wonder.cdc.gov/data2010. Accessed November 2003.

8. Smile Survey 2000. Olympia, WA: Washington State Department of Health, 2001. Available at: http://www.doh.wa.gov/Publicat/smilesurvey.pdf. Accessed November 2003.

9. Dental Sealants. National Oral Health Surveillance System, Centers for Disease Control and Prevention. Available at: http://www.cdc.gov/nohss. Accessed November 2003.

10. Selwitz RH, Winn DM, Kingman A, Zion GR. The prevalence of dental sealants in the U.S. population: findings from NHANES III, 1988–1991. J Dent Res 1996; 75 (Special Issue):652–660.

11. Winn DM, Brunelle JA, Selwitz RH, et al. Coronal and root caries in the dentition of adults in the United States, 1988–1991. J Dent Res 1996;75(Special Issue):642–651.

12. Brown LJ, Wall TP, Lazar V. Trends in caries among adults 18 to 45 years old. J Amer Dent Assoc 2002;133:827–834.

13. Lamkin MS, Oppenheim FG. Structural features of salivary function. Crit Rev Oral Biol Med 1993;4:251–259.

14. Featherstone JDB. The science and practice of caries prevention. J Am Dent Assoc 2000;131:887–899.

15. Loesche WJ. Role of *Streptococcus mutans* in human dental decay. Microbiol Rev 1986;50:353–380.

16. Shuler CF. Inherited risks for susceptibility to dental caries. J Dent Educ 2001;65:1038–1045.

17. National Institutes of Health. Diagnosis and management of dental caries throughout life. NIH Consensus Statement 2001;18:1–23.

18. Brunelle JA. The prevalence of dental fluorosis in U.S. children, 1987 [Abstract]. J Dent Res 1989;68(Special Issue):995.

19. Rozier RG. The prevalence and severity of enamel fluorosis in North American children. J Public Health Dent 1999;59:239–246.

20. Everett ET, McHenry MA, Reynolds N, et al. Dental fluorosis: variability among different inbred mouse strains. J Dent Res 2002;81:794–798.

21. Stamm JW. Epidemiology of gingivitis. J Clin Periodontol 1986;13:360–370.

22. Brown LJ, Brunelle JA, Kingman A. Periodontal status in the United States, 1988–1991. Prevalence, extent and demographic variation. J Dent Res 1996;75(Special Issue): 672–683.

23. Anonymous. Epidemiology of periodontal diseases [Position paper]. J Periodontol 1996;67:935–945.

24. Tomar SL, Asma S. Smoking-attributable periodontitis in the United States: findings from NHANES III. J Periodontol 2000;71:743–751.

25. Weintraub JA, Burt BA. Oral health status in the United States: tooth loss and edentulism. J Dent Educ 1985; 49:368–378.

26. U.S. Public Health Service. Loss of teeth: United States, June 1957–June 1958. PHS Pub. No. 584-B22, Series B No. 22. Washington DC: Government Printing Office, 1960.

27. Complete tooth loss, United States. National Oral Health Surveillance System, Centers for Disease Control and Prevention. Available at: http://www.cdc.gov/nohss. Accessed November 2003.

28. Marcus SE, Drury TF, Brown LJ, Zion GR. Tooth retention and tooth loss in the permanent dentition of adults: United States, 1988–1991. J Dent Res 1996;75(Special Issue):684–695.

29. Silverman S. Oral Cancer. Hamilton, London: BC Decker, 1998.

30. Greenlee RT, Hill-Harmon MB, Murray T, Thun N. Cancer statistics, 2001. CA Cancer J Clin 2001;55:15–36.

31. Day GL. Cancer rates and risks: oral cavity and pharynx. National Institutes of Health, National Cancer Institute. Available at: http://seer.cancer.gov/publications/raterisk/risks175.html. Accessed July 2003.

32. Surveillance, Epidemiology, and End Results (SEER) Program (www.seer.cancer.gov) SEER*Stat Database: Incidence–SEER 9 Regs Public-Use, Nov. 2002, Sub (1973–2000), National Cancer Institute, DCCPS, Surveillance Research Program, Cancer Statistics Branch, released April 2003, based on the November 2002 submission.

33. Day GL, Blot WJ, Austin DF, et al. Racial differences in risk of oral and pharyngeal cancer: alcohol, tobacco, and other determinants. J Nat Cancer Inst 1993;85:465–473.

34. Blot WJ, McLaughlin JK, Winn DM, et al. Smoking and drinking in relation to oral and pharyngeal cancer. Cancer Res 1988;48:282–287.

35. The health consequences of using smokeless tobacco. NIH Pub. No. 86-2874. Bethesda, MD: Department of Health and Human Services, 1986.

36. Blot WJ, McLaughlin JK, Devessa SS, Fraumeni JF. Cancers of the oral cavity and pharynx. In: Schottenfeld D, Fraumeni JFJ, eds. Cancer Epidemiology and Prevention. New York, NY: Oxford University Press, 1996.

37. Harras A, Edwards BK, Blot WJ, Ries LAG, eds. Cancer rates and risks. NIH Pub. No. 96-691. Bethesda, MD: National Cancer Institute, 1996.

38. Zang Z, Morgenstern H, Spritz MR, et al. Marijuana use and increased risk of squamous cell carcinoma of the head and neck. Cancer Epidemiol Biomarkers Prev 1999;8: 1071–1078.

39. McLaughlin JK, Gridley G, Block G, et al. Dietary factors in oral and pharyngeal cancer. J Nat Cancer Inst 1988; 80:1237–1243.

40. National Center for Health Statistics. FastStats: Birth Defects. Available at: http://www.cdc.gov/nchs/fastats/pdf/nvsr50_05t49.pdf. Accessed November 2003.

41. Cleft lip and cleft palate. March of Dimes. Available at http://www.marchofdimes.com. Accessed November 2003.

42. Lipton JA, Ship JA, Larach-Robinson D. Estimated prevalence and distribution of reported orofacial pain in the United States. J Am Dent Assoc 1993;124:115–21.

43. Vargas CM, Macek MD, Marcus SE. Sociodemographic correlates of tooth pain among adults: United States, 1989. Pain 2000;85:87–92.

Applying Epidemiology in Public Health Practice: Oral Health Surveillance

13

INTRODUCTION
VALIDITY AND RELIABILITY
SURVEILLANCE VERSUS CLINICAL DIAGNOSIS
MEASURING DENTAL CARIES
   Coronal Caries
   Root Caries
MEASURING PERIODONTAL STATUS
MEASURING DENTAL FLUOROSIS
MEASURING TREATMENT URGENCY

MEASURING TOOTH LOSS
MEASURING ORAL AND PHARYNGEAL CANCER
HOW TO COMPLETE A COMMUNITY-BASED
   ORAL HEALTH NEEDS ASSESSMENT
SUMMARY
LEARNING ACTIVITIES
RESOURCES
REVIEW QUESTIONS
REFERENCES

Objectives

After studying this chapter and completing the study questions and activities, the learner will be able to:

- Discuss the measures that can be used to assess the oral health status of a community.
- Compare and contrast the clinical measures used in oral health surveillance.
- Describe the basic steps necessary to complete an oral health needs assessment.

KEY TERMS

Basic Screening Survey (BSS)
Community Periodontal Index
   (CPI)
Dean's Fluorosis Index
df Index (df)
dmf Index (dmf)

DMF Index (DMF)
Gingival Index (GI)
Plaque Index (PlI)
Ramfjord Index Teeth
Reliability
Root Caries Index (RCI)

Simplified Oral Hygiene Index
   (OHI-S)
Surveillance
Tooth Surface Index of Fluorosis
   (TSIF)
Validity

The American Dental Education Association competencies addressed in this chapter include[1]:

C.7:   Provide quality assurance mechanisms for health services.

HP.4:   Identify individual and population risk factors and develop strategies that promote a health-related quality of life.

CM.1:   Assess the oral health needs of the community and the quality and availability of resources and services.

CM.6:   Evaluate the outcomes of community-based programs and plan for future activities.

Introduction

As described in earlier chapters, assessment is one of the three core public health functions, together with policy development and assurance. In public health dentistry, one key element of assessment is the ongoing monitoring of a community's oral health status. The process of ongoing monitoring is more commonly known as **surveillance,** defined by the Centers for Disease Control and Prevention as the ongoing systematic collection, analysis, and interpretation of outcome-specific data for use in the planning, implementation, and evaluation of public health practice.[2]

Information obtained through public health surveillance is used to assess public health status, define public health priorities, evaluate programs, and conduct research.[3] Simply, surveillance information tells you where the problems are, whom they affect, and where programmatic and prevention activities should be directed.

For an oral health surveillance system to be comparable between local, state, and national jurisdictions, it must be based on uniform data standards and measurements. This chapter presents standard methods for measuring dental caries, periodontal disease, dental fluorosis, treatment urgency, tooth loss, and other oral conditions in populations. The purpose of these measures is to describe the oral health of the community rather than the individual. For this reason, the methods outlined in this chapter are appropriate for public health practice but may have little value in a clinical setting with an individual patient. In addition, certain oral health measures or indices are useful in a clinical setting but are of little use in a community setting because they are too time consuming or have low reliability. Descriptions of indices for individual patients (e.g., Plaque Control Record, Eastman Interdental Bleeding Index) can be found in most clinical dental hygiene textbooks.

National and state level oral health surveillance data is maintained in the National Oral Health Surveillance System (NOHSS). NOHSS is a collaborative effort between the Association of State and Territorial Dental Directors (ASTDD) and the Centers for Disease Control and Prevention (CDC). Currently, there are eight oral health indicators included in NOHSS: caries experience, untreated caries, dental sealants, tooth loss, annual dental visits, teeth cleaning, fluoridation, and oral and pharyngeal cancer.

VALIDITY AND RELIABILITY

Most measures presented in this chapter are referred to as an "index." An index is a graduated, numeric scale that has upper and lower limits, with scores on the scale corresponding to specific criterion for individuals or populations. In general, the higher the index score, the more disease present. For an index to be useful in public health practice, it must be both valid and reliable (also referred to as **validity** and **reliability**). To be valid, it must measure what it is intended to measure. For this reason, levels of the index should correspond with the stages of the disease under study. For a gingivitis index to be valid, it must measure the prevalence and severity of gingivitis rather than the prevalence and severity of some other condition.

Reliability refers to the ability of an index to consistently measure the same level of disease at different times by different examiners under various conditions. Reliability can also be thought of as repeatability, reproducibility, and consistency. For an index to be considered reliable, two different examiners should be able to obtain the same score for the same person being examined.

All of the indices presented in this chapter are considered valid. They are also considered to be reliable if the examiners are trained and calibrated. Training and calibration is an essential component of any community-based oral health needs assessment. The purpose of training examiners is to ensure that each person involved in the assessment is making consistent clinical judgments and to ensure uniform interpretation, understanding, and application of the codes and criteria for the various indices used.

To better understand the concept of reliability, consider each of your clinical dental hygiene instructors. Most hygiene students would agree that some instructors view (or grade) a clinical case differently from other instructors. To make each instructor grade a case in a similar manner (i.e., reliably), the instructors must have extensive training and regular calibration.

SURVEILLANCE VERSUS CLINICAL DIAGNOSIS

Although dental public health surveillance activities often include an open-mouth examination, the examination process for surveillance and research differs significantly from a comprehensive clinical examination for the purpose of diagnosis and treatment planning. In most cases, a surveillance activity uses an abbreviated open-mouth examination, often referred to as a screening. A screening examination rarely includes radiographs and often looks at just one disease process, such as dental caries in children or periodontal disease in adults. In addition, most screenings do not include the use of a dental explorer and many only use a tongue blade and flashlight. For this reason, it is not appropriate to use screening examinations for the purpose of diagnosis or treatment planning. If a potential problem is identified during a screening, the individual should be referred to a dentist for a comprehensive examination.

It is also important to understand that surveillance activities can collect different levels of information at varying costs. For this reason, program budgets must be considered when deciding what type of information to collect. The more information collected, the more it will cost in terms of time for data collection, data entry, and data analysis.

MEASURING DENTAL CARIES

Dental caries is an infectious disease process that results in loss of tooth minerals (demineralization) on the outer surface of the tooth. If not controlled or remineralized at an early stage, caries can progress through the enamel, into the dentin, and eventually into the pulp. Dental caries occurs in both the primary and permanent dentitions and on both the coronal and root surfaces. Because of differences in the measurement of caries on coronal versus root surfaces, the measurement of each surface type will be addressed separately.

Coronal Caries

The traditional method for measuring caries experience—both present and past—on the coronal surface of the permanent dentition is the decayed, missing, and filled (DMF) Index. The **DMF Index,** which usually excludes the four third molars, counts either the number of teeth with a history of caries (DMFT: decayed, missing, and filled teeth) or the number of surfaces with a history of caries (DMFS: decayed, missing, and filled surfaces). After a systematic evaluation using a mouth mirror and good light source, each tooth or surface is scored as decayed, missing, or filled using the following diagnostic criteria: Decayed—loss of tooth structure at the enamel surface; Missing—tooth loss due to caries; and Filled—restorative treatment resulting from caries. Note that because teeth lost as a result of orthodontic extraction or injury are missing for reasons other than caries, they are not counted as missing in the DMF Index.

An individual's DMFT score will be a whole number, ranging from 0–28 (if third molars are excluded); an individual's DMFS score will also be a whole number, ranging from 0–128. When calculating a DMFS score, the 16 posterior teeth are considered to have five surfaces and the 12 anterior teeth to have four surfaces ($[16 \times 5] + [12 \times 4] = 128$). The mean DMF score for a community is the total DMF score for all individuals divided by the number of people in the community $([DMF^1 + DMF^2 + DMF^3 + ... + DMF^n] / n)$.

Although the DMF Index was designed to assess the coronal aspect of permanent dentition, it has been modified for use in primary dentition. The standard caries indices currently used in the primary dentition are the **df Index** and the **dmf Index.** The df Index counts either the number of decayed and filled primary teeth (dft) or the number of decayed and filled primary surfaces (dfs) (Box 13-1).

Because it is difficult to determine whether a primary tooth has been lost because of caries or natural exfoliation, missing teeth are not included in this index. The df Index is generally used in children who are beginning to exfoliate their primary teeth (≥5 years). Occasionally, you may see reference to the def (decayed, indicated for extraction, and filled) Index for caries in the primary dentition. The def Index will always have the same score as the df Index because the df Index combines decayed and indicated for extraction teeth into the same category. Most oral health surveillance programs will report a dft or dfs score rather than a deft or defs score.

The dmf Index can be used in children who have not yet reached the age of natural exfoliation (<5 years) to assess the number of teeth (dmft) or surfaces (dmfs) that are decayed, missing because of dental caries, or filled. The original description of the dmft/dmfs Index, published in 1944, described the index as only being used in children aged 7–12 years.[4] Today, the dmft/dmfs Index is generally used in preschool children, and the dft/dfs Index is used in children with mixed dentition. If you see reference to the dmft/dmfs only being used in older children, please note that this is no longer the case for oral health surveillance systems.

The benefit of using a DMF Index to measure dental caries is that it provides a measure of disease severity in addition to an estimate of disease prevalence. However, a dental public health program is usually only interested in prevalence rather than severity of dental caries. The appropri-

BOX 13-1 Use of Upper and Lower Case Letters for Dental Caries Indices

- Upper case letters are used when caries indices refer to permanent dentition, (e.g., DMFT, DMFS).
- Lower case letters are used when caries indices refer to primary dentition (e.g., dft, dfs, dmft, dmfs).

ate tool for measuring dental caries prevalence in a community is the **Basic Screening Survey (BSS),** developed by the Association of State and Territorial Dental Directors in 1999.[5] The BSS gathers information at a level consistent with monitoring the national health objectives found in the U.S. Public Health Service's Healthy People 2010 document. In other words, the BSS gathers information on a per-person basis rather than on a per-tooth or per-tooth-surface basis. Each person screened is classified in a dichotomous manner (e.g., yes or no) as to whether or not they have caries experience (at least one decayed tooth, restored tooth, or missing tooth) or untreated dental caries. The oral health status for a community or population is then presented as the percentage of the population that has caries experience and untreated decay. For example, a recent statewide survey of second and third grade children in Washington State found that 56% had caries experience and 21% had untreated decay.[6] Although the DMF Index differentiates between permanent and primary teeth (DMF/dmf), the Basic Screening Survey model does not differentiate between the two. For example, if a child is classified as having caries experience, the caries experience may be in their primary and/or permanent dentition. Note that for state level oral health data to be included in the NOHSS (www.cdc.gov/nohss), it must be based on a survey that followed the Basic Screening Survey model—DMF/dmf data are not included in the surveillance system.

The Association of State and Territorial Dental Directors (ASTDD) Basic Screening Survey model does have one indicator for the primary dentition only—early childhood caries. This indicator is designed for children age 3 years or younger. The six maxillary anterior teeth (central incisors, lateral incisors, and canines) are examined to determine if the child has untreated decay, a filling, or a tooth missing because of caries. If any of the six maxillary anterior teeth have caries experience, that child is classified as having early childhood caries.

Root Caries

A classification system similar to the DFT/DFS Index can be used to measure the prevalence and extent of root caries on exposed root surfaces. Each root or root surface is classified as being either decayed or filled. Unlike the indices for coronal caries, missing roots are not included in the total score for an individual. The problem with counting the number of decayed and/or filled roots is that the individual's score does not take into account the number of roots or root surfaces at risk. The **Root Caries Index** (RCI) is a measure of root caries that includes the number of exposed root surfaces as the denominator.[7] The RCI is calculated by adding the number of decayed and filled root surfaces and then dividing this number by the number of root surfaces with gingival recession. This resulting number is then presented as a percentage, which means that it is multiplied by 100 (Box 13-2). If a person has an RCI of 12%, it means that of their teeth with gingival recession, 12% of the root surfaces are either decayed or filled.

MEASURING PERIODONTAL STATUS

The **Community Periodontal Index (CPI)** is a quick, easy method for assessing and describing the overall periodontal status of a community.[8] The CPI, which is promoted by the World Health Organization and used throughout the world, eval-

---

BOX 13-2 Calculating the Root Caries Index[7]

$$\frac{\text{Decayed Root Surfaces} + \text{Filled Root Surfaces}}{\text{Number of Surfaces with Gingival Recession}} \times 100$$

---

uates three indicators of periodontal status—gingival bleeding, calculus, and periodontal pockets. It does not evaluate clinical loss of attachment. Until recently, the CPI was known as the Community Periodontal Index of Treatment Needs (CPITN). Changing patterns of periodontal treatment, however, have invalidated the treatment needs portion of the original index. For this reason, the index is now used to evaluate periodontal status rather than periodontal treatment needs.

The CPI uses a specially designed lightweight probe with a 0.5 mm ball tip and black bands between 3.5 and 5.5 mm and rings at 8.5 and 11.5 mm from the ball tip. In adults aged 20 years and older, 10 index teeth are evaluated: 2, 3, 8, 14, 15, 18, 19, 24, 30, and 31. In those younger than age 20, only six index teeth are examined: 3, 8, 14, 19, 24, and 30. After gently probing the index teeth, each tooth is scored according to the codes outlined in Box 13-3 and Figure 13-1.

In the early 1990s, a modified version of the CPITN—the Periodontal Screening and Recording (PSR)—was introduced in the United States.[9] The PSR is designed for use with individual patients in a clinical setting rather than for community periodontal status assessment.

Another approach to evaluating the periodontal status of a community is to separately measure each individual aspect of periodontal disease. Using this approach, each of the following aspects of periodontal health would be measured—gingival bleeding, recession or loss of periodontal attachment, pocket depth, and plaque and calculus

BOX 13-3 Community Periodontal Index—Codes and Criteria[8]

0:	Healthy
1:	Bleeding observed, directly or by using a mouth mirror, after probing
2:	Calculus detected during probing, but all of the black band on the probe visible
3:	Pocket 4–5 mm (gingival margin within the black band on the probe)
4:	Pocket 6 mm or more (black band on probe not visible)
X:	Excluded segment (less than two teeth present)
9:	Not recorded

(as contributing disease factors). Because collecting each aspect of periodontal health is time consuming and expensive, this approach is rarely used by public health programs. This approach to measuring periodontal health in a community-based population is usually limited to research projects.

One of the most commonly used indices for assessing gingival bleeding is the **Gingival Index (GI).**[10] With the GI, a periodontal probe is inserted about 2–3 mm into the sulcus and gently "swept" around the tooth, rather than being "walked" around the tooth. The mesial, distal, buccal, and lingual surfaces of each tooth are then given a score of 0–3, based on the criteria described in Box 13-4.

There are no specific indices designed to measure loss of periodontal attachment or pocket depth. The tools used to measure these aspects of periodontal health in community-based surveys are the same as those used to measure periodontal status in a clinical practice. However, the World Health Organization (WHO) suggests the use of an ordinal scale for recording loss of periodontal attachment similar to the ordinal scale used for the Community Periodontal Index. Box 13-5 lists the codes and criteria recommended by the WHO for recording loss of attachment in community-based surveys.

Two indices have commonly been used to measure the presence of plaque and calculus: (1) the **Simplified Oral Hygiene Index (OHI-S),** and (2) the **Plaque Index (PlI).** The OHI-S evaluates both supragingival and subgingival plaque

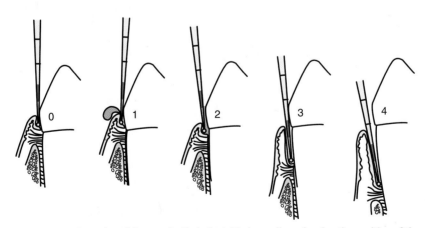

FIGURE 13-1 Examples of Community Periodontal Index coding, showing the position of the CPI probe (From: Oral Health Surveys Basic Methods. 4th Ed. Geneva, Switzerland; WHO, 1997. Reprinted by permission of the World Health Organization.)[8]

BOX 13-4 Gingival Index—Codes and Criteria[10]

0:   Normal gingiva
1:   Mild inflammation (slight edema and change in color; no bleeding on probing)
2:   Moderate inflammation (redness and edema; bleeding on probing)
3:   Severe inflammation (marked redness and edema; ulceration; tendency to spontaneous bleeding)

BOX 13-6 Plaque Index—Codes and Criteria[10]

0:   No plaque
1:   A film of plaque adhering to the free gingival margin and adjacent area of the tooth. The plaque may be recognized only by running a probe across the tooth surface.
2:   Moderate accumulation of soft deposits within the gingival pocket that can be seen with the naked eye or on the tooth and gingival margin.
3:   Abundance of soft matter within the gingival pocket and/or on the tooth and gingival margin.

and calculus on six teeth: 3, 11, 14, 19, 24, and 30. Although commonly used in the past, the OHI-S is becoming obsolete as periodontal research focuses more on subgingival rather than supragingival plaque and calculus as periodontitis risk factors.

The PlI was initially designed for use with the Gingival Index described earlier. As with the GI, the PlI scores the mesial, distal, buccal, and lingual surface of each tooth on a scale from 0–3, based on the thickness of plaque at the gingival margin. The scoring criteria for the PlI are shown in Box 13-6.

Completing a full-mouth periodontal status assessment on a group of individuals can be time consuming and cost prohibitive for many research projects and public health programs. For this reason, several methods have been developed that

BOX 13-5 Scoring Loss of Attachment (LOA)—Codes and Criteria[8]

0:   LOA, 0–3 mm
1:   LOA, 4–5 mm
2.   LOA, 6–8 mm
3:   LOA, 9–11 mm
4:   LOA, 12 mm or more
X: Excluded sextant
9:   Not recorded

evaluate only a subset of teeth in the mouth. One such method was developed in the 1950s by Dr. Sigurd P. Ramfjord.[11] Using this method, periodontal assessments are only completed on six teeth, known as the "Ramfjord Teeth" or the "**Ramfjord Index Teeth.**" These six teeth include the maxillary right first molar, left central incisor, left first premolar, mandibular left first molar, right central incisor, and right first premolar (or teeth 3, 9, 12, 19, 25, and 28).

The partial-mouth method used in the Third National Health and Nutrition Examination Survey (NHANES III) evaluated two randomly selected quadrants—one maxillary and one mandibular. For each tooth in these randomly selected quadrants, measures were taken at only two sites, the mesiobuccal and buccal. Although completing partial-mouth periodontal assessments are not appropriate for clinical settings because of the localized nature of periodontal disease, they do provide valuable and appropriate information for oral health surveillance and the monitoring of disease trends in populations.

When reading older dental literature regarding the prevalence and severity of periodontal disease, you may see references to periodontal indices not included in this section. Because our understanding of periodontal disease has changed significantly in the last 20 years, many previously used indices for measuring periodontal status are now obsolete. Three such obsolete indices are the Periodontal Index, Periodontal Disease Index, and the Papillary Marginal Attached (PMA) Index (although they may still be included in some dental hygiene textbooks).

MEASURING DENTAL FLUOROSIS

During tooth development, ingested fluoride becomes incorporated in the enamel structure of the tooth. If excessive amounts of fluoride are ingested, dental fluorosis can develop. Dental fluorosis is defined as hypomineralization of the dental enamel caused by excessive ingestion of fluoride during tooth development. The appearance of dental fluorosis varies, depending on the quantity and timing of fluoride ingestion. It can range from barely noticeable to noticeable brown staining and pitting of the enamel.

Several indices measure the prevalence and severity of dental fluorosis. The most common are Dean's Fluorosis Index[12] and the **Tooth Surface Index of Fluorosis (TSIF).**[13] With Dean's Fluorosis Index, the score for an individual is made on the basis of the two most affected teeth. If the two teeth are not equally affected, the score for the less affected of the two teeth is recorded. Although the Dean's Fluorosis Index only records the score for the two most affected teeth, the TSIF gives a score for each tooth surface in the mouth. The TSIF provides more comprehensive information on the amount and distribution of dental fluorosis for an individual; however, it is time consuming and the WHO recommends that community surveys use Dean's Fluorosis Index. The codes and criteria for Dean's Fluorosis Index and the TSIF are listed in Boxes 13-7 and 13-8.

MEASURING TREATMENT URGENCY

Many public health programs are not necessarily interested in the level of oral disease, but they may be interested in the proportion of the population that is in need of various levels of dental care. Two different organizations have developed criteria for quantifying treatment urgency. The first is the American Dental Association (ADA), which devel-

---

BOX 13-7   Dean's Fluorosis Index—Codes and Criteria[12]

0: **Normal**—The enamel surface is smooth, glossy, and usually a pale, creamy-white color.

1: **Questionable**—The enamel shows slight aberrations from the translucency of normal enamel that may range from a few white flecks to occasional spots.

2: **Very mild**—Small, opaque, paper-white areas scattered irregularly over the tooth but involving less than 25% of the labial tooth surface.

3: **Mild**—The white opacity of the enamel of the teeth is more extensive than for code 2, but covers less than 50% of the tooth surface.

4: **Moderate**—The enamel surfaces of the teeth show significant wear, and brown stain is frequently a disfiguring feature.

5: **Severe**—The enamel surfaces are badly affected and hypoplasia is so significant that the general form of the tooth may be affected. There are pitted or worn areas, and brown stains are widespread; the teeth often have a corroded appearance.

BOX 13-8 Tooth Surface Index of Fluorosis—Codes and Criteria[13]

0:    Enamel shows no evidence of fluorosis.

1:    Enamel shows definite evidence of fluorosis, namely areas with parchment-white color that total less than one third of the visible enamel surface. This category includes fluorosis confined only to incisal edges of anterior teeth and cusp tips of posterior teeth.

2:    Parchment-white fluorosis totals at least one third but less than two thirds of the visible surface.

3:    Parchment-white fluorosis totals at least two thirds of the visible surface.

4:    Enamel shows staining in conjunction with any of the preceding levels of fluorosis. Staining is defined as an area of definite discoloration that may range from light to dark brown.

5:    Discrete pitting exists of the enamel, unaccompanied by evidence of staining of intact enamel. A pit is defined as a definite physical defect in the enamel surface, with a rough floor surrounded by a wall of intact enamel. The pitted area is usually stained or differs in color from the surrounding enamel.

6:    Both discrete pitting and staining exist of the intact enamel.

7:    Confluent pitting exists of the enamel surface. Large areas of enamel may be missing, and the anatomy of the tooth may be altered. Dark brown stain is usually present.

oped a four-level treatment urgency scale in the 1950s.[14] The second organization is the Association of State and Territorial Dental Directors (ASTDD), which developed a three-level treatment urgency scale in 1999.[5] Most public health programs now use the ASTDD scale because of its improved reliability. Box 13-9 lists the criteria for each treatment urgency scale.

MEASURING TOOTH LOSS

Tooth loss is one of the few oral health conditions that can be reliably measured through an open-mouth examination or a self-administered questionnaire. When measuring tooth loss, however, a distinction must be made between loss of certain permanent teeth and total tooth loss. Total tooth loss, or loss of all natural teeth, is also referred to as edentulism.

A state-based, ongoing data collection program designed to measure behavioral risk factors in

U.S. adults—the Behavioral Risk Factor Surveillance System (BRFSS)—monitors tooth loss through a telephone survey. Each month, states select a random sample of adults for a telephone interview. This selection process results in a representative sample for each state so that statistical inferences can be made from the collected information.[15]

In 1999, all states asked a core set of oral health questions to obtain information on time since last dental visit, time since last tooth cleaning, and tooth loss. The following question was used to determine the prevalence and severity of tooth loss in U.S. adults.[16]

- Question: How many of your permanent teeth have been removed because of tooth decay or gum disease? Do not include teeth lost for other reasons, such as injury or orthodontics.
- Response: None; 5 or fewer; 6 or more, but not all; all.

BOX 13-9 ASTDD and ADA Treatment Urgency Scales—Codes and Criteria[5,14]

ASTDD Treatment Urgency Scale:

0:   No obvious problems. Routine dental care is recommended at next regular checkup.

1:   Early dental care is recommended within several weeks. Caries without accompanying signs or symptoms, individuals with spontaneous bleeding of gums, suspicious white or red soft tissue area, or ill-fitting dentures.

2:   Urgent/emergency care is recommended within 24 hours. Signs or symptoms include pain, infection, swelling, or soft tissue ulceration of more than 2 weeks' duration (determined by questioning).

ADA Treatment Urgency Scale:

1:   Apparently requires no dental treatment

2:   Requires treatment, but not of an urgent nature

3:   Requires early treatment

4:   Requires immediate dental treatment

MEASURING ORAL AND PHARYNGEAL CANCER

As with other cancers, oral and pharyngeal cancer is usually expressed as a rate or proportion. For example, the 1998 age-adjusted incidence rate for cancers of the oral cavity and pharynx was 15.4 per 100,000 population for White males and 19.8 per 100,000 population for Black males.[17] There are two primary methods for measuring mortality and morbidity from oral and pharyngeal cancer: (1) mortality rates, and (2) incidence rates. Mortality (death) rates from cancers of the oral cavity and pharynx are generated by the Centers for Disease Control and Prevention's National Center for Health Statistics (NCHS), which obtains data from death certificates collected through the National Vital Statistics System. Mortality data, together with other vital statistics data, can be obtained from the National Center for Health Statistics Web site.

Information for the calculation of cancer incidence rates is obtained through a network of local and state cancer registries that receives reports of new cancer cases from physicians and hospitals. Twelve such population-based cancer registries (Atlanta, Connecticut, Detroit, Hawaii, Iowa, Los Angeles, Native Americans in Alaska, New Mexico, San Francisco-Oakland, San Jose-Monterey, Seattle-Puget Sound, and Utah) participate in the Surveillance, Epidemiology, and End Results (SEER) program, which is conducted by the National Institutes of Health, National Cancer Institute. SEER is the primary source of all cancer incidence data in the United States.

HOW TO COMPLETE A COMMUNITY-BASED ORAL HEALTH NEEDS ASSESSMENT

Although this chapter provides basic information on dental indices and other measures of oral health, it does not provide detailed information on how to complete an oral health survey. Planning and implementing a comprehensive community-level oral health survey is an arduous task that is beyond the scope of this text. There are, however, three guides that give detailed information on how to complete an oral health assessment. The first is

Assessing Oral Health Needs: ASTDD Seven-Step Model developed and produced by the Association of State and Territorial Dental Directors.[18] The Seven-Step Model was described in Chapter 5 and gives detailed information on how to conduct a comprehensive needs assessment, ranging from the evaluation of existing data to the collection of new data.

Two other resources provide detailed information on how to implement an open-mouth survey. They are Oral Health Surveys: Basic Methods,[8] published by the WHO, and Basic Screening Surveys: An Approach to Monitoring Community Oral Health,[5] published by the ASTDD. Both references are extremely useful; however, Basic Screening Surveys: An Approach to Monitoring Community Oral Health provides the most practical information for monitoring the Healthy People 2010 oral health objectives. Basic Screening Surveys: An Approach to Monitoring Community Oral Health, together with a detailed BSS Planning Guide, are available for downloading from the ASTDD Web site.

SUMMARY

This chapter introduced the concept of oral health surveillance and described methods commonly used to measure the prevalence of dental caries, periodontal disease, dental fluorosis, tooth loss, and treatment urgency in a community setting. Using these methods, together with the needs assessment information presented in earlier chapters, you will be able to evaluate the oral health status of the community that you serve.

RESOURCES

National Center for Health Statistics
    http://www.cdc.gov/nchs
Surveillance, Epidemiology, and End
    Results (SEER) Program
    http://www.seer.cancer.gov
National Oral Health Surveillance System
    http://www.cdc.gov/nohss
ASTDD Basic Screening Surveys: An Approach
    to Monitoring Community Oral Health
    http://www.astdd.org

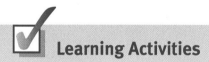 **Learning Activities**

1. Go to the National Oral Health Surveillance System Web site (www.cdc.gov/nohss). Look up the proportion of adults ≥18 who have lost one or more permanent teeth and the proportion of adults ≥65 who have lost all of their teeth. Compare the prevalence of tooth loss in your state with the national prevalence.

2. Go to the Centers for Disease Control and Prevention's, National Center for Health Statistics Web site (www.cdc.gov/nchs). Look up the age-adjusted death rate for malignant neoplasms of the lip, oral cavity, and pharynx. Has the age-adjusted death rate changed over time?

3. Download the Basic Screening Survey manual from the Association of State and Territorial Dental Director's Web site (www.astdd.org). Conduct an oral health survey of your class. What proportion of the class has a history of dental caries? What proportion of the class has dental sealants on their permanent molars?

Periodontal Screening and Recording (PSR)
procedure http://www.ada.org
Oral Health Surveys: Basic Methods
Order at: http://www.who.int
Behavioral Risk Factor Survey System
http://www.cdc.gov/brfss

Review Questions

1. What does the abbreviation DMFS mean?
   a. Decayed, missing, and filled tooth surfaces
   b. Decayed, missing, and filled permanent teeth
   c. Decayed, missing, and filled primary tooth surfaces
   d. Decayed, missing, and filled permanent tooth surfaces
   e. Decayed, missing, and filled primary teeth

2. A 16 year old has occlusal decay on #2 and #15, occlusal fillings on all four first molars, an MOD filling on #18, and an MO filling on #31. Teeth #5 and #12 are missing. What are the DMFT and DMFS scores for this adolescent?
   a. DMFT = 10; DMFS = 21
   b. DMFT = 7; DMFS = 12
   c. DMFT = 8; DMFS = 11
   d. DMFT = 4; DMFS = 4

3. DMFS measures caries experience in permanent teeth, and dmfs measures caries experience in the primary dentition.
   a. True
   b. False

4. If a person has a Root Caries Index of 25%, it means that 25% of their teeth have decay or fillings on the roots.
   a. True
   b. False

5. The Community Periodontal Index evaluates three indicators of periodontal status. What are they?
   a. Plaque, calculus, and attachment loss
   b. Plaque, calculus, and periodontal pockets
   c. Gingival bleeding, plaque, and attachment loss
   d. Gingival bleeding, calculus, and periodontal pockets
   e. Gingival bleeding, calculus, and attachment loss

6. For adults, how many teeth does the Community Periodontal Index evaluate?
   a. 6
   b. 8
   c. 10
   d. 14
   e. 28

7. The Simplified Oral Hygiene Index (OHI-S) is the best index for evaluating plaque and calculus.
   a. True
   b. False

8. A 12-year-old child is being examined for dental fluorosis using Dean's Fluorosis Index. She has mild fluorosis on teeth #8 and #9 and very mild fluorosis on teeth #3, 14, 18, and 30. How would she be classified in terms of fluorosis?
   a. Questionable
   b. Very mild
   c. Mild
   d. Moderate
   e. Severe

9. Which of the following can be easily measured through a questionnaire or survey?
   a. Untreated decay
   b. Caries experience
   c. Tooth loss
   d. Treatment urgency
   e. Dental sealants

10. What are the two primary methods for measuring mortality and morbidity from oral and pharyngeal cancer?
    a. Morbidity rates and prevalence rates
    b. Mortality rates and prevalence rates

c. Morbidity rates and incidence rates
d. Mortality rates and incidence rates
e. Mortuary rates and incidence rates

REFERENCES

1. American Dental Education Association. Competencies for entry into the profession of dental hygiene, exhibit 7. J Dent Ed 2003; July;67(7):1–5. Available at: http://www.adea.org/cepr. Accessed January 2004.
2. Healthy People 2000. National health promotion and disease prevention objectives, 1991. DHHS Pub. No. (PHS) 91-50212. Washington, DC: U.S. Department of Health and Human Services, Public Health Service, 1991.
3. Thacker SB. Historical development. In: Teutsch SM, Chutchill RE, eds. Principles and Practice of Public Health Surveillance. Oxford: Oxford University Press, 2000.
4. Gruebbel AO. A measurement of dental caries prevalence and treatment service for deciduous teeth. J Dent Res 1944;23:163–168.
5. Basic screening surveys: An approach to monitoring community oral health. Association of State and Territorial Dental Directors, 2003. Available at: www.astdd.org.
6. Smile Survey 2000. Washington State Department of Health, Maternal and Child Health, 2001. Available at: http://www.doh.wa.gov/Publicat/smilesurvey.pdf.
7. Katz RV. Assessing root caries in populations: The evolution of the Root Caries Index. J Public Health Dent 1980; 40:7–16.
8. World Health Organization. Oral Health Surveys: Basic Methods. 4th Ed. Geneva, Switzerland: WHO, 1997.
9. Nasi JH. Background to, and implementation of, the Periodontal Screening and Recording (PSR) procedures in the USA. Int Dent J 1994;44:585–588.
10. Loe H, Silness J. Periodontal disease in pregnancy. I. Prevalence and severity. Acta Odont Scand 1963;21:533–551.
11. Ramfjord SP. Indices for prevalence and incidence of periodontal disease. J Periodontol 1959;30:51–59.
12. Dean HT. The investigation of physiological effects by the epidemiological method. In: Moulton FR, ed: Fluorine and Dental Health. Washington DC: American Association for the Advancement of Science, 1942.
13. Horowitz HS, Driscoll WS, Meyers RJ, et al. A new method for assessing the prevalence of dental fluorosis—the Tooth Surface Index of Fluorosis. J Am Dent Assoc 1984;109:37–41.
14. Council on Dental Health and Bureau of Dental Health Education. A dental health program for schools. Chicago, IL: American Dental Association, 1956.
15. Behavioral Risk Factor Surveillance System. Centers for Disease Control and Prevention, National Center for Chronic Disease Prevention and Health Promotion. Available at: http://www.cdc.gov/brfss. Accessed July 2003.
16. Behavioral risk factor surveillance system questionnaire. Centers for Disease Control and Prevention, National Center for Chronic Disease Prevention and Health Promotion, 1999. Available at: http://www.cdc.gov/brfss/questionnaires/pdf-ques/99brfs.pdf. Accessed July 2003
17. National Center for Health Statistics. FastStats A to Z: Cancer. Available at: http://www.cdc.gov/nchs/fastats/cancer.htm. Accessed July 2003.
18. Assessing Oral Health Needs: ASTDD Seven-Step Model. Association of State and Territorial Dental Directors, 2003. Available at: www.astdd.org.

Biostatistics

14

Objectives

After studying this chapter and completing the study questions and activities, the learner will be able to:
- Explain the use of biostatistics in dental public health.
- Describe the purpose for data analysis.
- Describe the rationale for sampling methods.
- Select an appropriate statistical test to analyze a data set.
- Define common statistical terms.
- Compute central tendency measures from a data set.
- Use graphs and tables to describe data.
- Interpret the results of statistical tests.

KEY TERMS

Alternative hypothesis
Analysis of Variance (ANOVA)
Bar chart
Bias
Cluster sampling
χ^2 test (chi-square test)
Confidence intervals
Confounding
Convenience sample

Correlation coefficient
Degrees of freedom
Dependent variables
Descriptive statistics
Frequency table
Histogram
Hypothesis testing
Independent variables
Inferential statistics

Interval variables
Linear regression
Logistic regression
Mean
Median
Mode
Nominal variables
Nonprobability samples
Normal distribution

Null hypothesis	Quota sample	Statistical inference
Ordinal variables	Ratio variables	t-test
p-value	Sample	2×2 table
Parameter	Simple random sampling	Type I error
Percentile	Standard deviation	Type II error
Power	Statistics	Variables
Probability sample	Stratified random sample	Variance
Quartile	Standard error	

The American Dental Education Association competencies addressed in this chapter include[1]:

CM.1: Assess the oral health needs of the community and the quality and availability of resources and services.

CM.6: Evaluate the outcomes of community-based programs and plan for future activities.

Introduction

Statistics is the science of making statements about an entire population from a limited sample of that population. It involves analyzing data and drawing conclusions, taking variation and uncertainty into account. Biostatistics is simply the application of these methods in biologically relevant areas. The appropriate use and interpretation of biostatistical measures and tests are essential to every stage of a dental public health initiative. To define a problem in a community, you first must quantify it using descriptive statistics and measures of disease. As it often is impractical to evaluate the entire population, this requires that you take an appropriate **sample** of the population. You should be able to present your findings clearly, through the appropriate use of tables and graphs. During the planning (Chapter 6) and implementation of the initiative, you must have a sound understanding of data analysis, so that you will be sure to collect sufficient data to allow for program evaluation. For this reason, data analysis should always be planned prior to beginning your data collection. Finally, you should evaluate the success of your program (Chapter 7). As in the definition of

the problem, descriptive statistics and biostatistical tests play a central role in this important stage of a dental public health intervention.

This chapter shows that epidemiology and biostatistics are intimately connected. A thorough description of concepts in epidemiology (Chapter 11) and their application (Chapter 13) serve as important bases for understanding the information presented here. A referenced, published, dental public health cohort study will make abstract concepts more concrete. This study concerned the effectiveness of a dental health program in the town of Móstoles, Spain, to prevent dental caries in a population of schoolchildren.[2] A more complete description of the study may be found in Box 14-1. Further relevant details about this study will be revealed in the appropriate sections of this chapter.

SAMPLING FROM A POPULATION

In the example study, the authors did not assess every child in their population of interest (i.e., all 6-year-old Spanish schoolchildren followed from first grade). Instead, they examined a subset of this population, the 6-year-old, public and private, first grade schoolchildren of Móstoles, Spain, who

> ### BOX 14-1   Example Study
>
> The example study was a prospective cohort study to assess the effectiveness of a Spanish dental public health program after 7.5 years of follow-up. A1985 report established the problem: 75% of Spanish schoolchildren between the ages of 6 and 12 were found to experience carious lesions. In 1987, a preventive program was established by the Ministry of Health. The program included health education, a weekly mouth rinse using sodium fluoride (NaFl) at 0.2% concentration, sealant placement on first permanent molars, and topical application of fluoride gel. To evaluate the effectiveness of the initiative in Móstoles, Spain, 547 children who had received the program and 237 children who had not received the preventive program were assessed. Dental examinations used World Health Organization criteria, using a mouth mirror, a sharp explorer, and natural light. DMFT (number of decayed, missing, or filled permanent teeth) and DMFS (number of decayed, missing, or filled permanent tooth surfaces) were compared using the Mann-Whitney μ test. A multivariate logistic regression was conducted to compare the odds of incident caries between the groups during the 7.5 years of follow-up, controlling for clinical and demographic variables. Significant differences between the groups were found in each case. The authors concluded that the preventive program had a protective effect.
>
> Source: Tapias MA, DeMiguel G, Jimenez-Garcia R, Gonzalez A, and Dominguez V. Incidence of caries in an infant population in Móstoles, Madrid. Evaluation of a preventive program after 7.5 years of follow-up. Int J Paediatr Dent 2001; 11:440–446.[2]

had been followed for 7.5 years. To be included in the study, both study and control children must have been examined in first and eighth grades, been born in 1982, and have provided parental informed consent. In statistical language, this subset is called a sample. Usually, we wish to draw conclusions about some numeric aspect of the population. In statistical terms, a **parameter** is a numeric characteristic of the *population*. A parameter has a set value, but we usually do not know that value. A *statistic* is a numeric characteristic of the *sample*. We can know the value of a statistic in our sample, but the value will change from sample to sample. It is important that the sample be representative of the population of interest from which it was drawn because the statements (or inferences) about the whole population may be made from the measurements taken on the sample. If a sample is not representative of the population of interest, it is a biased sample. For example, in caries prevalence measures, schoolchildren living in a fluoridated community would be a biased sample of all children because, as a group, they would have a lower prevalence than the entire population of interest.

The best way to ensure a representative, unbiased sample is to perform **simple random sampling.** A simple random sample is one in which every item or person in the population has an equal and independent chance of being selected. A simple random sample is an example of a **probability sample.** Probability samples are those drawn when you are able to identify and have access to all members of the population of interest. A **stratified random sample,** another type of probability sample, is a variant of the simple random sample. This sampling scheme is random sampling carried out in subgroups of a population to ensure that selections will be made from each level of the subgroup. For example, you may take steps to ensure that every age, sex, race, or social stratum subgroup is represented in sufficient numbers in the sample. This approach may be used for two reasons: (1) a simple random sample may allow an unrepresentative sample to be chosen because all possible combinations, including unrepresentative combinations, can occur in a simple random sample, or (2) you want to have sufficient numbers of people in a given subgroup to analyze.

At times, a probability sample may not be possible or warranted. For example, you may not have access to the entire population of interest or variability may be low enough that the effort and cost of probability sampling outweighs the risk of drawing a biased sample. There are several subtypes of **nonprobability samples. Cluster sampling** divides the population into small groups (clusters), draws a simple random sample of clusters, and assesses every subject in the sampled clusters. This may be a good approach when cost and time to travel between randomly selected subjects would be prohibitive. A **quota sample** is drawn by selecting items or people in a block of predetermined size. For example, you may select the first 10 women, without regard for the pool

they may represent. Finally, a **convenience sample,** as its name suggests, is selected on the basis of convenience to the researcher, with little concern for representativeness. The types of samples are summarized in Box 14-2.

Applying this information to our example study, if the population of interest is Móstoles, then (not considering nonparticipation and loss to followup) we can think of the authors as having examined the entire population of interest, rather than a sample of the population. However, if all 6-year-old Spanish schoolchildren were the population of interest, which would be of broader interest, the children of Móstoles would represent a convenience sample of that population. In this case, one may argue that the effect of the preventive program in these children would not be representative of the effect in all Spanish schoolchildren.

DEFINITION AND COLLECTION OF DATA

The population of interest is sampled for the purpose of making inferences from the data drawn. Raw data are organized into **variables,** anything that can be measured or manipulated in the

---

BOX 14-2 Types of Samples

Probability Sample: A sampling from a population that you can identify and to which you have access to all members.

Simple Random Sample: Each item or person in the population of interest has an equal and independent chance of being selected.

Stratified Random Sample: Random sampling carried out in subgroups of a population to ensure that selections will be made from each level of the subgroup.

Nonprobability Sample: A sampling when you cannot identify or do not have access to the entire population of interest.

Cluster Sample: Drawing a simple random sample of small groups (clusters) of the population and assessing each subject in the sampled cluster.

Quota Sample: Sampling items or people in a block of predetermined size.

Convenience Sample: A sampling scheme in which the subjects are selected, partly or entirely, at the convenience of the researcher.

study.[3] Often, variables are described as being independent or dependent. **Dependent variables** essentially can be considered as the variables that define the outcome of interest, whereas the **independent variables** are those that may determine outcome. For example, in the example study, there were several dependent variables: DMFT (decayed, missing, or filled permanent teeth), DMFS (decayed, missing, or filled permanent tooth *surfaces*), and the presence or absence of carious lesions. The primary independent variable in the study was exposure to the preventive program.

Another way of classifying variables is by form (Box 14-3). Understanding this classification is essential to selecting the appropriate statistical test to analyze data. Broadly, variables can be classified into categorical and continuous variables.

Categorical variables can be further divided into **nominal** and **ordinal variables.** In a nominal scale, discrete categories do not have a quantitative relationship with each other. A nominal scale, for example, records eye color as blue/green/brown/hazel or answers to a question as yes/no. As implied, ordinal variables consist of ordered categories; however, the difference between the categories is not specified. The use of *A, B,* and *C* letter grades is an example of an ordinal scale. Unless specific numeric quantities are assigned, the difference between a *C* and a *B* is not necessarily the same as the difference between a *B* and an *A.*

Continuous variables represent measured quantities (e.g., blood pressure and temperature). Continuous variables may be divided into **interval** and **ratio variables.** The points on an interval scale are equally spaced, and the difference between two points is meaningful (e.g., the difference between 30°C and 31°C is the same as 89°C and 90°C). However, 100°C is not twice as hot as 50°C. As you may guess, the ratio between points on a ratio scale has meaning. Age is an example of a ratio scale. Therefore, David, who is 18, is twice as old as his brother Michael, who is 9. It should be noted that continuous variables, whether interval or ratio, are analyzed in the same way.

BOX 14-3 Classification of Variables

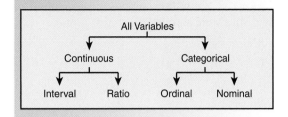

Returning to our example study, you now can see that the DMFT and DMFS outcomes are continuous, interval-scale variables, whereas presence or absence of carious lesions is a nominal categorical variable.

FREQUENCY TABLES AND DESCRIPTIVE STATISTICS

There are two steps in data analysis. The first is to calculate **descriptive statistics,** the characteristics of the data found within the sample of individuals in whom the study was conducted. The second step is to calculate inferential statistics. The purpose of generating **inferential statistics** is to determine whether the results found in the sample may be a result of chance or, assuming no other threats to validity, whether we can generalize our results to the general population of interest. First, we will consider descriptive statistics and then move on to inferential statistics.

Frequency Tables

A study yields raw data that is organized into variables, which are distributed in some way among the various categories (categorical variables) or across the various possible values (continuous variables). To enhance the communication of results, visual and mathematical simplification is necessary. There are several techniques available for displaying data. Here, we will discuss the **frequency table,** relative frequency table, **histogram,** and **bar chart.**

The investigators in our example study measured DMFT for each child in the sample. For the purposes of illustration, suppose that a subset of the results were as follows:

0	2	3	1	0
0	9	4	1	4
1	2	2	8	0
0	5	5	1	1
6	0	1	0	2
2	0	7	4	4

The first step you may take would be to organize the data in ascending order:

0	0	0	0	0
0	0	0	1	1
1	1	1	1	2
2	2	2	2	3
4	4	4	4	5
5	6	7	8	9

One way of summarizing the measurements is a frequency table, shown in Table 14-1. To create the table, appropriate intervals were chosen for DMFT, and a number was computed for measurements falling within each interval. In this case, the intervals are of equal width, which, although not strictly necessary, is often desirable. The width of each class interval determines the number of intervals and, thus, the level of detail with which the data will be reported. As a rule of thumb, about 5–10 intervals are appropriate for most purposes. With fewer intervals, too much information may be lost. A greater number of intervals may give too much detail, losing the ability to obtain an overall feel for the distribution. In some cases, you may select intervals on the basis of precedence—if other investigators have reported findings with certain intervals, using the same intervals would facilitate comparison. Of course, in the case of categorical variables, the information is already organized into categories, although you may choose to combine two or more levels of a category. For example, if information was collected about a subject's smoking history as "never smoker/past smoker," "quit ≥2 years ago/past smoker," "quit <2 years ago/current smoker," depending on the aim of your analysis, you may decide to combine the two "past smoker" categories, leaving "never smoker/past smoker/current smoker."

TABLE 14-1 HYPOTHETICAL FREQUENCY TABLE OF DMFT IN SPANISH SCHOOL-CHILDREN AT AGE 13

DMFT	FREQUENCY*
0–1	14
2–3	6
4–5	6
6–7	2
8–9	2

* Frequency is the number of subjects with the corresponding DMFT range

By dividing actual frequency by the total number of observations and, subsequently, multiplying by 100, the percentage of subjects in each interval can be obtained. By doing so, you have calculated a relative frequency distribution. As a math check, the relative frequencies should total approximately 100%, allowing for some error due to rounding. The relative frequency distribution for the frequency table presented as Table 14-1, "Hypothetical Relative Frequency Table of DMFT in Spanish School-children at Age 13," is shown in Table 14-2.

A histogram or bar chart can be constructed from a relative frequency distribution. Histograms are used for continuous variables, and bar charts are used for categorical variables. A bar should be drawn for each interval or category; the height of the bar is determined by the relative frequency of occurrence of measurements in that interval. The data from Table 14-2 are represented in Figure 14-1. Assuming that every interval of the continuous variable has at least one subject, there are no spaces between the bars of a histogram.

In a bar chart, the bars are of equal width and may be vertical or horizontal. There are spaces between the bars representing each category. In the

TABLE 14-2. HYPOTHETICAL RELATIVE FREQUENCY TABLE OF DMFT IN SPANISH SCHOOLCHILDREN AT AGE 13

DMFT	FREQUENCY	RELATIVE FREQUENCY (%)
0–1	14	46.67
2–3	6	20.00
4–5	6	20.00
6–7	2	6.67
8–9	2	6.67
Total	30	100.01

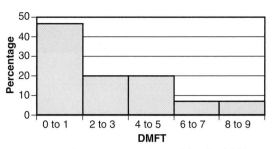

FIGURE 14-1 Histogram—DMFT in Spanish Schoolchildren.

example study, the investigators assessed the social class of the study subjects at the beginning of the study. To assess whether exposure to the preventive programs varied by social class, the authors may have presented a bar chart, such as shown in Figure 14-2.

Despite similarities, do not confuse histograms and bar charts. Histograms need to be constructed more precisely because the area of the bar (height × width) represents the frequency distribution of the data. If the intervals are equally spaced, the bars are of equal width; however, you must be more careful when using unequally spaced intervals. As previously mentioned, there are no spaces between the bars of a histogram.

Descriptive Statistics

Although frequency distributions are convenient ways to summarize data, they do have disadvantages. For example, it would be easier to compare a single summary value than to try to compare distributions from two different samples. As a result, we rely on mathematical approaches to summarizing the data through two types of descriptive statistics: (1) measures of central tendency, and (2) measures of spread.

MEASURES OF CENTRAL TENDENCY

Measures of central tendency attempt to identify the middle of a distribution to provide one sample

statistic that describes the character of an entire data set. Three measures of central tendency—the **mode,** the **median,** and the **mean**—are introduced here. The sample mean of a data set is the arithmetic average, which is the sum of observations divided by the number of observations. For example, if you measured dmfs (decayed, missing, or filled primary tooth surfaces) among five first grade schoolchildren and obtained the following data: 0, 3, 1, 2, and 4, the mean, or average, dmfs would be $(0 + 3 + 1 + 2 + 4)/5 = 2.0$. By substituting symbols for these numbers, we can represent the general formula for the mean. Each symbol, x_1, x_2, x_3 . . . , etc., to x_n, represents an individual observation, where n is the total number of observations. The mean of the sample is represented by the symbol $\bar{x}$ (x-bar). Thus, the formula for the mean would be:

$$\bar{x} = \frac{x_1 + x_2 + \dots x_n}{n}$$

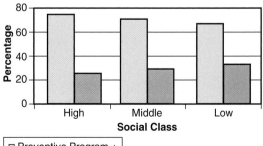

FIGURE 14-2 Bar Chart—Exposure to Preventive Program by Social Class.

Median is a second measure of central tendency. The median of a sample is the middle item of a data set, which will divide a data set arranged in order in half. To find the median, the data must first be arranged in order of increasing value. Continuing the example from the previous paragraph, this results in 0, 1, 2, 3, and 4. In this case, the median is 2. This example was straightforward because there were an odd number of observations, with a single observation in the middle to serve as the median. If there is an even number of observations, then the median is the mean of the middle *pair* of observations. To illustrate, if you had collected dmfs data on one additional child, you would have the following observations: 0, 1, 2, 3, 3, and 4. The middle pair of observations is formed by 2 and 3, and the mean of this pair is $(2+3)/2 = 2.5$. Thus, the median in this case is 2.5. Note that three observations fall below 2.5 and three observations fall above 2.5. Because it would be impossible to visually judge the location of the middle point in a large data set, out of n ordered observations, the $((n + 1)/2)$th observation is the median. Using this technique to identify the median in an odd number of observations is straightforward, so we will illustrate this technique on the data set with an even number of observations: 0, 1, 2, 3, 3, and 15. There are six observations, so the $(6 + 1)/2 = 3.5$th observation should be the median. The 3.5th observation is midway between 2 and 3, or 2.5, agreeing with what was concluded previously.

The final measure of central tendency to be considered is the mode, which is the most frequently occurring value in a set of observations. Again, it is convenient to arrange the observations in increasing order to judge how often a value occurs. For example, the mode of the 0, 1, 2, 3, 3, 4 data set is 3 because this value occurs twice and all other values occur only once. If our data set were 0, 1, 1, 2, 3, 3, 4, there would be two modes, 1 and 3, and this data set would be called bimodal. When all values occur with the same frequency, the data set is said to have no mode.

BOX 14-4 Definition of Measures of Central Tendency

Mean: The mean of a set of n observations is the arithmetic average, which is the sum of the observations divided by the number of observations.

Median: The median is the midpoint of a set of observations when they are arranged in increasing order.

Mode: The mode is the most frequent value in a set of observations.

The definitions of the measures of central tendency are located in Box 14-4 to assist in review. We will now discuss their use. The chief advantage of mode is that it is the only measure of central tendency that makes sense for nominal categorical variables, such as eye color. It would not make sense to place eye color in ascending order to identify the median, nor would it make sense to identify the average eye color. It would, however, be perfectly sensible to say that the most frequent eye color in a given sample is brown. Otherwise, mode is not often used, as it records only the most frequent value, which may be far from the center of the distribution of values. Median is based only on the order of information in the data (i.e., how many observations are above and below a given point). Therefore, median is useful for describing the central tendency of ordinal categorical variables, as well as continuous variables. Median is not influenced by and does not convey the actual numeric values of the observations. In some cases (e.g., when a single observation has an unusually high or low value), this may be advantageous because this observation will not influence the median. This can be illustrated using the example used in this section. The observations of dmfs were 0, 1, 2, 3, 3, and 4, with a mean of 2.16 and a median of 2.5. Suppose, however, that instead of a dmfs of 4, the child with the highest dmfs had 15 decayed, missing, or filled primary tooth surfaces. Clearly, this child had an unusually high dmfs. The mean dmfs in this sample would be 4.2, whereas the median would remain 2.5. Despite this, because the additional information about numeric values of the observations is useful in most cases, the mean is the most commonly used measure of central tendency. The mean only makes sense in the context of continuous variables; however, in practice, the mean is also frequently calculated for ordinal variables.

The relationship between mean, median, and mode may be graphically appreciated through the frequency curve of a distribution. The frequency curve is simply a smooth version of the histogram. The mode is the highest point of the curve; the median is the value that divides the area under the curve in half. The location of the mean is slightly more difficult to conceptualize. If you think of the curve as a solid object, the mean would be the point at which the shape would balance. The mean, median, and mode coincide on a symmetrical frequency curve. If, however, the distribution is skewed, the mean is drawn toward the long tail of the distribution, again demonstrating how sensitive the mean is to extreme values. These points are illustrated in Box 14-5.

BOX 14-5 Graphical Relationships Between Mean, Median, and Mode

The mode is located at the highest point of the frequency distribution, whereas the median is the point that divides the area under the curve into two equal parts, to the left and the right. The mean is the point at which the curve would balance on a pivot placed beneath the curve.

In a symmetric distribution, the mean, median, and mode coincide:

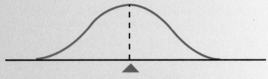

Mean, Median, and Mode

In a skewed distribution, the mean is located farther toward the long tail than is the median.

Positive (towards the right) Skew:

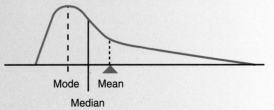

Mode | Mean
Median

Negative (towards the left) Skew:

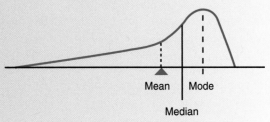

Mean | Mode
Median

MEASURES OF SPREAD

By itself, a measure of center is an incomplete descriptor of data because it says nothing about the variability among the data. For example, knowing that the median real income of U.S. households in 1999 was $40,816 does not reveal that 20% of households earned less than $17,196 or that the top 5% of households earned more than $142,021. To provide a more complete description, the second category of descriptive statistics—measures of spread—is required.[4] The measures of spread presented depend on the measure of central tendency.

When the median is the measure of central tendency, both the variability and the shape of a distribution can be described by giving several percentiles and the extreme values of a data set. The xth percentile of a distribution of numbers is a value in which "x" percent of numbers fall below it and the remainder fall above it. You may have encountered percentiles in reviewing the results of standardized tests, such as the standard achievement tests (SAT). For example, your score may have been reported as "Raw score, 640; percentile, 88," meaning that you scored 640 and that 88% of those taking the exam had scores lower than yours. Certain percentiles are used so often for describing data that they have specific names: the 50th **percentile** is the median; the lower **quartile** is the 25th percentile, and the upper quartile is the 75th percentile. To completely describe a data set when presenting the median as the measure of central tendency, you should report four other values: the lower quartile, the upper quartile, and the two extremes (the smallest and largest individual observations). Each measure fulfills some function in describing the data. The extremes convey the overall spread of the data, but they clearly are sensitive to outliers. The upper quartile, lower quartile, and median divide the data into quarters. The area bound by the upper and lower quartiles shows the spread of the middle of the data, and the distance of the upper and lower quartiles from the median gives an indication of the symmetry of

distribution. With symmetric distribution, the upper and lower quartiles will be equidistant from the median.

To illustrate this, suppose that we conducted a survey of 30 dental hygienists regarding their yearly income, with the obtained results listed below:

$30,017	$30,028	$30,780	$31,889	$32,345
$33,222	$33,947	$35,816	$36,989	$37,734
$38,478	$38,725	$39,431	$40,567	$40,941
$41,789	$42,199	$44,157	$44,275	$45,000
$45,601	$46,050	$46,872	$47,378	$48,722
$48,999	$49,756	$50,102	$51,341	$54,073

The results have been arranged in ascending order to simplify the identification of the percentiles. As there are 30 results, the median should be the mean of the 15th and the 16th values, or $41,365. To find the lower quartile, compute the median of all observations falling below the location of the overall median. Because there are 15 incomes below $41,365, the 8th value should be the median. Thus, the lower quartile is demarcated by $35,816. To find the upper quartile, compute the median of all observations falling above the location of the overall median. In this case, it is $46,872. The smallest individual observation is $30,017, whereas the largest individual observation is $54,073. Graphically, we can represent these values in a box plot, as illustrated in Figure 14-3. The ends of the central box are marked by the quartiles, and the median of the distribution is marked by the line within the box. The "whiskers" at either end extend to the extremes.

When using the mean as a measure of central tendency, the measure of spread presented is either the **standard deviation** or the **variance.** The standard deviation is sometimes abbreviated as s, and the variance sometimes is abbreviated as s^2. The standard deviation is simply the square root of the variance. To calculate variance, you first must determine the mean of the observations. The next step is to determine the deviation of each

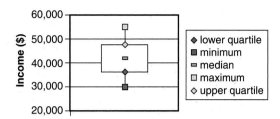

FIGURE 14-3 Box Plot—Income Levels of Dental Hygienists.

observation from the mean (difference between each observation and the mean); for each observation, you then square this deviation. Finally, you find the mean squared deviation. This is the variance. These points are illustrated in Box 14-6. You can interpret the standard deviation as a type of average deviation of the observations from their mean. If the observations are close together, the

---

BOX 14-6 Illustration of Variance and Standard Deviation

You want to find the variance and standard deviation of the five observations: 2, 7, 5, 3, and 10. To do so, you would follow four steps.

1. Compute the mean of the observations:

$$\bar{x} = \frac{2 + 7 + 5 + 3 + 10}{5} = \frac{27}{5} = 5.4$$

2. Determine the squared difference (deviation) between each observation x and the mean $\bar{x}$.

Observation x	Deviation $x - \bar{x}$	Squared Deviation $(x - \bar{x})^2$
2	$2 - 5.4 = -3.4$	$(-3.4)^2 = 11.56$
3	$3 - 5.4 = -2.4$	$(-2.4)^2 = 5.76$
5	$5 - 5.4 = -0.4$	$(-0.4)^2 = 0.16$
7	$7 - 5.4 = 1.6$	$(1.6)^2 = 2.56$
10	$10 - 5.4 = 4.6$	$(4.6)^2 = 21.16$
Total:	0	41.20

3. Calculate the variance by determining the mean squared deviation:

$$\text{variance} = \frac{\text{sum of squared deviations}}{\text{number of observations}} = \frac{41.20}{5} = 8.24$$

4. Determine the standard deviation by taking the square root of the variance:

$$\text{standard deviation} = \sqrt{\text{variance}} = \sqrt{8.24} = 2.87$$

standard deviation is small. In the extreme case, in which all observations have the same value, the standard deviation will be zero. As the observations become more spread out, the standard deviation increases. Like the mean, the standard deviation may be strongly influenced by unusually high or low values (outliers). Finally, the standard deviation is not useful in describing strongly skewed distributions. Because the two sides of a skewed distribution have different spreads, the standard deviation, being a single number, cannot adequately describe the spread. In these cases, the previously described median, quartiles, and extremes would serve as better descriptors.

THE STANDARD NORMAL DISTRIBUTION

The previous section discussed frequency distributions. This section pays special attention to a particular type of frequency distribution: the standard **normal distribution.** This distribution is important because it plays a central role in many statistics. Thus, you should know its general characteristics and feel comfortable using it to calculate probabilities. There are several types of normal distributions, and they share several characteristics. All normal distributions are a symmetrical bell-shape; the mean, median, and mode are identical. Because the tails of the normal distribution drop off quickly, the normally distributed data set has few extreme values. In fact, 95% of the data fall within two standard deviations from the mean. More explicitly: (1) 68% of the observations lie within one standard deviation from the mean; (2) another 27% of the observations fall between one and two standard deviations from the mean; and (3) in all, 99.7% of the observations fall within three standard deviations from the mean (Fig. 14-4).

Given this information, if you know that a variable follows a normal distribution, you can calculate the probability that an event will fall within a specified range of values of that variable. Specifically, the probability is governed by the mean and the standard deviation. The standard normal

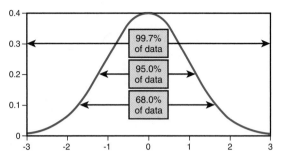

FIGURE 14-4 Properties of Normal Distribution. In a normal distribution, 68% of the data lies within one standard deviation (sd) of the mean, 95% falls within 2 sd of the mean, and 99.7% falls within 3 sd of the mean. In the standard normal distribution with mean = 0 and sd = 1, the data would be distributed as shown here.

distribution is a normal distribution in which the mean = 0, and the standard deviation = 1. It is customary to use the capital letter Z to designate the variable associated with this distribution and to use a small letter z to denote a particular value taken by Z.

As mentioned, the shape of the standard normal distribution governs the probability with which Z takes on a particular value z. Tables have been prepared to enable us to read the area under the standard normal curve. One such table is presented as Table 14-3. It gives the area to the left of a point on the x-axis, for many potential values of z (Fig. 14-5).

Consult Table 14-3 to determine the probability that Z will be equal to or less than 1.0. You

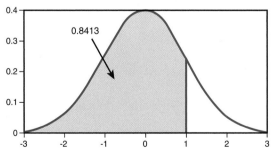

FIGURE 14-5 Determining the Probability of Z ≤1 from the Standard Normal Curve.

TABLE 14-3 STANDARD NORMAL DISTRIBUTION

z	P(Z<z)	z	P (Z<z)	z	P (Z<z)	z	P (Z<z)
0.0000	0.5000	0.8416	0.8000	1.6000	0.9452	2.4000	0.9918
0.1000	0.5398	0.9000	0.8159	1.6450	0.9500	2.5000	0.9938
0.1257	0.5500	1.0000	0.8413	1.7000	0.9554	2.5760	0.9950
0.2000	0.5793	1.0364	0.8500	1.7510	0.9600	2.6000	0.9953
0.2533	0.6000	1.1000	0.8643	1.8000	0.9641	2.7000	0.9965
0.3000	0.6179	1.2000	0.8849	1.8810	0.9700	2.8000	0.9974
0.3853	0.6500	1.2816	0.9000	1.9000	0.9713	2.9000	0.9981
0.4000	0.6554	1.3000	0.9032	1.9600	0.9750	3.0000	0.9987
0.5000	0.6915	1.3410	0.9100	2.0000	0.9773	3.0900	0.9990
0.5244	0.7000	1.4000	0.9192	2.0540	0.9800	3.2000	0.9993
0.6000	0.7257	1.4050	0.9200	2.1000	0.9821	3.2910	0.9995
0.6745	0.7500	1.4760	0.9300	2.2000	0.9861	3.4000	0.9997
0.7000	0.7580	1.5000	0.9332	2.3000	0.9893	3.6000	0.9998
0.8000	0.7881	1.5550	0.9400	2.3260	0.9900	3.7190	0.9999

For negative values of z, $P(Z \leq -z) = 1 - P(Z<z)$.

should have obtained a 0.8413, or 84.13%. Figure 14-5 illustrates this probability on the standard normal curve. The probability gives both the likelihood that a single random drawing from a population has the specified property (such as z ≤1.0), as well as the proportion of the entire population that has that property. In a standard normal population, 84.13% of the members of the population have z measurements of ≤1.0.

The Standard Normal Distribution Table (Table 14-3) does not give the probabilities for negative values of Z. Nevertheless, you can obtain these probabilities with the information in the table. For example, the probability that Z is −0.5 or less is [1 − (probability that Z <0.5)]. We can consult the table to determine that the probability that Z is less than 0.5 is 0.6915, and we can then quickly calculate that the probability that Z is −0.05 or less = 1 − 0.6915 = 0.3085.

Using this same table, we can calculate the probability that Z would take on a value within an interval of z values. For example, let us determine the probability that Z will lie between −1 and 0. To do this, we need to accomplish three steps, represented in Figure 14-6: (1) determine the probability of Z <0, (2) determine the probability of Z <−1, and (3) subtract the answer obtained in (2) from the answer obtained in (1). Following these procedures, you can determine that the answer to step 1 is 0.50, and the answer to step 2 is 0.1587. Therefore, the probability that −1<Z<0 is 0.3413.

To obtain probabilities from a *nonstandard* normally distributed variable X, you first transform the nonstandard distribution into standard normally distributed Z. The transformation formula is $Z = \dfrac{(X - \overline{X})}{s}$, where X is the variable that follows the nonstandard normal distribution, $\overline{X}$ is the estimated mean of this distribution, and s is the estimated standard deviation of the distribution.

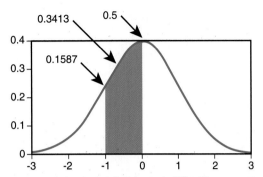

FIGURE 14-6 Determining the Probability That −1< Z < 0 on the Standard Normal Distribution.

You may then determine probabilities in the manner just discussed.

Let us consider an example: You are treating an 8.7-year-old child. His parents are concerned because he does not yet have his first permanent molars. A recent article reported that the eruption age of first permanent molars is normally distributed, with a mean of 6.0 years and a standard deviation of 1.5 years. Designating X as age of eruption of the first permanent molars, we have $\overline{X} = 6.0$ and $s = 1.5$, so the conversion formula is:

$$Z = \frac{(X - 6.0)}{1.5}$$

We want to know whether an eruption age of 8.7 years is particularly late. In other words, what fraction of first permanent molars erupts at 8.7 years or later? In symbols, we are asking what is $P(X \geq 8.7)$?

If this question were asked in terms of Z, we could go directly to Table 14-3 to get the answer. Because our distribution does not have a mean of zero and a standard deviation of 1, we must convert X to Z by subtracting $\overline{X}$ from X and dividing by s:

$$P(X \geq 8.7)$$

$$= P\left[\frac{(X - 6.0)}{1.5} \geq \frac{(8.7 - 6.0)}{1.5}\right]$$

$$= P\left[Z \geq \frac{(8.7 - 6.0)}{1.5}\right]$$

$$= P[Z \geq 1.80]$$

Consulting Table 14-3, we see that the probabilities are given for $Z < z$. We want a probability of $Z \geq z$—it is simple to obtain. First, we see probability of $Z < 1.80$ is 0.9641. The probability of $Z \geq 1.80$ is simply $1 - 0.9641 = 0.0359$, or 3.59%. This is the answer to our original question. In this population, the probability that a child of 8.7 years would not have erupted first permanent molars is 3.59%. Thus, it does seem that the parents' concern is justified.

ASSESSING RELATIONSHIPS BETWEEN TWO VARIABLES

Our example study, summarized in Box 14-1, found that schoolchildren who were "exposed" to a preventive program had a lower DMFT than those who were not exposed to this program. The purpose of many studies is to identify the relationship between two variables in a data set, and from this, to make inference about the relationship between these two variables in a more general population. Here, we will discuss how to describe the relationships, and in the next section, we will move on to statistical inference.

The first goal in exploring the relationship between two variables is to describe the relationship. When both variables are categorical, a frequency table is used to describe the association between them. If both categorical variables have only two levels (binary variables), we can further calculate a risk ratio or an odds ratio, as appropriate, to summarize the relationship. When both variables are continuous, we can convey the relationship in a type of graph, often called a scatter diagram. We can then determine the presence, strength, and direction of any straight-line pattern to the relationship using the **correlation coefficient.** If the outcome is continuous and the exposure is categorical, we can report measures of central tendency

TABLE 14-4 CROSS-TABULATION OF EXPOSURE TO PREVENTIVE PROGRAM AND PRESENCE OF CARIOUS LESIONS IN THE PERMANENT TEETH

	CARIOUS LESIONS IN PERMANENT TEETH	NO CARIOUS LESIONS IN PERMANENT TEETH	TOTAL
Exposed	289	258	547
Nonexposed	169	68	237
Total	458	326	

and spread of the continuous outcome variable for each level of the categorical exposure variable. Each of these concepts will be discussed in the following sections.

Cross-Tabulated Data

One outcome examined in the example study described in Box 14-1 was the prevalence of carious lesions in the permanent dentition in those exposed and not exposed, respectively, to a dental preventive program. The two variables being considered here are presence of carious lesions and exposure status. The findings can be depicted in a **2×2** (two-by-two) **table,** as shown in Table 14-4.

Because 2×2 tables are commonly used, you should have a good understanding of the information they contain. Table 14-4 shows that 547 subjects were exposed and 237 subjects were not exposed to the program. Additionally, 458 had carious lesions in their permanent teeth, whereas 326 did not. Finally, we can see how many of the exposed and the nonexposed had carious lesions in their permanent teeth. By using this information to calculate the percentage of the exposed and the nonexposed, respectively, who had carious lesions in the permanent teeth, we can begin to describe the relationship between the preventive dental program and the presence of carious lesions. 52.8% (289/547) of those who received the pro-

gram had carious lesions in their permanent teeth, whereas 71.3% (169/237) of those who did not receive the program had carious lesions in their permanent teeth. Restated, the risk for carious lesions in the permanent teeth is 52.8% in the exposed and 71.3% in the nonexposed—a larger percentage of the nonexposed than the exposed had carious lesions in their permanent teeth. Because both the exposure and the outcome variables are binary, we can summarize the relationship in a single number—the risk ratio. To calculate risk ratio, you simply take the risk in the exposed and divide it by the risk in the nonexposed. In our example, it is 52.8/71.3%, which is 0.74, indicating that the exposed are 26% less likely to have carious lesions than the nonexposed. The risk ratio always has a positive value, which can range from 0 to infinity. A risk ratio of 1 indicates that there is no relationship between exposure and outcome. This is easier to understand through an example. Suppose that the exposed and the nonexposed cohorts had the same risk for having permanent carious lesions and that this risk was 60%. The risk ratio would then be 60/60%, which is 1. A risk ratio below 1 indicates that the exposed group is at lower risk for the outcome than the nonexposed group, whereas a risk ratio above 1 indicates that the exposed group is at higher risk for the outcome than the nonexposed group.

Here, we examined results from a cohort study. From data collected through cohort studies or experimental studies, you can calculate a risk ratio. You cannot calculate a risk ratio from data collected through a case-control study, but you can calculate what we interpret as an approximation to the risk ratio—the odds ratio. The reasoning behind the inability to directly calculate the risk ratio from case-control studies is beyond the scope of this chapter. For further information, you may consult the excellent book, *Modern Epidemiology* (Lippincott Williams & Wilkins, 1998).[5]

The general formulae for the risk ratio and the odds ratio may be found in Box 14-7. Suppose we conduct a retrospective case-control study to ex-

BOX 14-7 Relative Risk and Odds Ratio

	Outcome +	Outcome −
Exposed	a	b
Nonexposed	c	d

1. Calculation of the risk ratio:

   a. Risk in the exposed $= \dfrac{a}{a+b}$

   b. Risk in the nonexposed $= \dfrac{c}{c+d}$

   c. Risk Ratio $= \dfrac{a/(a+b)}{c/(c+d)}$

2. Calculation of the odds ratio:

   a. Odds of exposure among outcome $+ = \dfrac{a/(a+c)}{c/(a+c)}$

   b. Odds of exposure among outcome $- = \dfrac{b/(b+d)}{d/(b+d)}$

   c. Odds Ratio $= \dfrac{\left(\dfrac{a/(a+c)}{c/(a+c)}\right)}{\left(\dfrac{b/(b+d)}{d/(b+d)}\right)} = \dfrac{\dfrac{a}{c}}{\dfrac{b}{d}} = \dfrac{a \times c}{b \times d}$

Note: The odds ratio is interpreted as an approximation to the risk ratio.

amine the relationship between oral cancer and a history of heavy alcohol intake. This means that we identified people from the same population with (case) and without (control) oral cancer and determined their alcohol intake history. Suppose that this yielded the 2×2 table shown as Table 14-5.

The odds of exposure to heavy alcohol intake among the cases is:

$$\frac{a/(a+c)}{c/(a+c)} = \frac{a}{c} = 0.22$$

The odds of exposure to heavy alcohol intake among the controls is:

$$\frac{b/(b+d)}{d/(b+d)} = \frac{b}{d} = 0.15$$

The odds ratio, then, is:

$$\frac{a/c}{b/d} = \frac{0.22}{0.15} = 1.47$$

This answer is nearly the same as by using the $(a \times c)/(b \times d)$ formula. They differ slightly because of a rounding error. Interpreting this as an approximation to the risk ratio, it can be concluded that those exposed to heavy alcohol intake are 47% more likely to develop oral cancer than those not exposed to heavy alcohol intake.

TABLE 14-5 CROSS-TABULATION OF HEAVY ALCOHOL INTAKE AND PRESENCE OF ORAL CANCER

		ORAL CANCER		
		+	−	TOTAL
Heavy Alcohol Intake	+	18	13	31
	−	82	87	169
Total		100	100	200

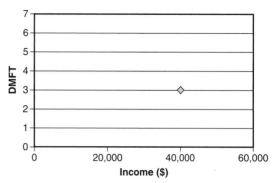

FIGURE 14-7 Plotting the Point (Income = $40,000; DMFT = 3) in a Scatter Diagram.

Scatter Diagrams and Correlation

When the exposure and the outcome variables are continuous or ordinal, a scatter diagram can be used to visually depict the relationship and a correlation coefficient can be calculated to numerically describe the relationship. Exposure and outcome are positively associated when larger values of one tend to be associated with larger values of the other (e.g., height and weight are positively associated because taller people tend to weigh more). However, an exposure and an outcome are negatively associated when larger values of one tend to be associated with *smaller* values of the other (e.g., you may suppose that DMFT would decrease with increasing income).

This hypothetical relationship between DMFT and income can be visually conveyed through a scatter diagram. In a scatter diagram, the exposure units are marked on the x-axis (horizontal), and the outcome units are marked on the y-axis (vertical). Each observation is represented by a point with a horizontal coordinate equal to the value of the exposure and a vertical coordinate equal to the value of the outcome. Therefore, for a person with an annual income of $40,000 and a DMFT of 3, the point shown in Figure 14-7 would be plotted. Continuing this procedure for each observation, you may end up with a similar scatter diagram as the one shown in Figure 14-8. Through the scatter diagram, you can appreciate the relationship between continuous exposure and outcome, and you can identify individual observations that deviate from the overall relationship. These observations are called outliers. Figure 14-8 shows that the person with an annual income of about $35,000 had an unusually low DMFT of 1.

A **correlation coefficient** (r) numerically describes the relationship between continuous exposure and continuous outcome. It should not be calculated for ordinal variables; however, in practice, it often is. The calculation of the correlation coefficient is algebraically intensive; nevertheless, the formula for the Pearson correlation coefficient is included in Box 14-8. In practice, this and most other statistical calculations are done with a computer or statistical calculator.

The following points help to understand and properly interpret the correlation coefficient:

1. The correlation coefficient has a range from −1 to +1. It is positive when the association is

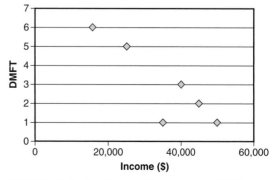

FIGURE 14-8 Scatter Diagram of Income versus DMFT.

BOX 14-8 Formula for the Pearson Correlation Coefficient

For each of the n subjects you ascertained, you gathered information on exposure (x; for example, income) and outcome (y; for example, DMFT). Therefore, for the first subject, you collected observation x_1, y_1; for the second subject, you collected observation x_2, y_2; and for the nth subject, you collected observation x_n, y_n. To compute the correlation coefficient, follow these steps:

1. Find the mean $\bar{x}$ and standard deviation s_x of the values $x_1, x_2, ..., x_n$ of the exposure variable.
2. Find the mean $\bar{y}$ and standard deviation s_y of the values $y_1, y_2, ..., y_n$ of the outcome variable. The correlation coefficient r is:

$$r = \frac{\frac{1}{(n-1)}[(x_1 - \bar{x})(y_1 - \bar{y}) + (x_2 - \bar{x})(y_2 - \bar{y}) + ... + (x_n - \bar{x})(y_n - \bar{y})]}{s_x s_y}$$

positive (as the value of the exposure variable increases, the value of the outcome variable increases), and it is negative when the association is negative (as the value of the exposure variable increases, the value of the outcome variable decreases).

2. The correlation coefficient measures how tightly the points on the scatter diagram cluster around a straight line. The extreme values of the correlation coefficient, -1 and $+1$, indicate that all points fall *perfectly* on a straight line. If the r $= -1$, the straight line would have a negative slope; if r $= +1$, the straight line would have a positive slope. As a rule of thumb, there is a strong linear association if the absolute value of r, $|r| \geq 0.7$; there is a moderate linear association if $0.3 \leq |r| < 0.7$; and there is a weak linear association if $|r| < 0.3$. Weak, moderate, and strong correlations between height (inches) and weight (pounds) are illustrated in Figure 14-9.

3. To understand how the correlation coefficient is strongly influenced by outliers, consider the relationship shown in Figure 14-8. Based on the data shown, the correlation coefficient is -0.82, indicating a strong, negative linear relationship. If we were to delete the outlier with the income of $35,000 and the DMFT $= 1$, the

correlation coefficient would become -1.0, indicating a perfect negative linear relationship.

Comparing Means

Another outcome examined in the example study (detailed in Box 14-1) was DMFT in those exposed and not exposed to the dental preventive program. Here, the two variables being considered are number of decayed, missing, or filled permanent teeth and exposure status. DMFT may be considered a continuous variable, whereas exposure status is binary categorical. We begin to understand the relationship between exposure to the program and DMFT by reporting the measure of central tendency and spread of DMFT for each level of exposure. The authors provided the mean, as well as information that allowed us to determine standard deviation. Such information may be summarized in a table, as shown in Table 14-6.

STATISTICAL INFERENCE

In our example study, 52.8% of the children exposed to the preventive program and 71.3% of the children not exposed, respectively, had carious lesions in their permanent teeth. In this sample, a larger percentage of nonexposed than the exposed

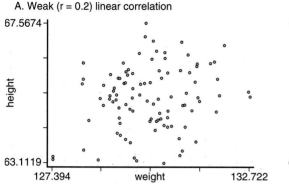

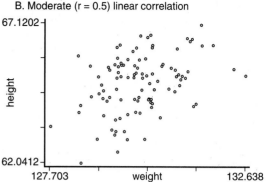

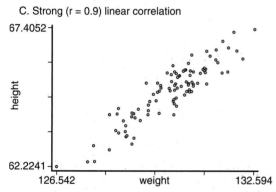

FIGURE 14-9 Graphical Representation of Weak, Moderate, and Strong Linear Correlations Between Height (Inches) and Weight (Pounds).

had carious lesions in their permanent teeth. Possibly, however, this difference may just be caused by chance variation. **Statistical inference** can determine this, provided that you have chosen the appropriate study design and statistical approaches. Statistical inference consists of formal methods to draw conclusions from data taking into account chance variation. There are two major types of statistical inference: confidence intervals and hypothesis testing.

Confidence Intervals

Confidence intervals are used when we are estimating a population parameter. For example, we want to estimate the proportion of children not re-

ceiving the preventive program who have carious lesions in their permanent teeth in the entire study population of interest. This is the population parameter. However, we only have a sample of the population from which we generated a statistic. Based on our sample of 237 children not exposed to the program, this proportion is 71.3%; however, a different sample may have produced a different proportion. By calculating confidence interval, we can construct a margin of error around the statistic of 71.3%. Additionally, we can state how confident we are that the true population parameter will fall within the margin of error. Most often, a 95% confidence interval is constructed, which is the range of values that would cover the true population parameter 95% over time. Using a formula not

TABLE 14-6 MEAN ± SD DMFT IN THOSE EXPOSED AND THOSE NOT EXPOSED TO THE PREVENTIVE PROGRAM

	N	MEAN DMFT (SD)
Exposed to preventive program	547	1.52 (2.03)
Not exposed to preventive program	237	3.07 (2.91)

shown here, the 95% confidence interval can be determined for the population proportion of children not exposed to the preventive program that have carious lesions in the permanent teeth to range from 65.5 to 77.1%. Or, we are "95% confident" that the 65.5 to 77.1% of the children not exposed to the preventive program have carious lesions in their permanent teeth. This chapter does not detail how confidence intervals are calculated. There is no standard formula—it will depend on the parameter being estimated (e.g., proportion, mean, median), as well as the sampling design.

Essential to the calculation of all confidence intervals is the **standard error.** Suppose that we need to estimate the mean income of dental hygienists in the United States. To accomplish this goal, we took a random sample of hygienists. If we sampled two or three hygienists, the chances are good that some may earn little or some may earn a lot; therefore, our calculated mean may be far from the truth. By contrast, if we randomly sampled hundreds of hygienists, the sample mean income should fall close to the true population mean. The mean values determined from repeated samples of the same size are distributed around the true population mean in a bell-shaped curve with a standard deviation (of the sample estimates of the *mean incomes*) equal to the standard deviation of the *incomes* divided by the square root of the sample size. We call this standard deviation of the sample estimates of the

mean incomes, the standard error. In practice, this implies a few points:

1. As a result of random variation, every sample mean calculated will be somewhat different. Most sample means will be close to the population mean; however, at times, we will obtain a sample mean that differs greatly from the true population mean purely by chance.
2. The larger the sample size, the more tightly you expect the sample means to cluster around the population mean.

Hypothesis Testing

The second approach to statistical inference is **hypothesis testing.** The goal of hypothesis testing is to judge the evidence for a hypothesis. Hypothesis testing can be divided into four discrete steps: (1) formally stating the null and alternative hypotheses; (2) choosing an appropriate statistical test; (3) conducting the statistical test to obtain a p-value; and (4) comparing the p-value against a fixed cutoff for statistical significance—α (alpha). Typically, this value is set to 0.05. If a researcher is particularly rigorous, he or she may set it to 0.01.

We will discuss basic concepts and definitions and review the application of statistical testing to the various relationships discussed in the previous section. Note that Box 14-9 summarizes choosing among the statistical tests reviewed in this chapter; it does not include all possible statistical tests.

Essential to the concept of hypothesis testing is the **p-value.** The objective of hypothesis testing is to formally weigh the evidence against a **null hypothesis.** Usually, the null hypothesis (H_0) is a statement of no difference between or no effect of exposures (e.g., using the study in Box 14-1, H_0 may be that children who received the preventive program have the same mean DMFT as children who did not receive the preventive program). By contrast, the **alternative hypothesis**—H_A—is a statement of effect of exposure. In our example, the alternative hypothesis may be that the children who received the preventive program do not have the same mean DMFT as the children who did

BOX 14-9 Choice of Statistical Test for Independent Observations

		OUTCOME			
	BINARY	**NOMINAL CATEGORICAL (>2 CATEGORIES)**	**ORDINAL CATEGORICAL (>2 CATEGORIES)**	**NON-NORMAL CONTINUOUS**	**NORMAL CONTINUOUS**
EXPOSURE **BINARY**	χ^2 (chi-square) or Fisher's exact	χ^2 or Fisher's exact	χ^2, Fisher's exact, or Mann-Whitney μ	Mann-Whitney μ	t-test
NOMINAL CATEGORICAL (>2 categories)	χ^2, or Fisher's exact	χ^2 or Fisher's exact	χ^2, Fisher's exact, or Kruskal-Wallis	Kruskal-Wallis	ANOVA/F-test
ORDINAL CATEGORICAL (>2 categories)	χ^2 or Fisher's exact	χ^2 or Fisher's exact	Spearman rank or χ^2	Spearman rank or Kruskal-Wallis	Spearman rank or Linear regression
NON-NORMAL CONTINUOUS	Logistic regression	Not covered in this chapter	Spearman rank	Spearman rank	Spearman rank or Linear regression
NORMAL CONTINUOUS	Logistic regression	Not covered in this chapter	Spearman rank or Linear regression	Spearman rank or Linear Regression	Pearson correlation or Linear regression

not receive the program. The p-value is the probability of a result being as far or further from what would be expected if the null hypothesis were true. Simply, you can think of the p-value as the probability that the results were obtained by chance. The smaller the p-value, the stronger the evidence in the data against the null hypothesis. Our decision about whether to reject the null hypothesis is based upon the p-value. Below a certain p-value, we will reject the null hypothesis. This certain value, the significance level, is denoted by the symbol α.

Hypothesis testing requires that we make a decision about whether to reject the null. As in any other decision-making process, errors may occur. Figure 14-10 depicts the two types of errors that may occur purely by chance. If the P value is less than our cutoff α (usually 0.05 or 0.01), we will reject the null hypothesis. Suppose we conducted a hypothesis test of the H_0 that children who received the preventive program have the same mean DMFT as the children who did not receive the program. We set α to be 0.05 and received a P value of 0.04, so we rejected the null hypothesis. Two things could have happened. First, there could be a true difference in the mean DMFTs of those who did and did not receive the preventive program. In this case, we correctly rejected the null hypothesis. Second, there may not be a true difference in the mean DMFTs of those who did and did not receive the program. In this case, we have incorrectly rejected the null hypothesis. We have committed an error, and this error has a name. If by chance we reject the null hypothesis when the null hypothesis is true, we have committed **Type I error,** also called α error (alpha error). It is called an α error because it is equivalent to the significance level discussed in the previous section.

If our significance level is set at the typical value of 0.05, we will reject the null hypothesis 5% of the time when it really is true. Clearly, a Type I error is a concern only when we have rejected the null hypothesis. Now consider the opposite circumstance. Suppose that alpha is set to 0.05 with an obtained p-value of 0.09, failing to reject the null. Again, two things could have happened. If there is no difference between the mean DMFTs of children who did and did not receive the preventive program, then we were correct in failing to reject the null. However, if we simply failed to detect a true difference between the mean DMFTs, we have committed another type of statistical error. When we fail to reject the null, we are concerned about **Type II error,** the β error (beta error). β errors occur when you fail to reject the null when the null is true. A related term is **power.** Power is simply $1-\beta$, the probability that you will reject the null, given that the alternative is true (Fig. 14-10).

CROSS-TABULATED DATA

Let us return to our example study. Suppose that we would like to *compare* the proportions of children exposed and not exposed to the preventive program who have carious lesions in their permanent teeth. First, we should state the null hypothesis. Usually, the null hypothesis is that the observations are a result of chance. In this case, it would be that any observed differences in the proportion of children with carious lesions in their permanent teeth are by chance; in other words, an equal proportion of children exposed and not exposed to the preventive program, respectively, have decay in their permanent teeth. By contrast, the alternative hypothesis is that there is a true effect of exposure. In this case, our alternative hypothesis would be

		Truth about the study population of interest	
		Null true	Alternative true
Decision based upon data from sample	Reject null	Type I Error (α)	Correct
	Fail to reject null	Correct	Type II Error (β)

FIGURE 14-10 Statistical Errors.

that children exposed and not exposed to the preventive program are not equally likely to have decay in their permanent teeth.

Having explicitly stated the null and alternative hypotheses, we need to identify a statistical test that will help weigh the evidence against the null hypothesis. There are many statistical tests. Generally, you should follow three steps in selecting a test: (1) specifically state the hypothesis to be tested; (2) determine whether the data are independent; and (3) determine the form of the exposure and outcome variables. We have completed step 1. Determining whether data are truly independent sometimes can be difficult. Usually, results from the same individual or from matched individuals should not be considered independent. The analysis of nonindependent data can be complex and is beyond the scope of this chapter. Finally, you should review the form of the exposure and outcome variables. In our example, the exposure variable (preventive program) is binary categorical (two categories) and the outcome (presence of carious lesions in the permanent teeth) also is binary. In this case, the χ^2 (**chi-square**) test would be the correct statistical test. The data corresponding to this example have been shown previously (Table 14-4). We can use the information in this table to evaluate the null hypothesis.

To better understand the test, we will first answer two questions. First, using the table, you should be able to identify the proportion of subjects in this sample (both groups combined) who had decay in their permanent teeth. There were 784 subjects and 458 had carious lesions in their permanent teeth; therefore, 458/784 = 58.4% who had carious lesions in their permanent teeth. If the null hypothesis is true, there is no difference in the proportion of subjects with carious lesions in their permanent teeth between the two groups. Each group should have approximately the same proportion of subjects with decay in their permanent teeth (i.e., 58.4%). Looking at the table, 547 subjects were exposed to the preventive program. If the null hypothesis were true, 319 children (58.4% × 547 = 319 children) exposed to the pre-

ventive program would be expected to have carious lesions in their permanent teeth. Similarly, 138 of the 237 children not exposed to the preventive program would be expected to have carious lesions in their permanent teeth. The chi-square statistic can be thought of as a quantitative comparison between what was calculated as expected under the null hypothesis and what was actually observed. To facilitate this calculation, the observed and expected values are shown in Table 14-7.

If the null hypothesis were true, there should be small differences between the observed and expected values. The chi-square statistic is based on this. To compute the chi-square statistic, you have to complete 3 steps for each category (cell):

1. Compute the difference between the observed and the expected values (O − E).
2. Square the difference (O − E)^2.
3. Divide the squared difference by the expected value (O − E)^2/E.

Finally, sum the values obtained in step three across all categories. The formula corresponding to these steps may be found in Box 14-10. The results of these steps are summarized in Table 14-8. Therefore, the chi-square statistic is 23.44. To interpret this statistic, recall that if the null hypothesis were true, the chi-square statistic should be small. If we observe a large value chi-square statistic, we tend to reject the null, whereas if we observe a small value, we fail to reject the null. To

TABLE 14-7 OBSERVED AND EXPECTED NUMBERS OF SUBJECTS WITH AND WITHOUT CARIOUS LESIONS IN THE PERMANENT TEETH BY EXPOSURE TO PREVENTIVE PROGRAM

CATEGORY	OBSERVED	EXPECTED
Exposed: no carious lesions	258	228
Exposed: carious lesions	289	319
Not exposed: no carious lesions	68	99
Not exposed: carious lesions	169	138

BOX 14-10 Chi-Square (χ^2) Test

The chi-square test is used to analyze R×C tables, provided you have a sufficient number of subjects in each cell. Its two steps are:

1. The chi-square statistic should be calculated using the following formula:

$$\chi^2 = \sum \frac{(Observed - Expected)^2}{Expected} = \sum \frac{(O - E)^2}{E}$$

where $(O-E)^2/E$ is calculated for each category or cell in the table.

2. The chi-square statistic calculated in step 1 is compared with a tabulated critical cutoff value corresponding to the degrees of freedom to determine whether we accept or reject the null hypothesis. For convenience, the 5 and 1% critical cutoffs of the chi-square distribution for degrees of freedom from 1 to 10 are listed below.

DEGREES OF FREEDOM (DF)	5% CRITICAL VALUE	1% CRITICAL VALUE
1	3.8415	6.6349
2	5.9915	9.2103
3	7.8147	11.3449
4	9.4877	13.2767
5	11.0705	15.0863
6	12.5916	16.8119
7	14.0671	18.4753
8	15.5073	20.0902
9	16.9190	21.6660
10	18.3070	23.2092

TABLE 14-8 CALCULATIONS NECESSARY TO DETERMINE THE CHI-SQUARE STATISTIC TO ASSESS THE RELATIONSHIP BETWEEN EXPOSURE TO THE PREVENTIVE PROGRAM AND CARIOUS LESIONS

CATEGORY	OBSERVED (O)	EXPECTED (E)	(O-E)	(O-E)²	(O-E)²/E
Exposed: no carious lesions	258	228	30	900	3.95
Exposed: carious lesions	289	319	−30	900	2.82
Not exposed: no carious lesions	68	99	−31	961	9.71
Not exposed: carious lesions	169	138	31	961	6.96
				Total:	23.44

make this objective, we rely on statistical tables that show the probability of chi-square being above certain values when the null hypothesis is true. Generally, we reject the null when the probability of the observed chi-square value being under the null is 5% or less, setting α error to 0.05. For a 2×2 table, such as discussed, the critical cutoff value corresponding to the 5% level is 3.84. As our chi-square statistic is far greater than 3.84, we reject the null hypothesis that the same proportions of children exposed and not exposed to the preventive program have carious lesions in their permanent teeth.

Because the chi-square statistic is obtained by summing $(O-E)^2/E$ over all cells, with greater numbers of categories, the chi-square statistic will tend to increase. Thus, to adjust for this, we need to change our critical cutoff value. This adjustment is related to another concept discussed later in this chapter—**degrees of freedom.** Degrees of freedom may be considered the number of unconstrained units of information in the data. This may seem a bit abstract; the idea is most easily conceptualized when applied to R×C tables. We have already discussed the simplest form of an R×C table: the 2×2 table.

Generally, a table with *R* rows and *C* columns is an R×C table. Suppose that our example study had three exposures: (1) no intervention, (2) sending educational materials home to the parents, and (3) a complete caries preventive program. Again, suppose that at the end of the programs we would like to compare the proportions of children with carious lesions in their permanent teeth across the levels of exposure. Because our exposure is multiple categorical and our outcome is binary, we would use the chi-square test to test the null hypothesis that those children receiving no preventive program, the educational program, and the full preventive program, respectively, are equally likely to have carious lesions in their permanent teeth. First, we would generate a 3×2 table to show the hypothetical results, as in Table 14-9, showing the row and column totals. To understand degrees of freedom, consider these totals to be

TABLE 14-9 HYPOTHETICAL CROSS-TABULATION OF EXPOSURE STATUS AND PRESENCE OF CARIOUS LESIONS IN PERMANENT TEETH

	CARIOUS LESIONS IN PERMANENT TEETH	NO CARIOUS LESIONS IN PERMANENT TEETH	TOTAL
Full preventive program	289	258	547
Education alone	287	156	443
No prevention	169	68	237
Total	745	482	

fixed quantities and the cells inside the table to be variable. You may see that when two inner cells are filled, restrictions would be placed on other cells—only two cells can be given numeric values freely. In general, an R×C table has $(r-1) \times (c-1)$ degrees of freedom; in this case, there are $(3-1)\times(2-1) = 2$ degrees of freedom.

To calculate the chi-square statistic, go through the previously outlined steps, adding the $(O-E)^2/E$ across all cells. The chi-square statistic would be 28.48. Then consult the chi-square table for degrees of freedom (DF) = 2. Looking at Box 14-10, you can see that 28.48 is greater than not only the 5% level critical cutoff (5.9915) but also the 1% critical cutoff (9.2103), giving strong evidence to reject the null hypothesis.

CORRELATION

Previously, we considered a hypothetical relationship between two continuous variables (income and DMFT). The scatter diagram shown as Figure 14-8 showed a negative relationship; as income increased, DMFT tended to decrease. The correlation coefficient (r) describing the relationship was −0.82. If there were no linear relationship between income and age, r would be 0, so it makes sense that our null hypothesis is r = 0. The alternative is simply that r ≠ 0, that there is a linear relationship between income and DMFT. Assuming that income and DMFT are normally distributed, we would then calculate a Pearson correlation coefficient and perform a statistical test to determine the probability that the difference between this correlation coefficient and 0 is a result of chance. This statistical test is a form of t-test (a one-sample t-test), which compares the correlation coefficient obtained to 0. The two-sample t-test is described in more detail in the next section. In running the test, we would obtain a p-value of 0.02. Comparing this to the customary cutoff of α = 0.05 (5%), we would reject the null hypothesis and conclude that there is a statistically significant, strong, negative linear relationship between income and DMFT.

COMPARING MEANS

In an earlier section (Table 14-6), we reviewed the mean DMFT in those exposed and not exposed to the dental preventive program described in the example study (Box 14-1). We will now illustrate how to conduct a statistical test when the exposure variable is binary and the outcome variable is continuous. If there was no relationship between the exposure to the preventive program and the mean DMFT, we would expect the difference between the mean DMFTs of those exposed to the preventive program (μ_p) and those not exposed to the preventive program (μ_{np}) to equal 0. Thus, we could state our null hypothesis, H_0, as $\mu_p - \mu_{np} = 0$. Our alternative hypothesis, H_A, would be that the difference between the two means is not equal to 0, or, $\mu_p - \mu_{np} \neq 0$. If DMFT were normally distributed, the two-sample **t-test** would be used to evaluate this null hypothesis. The t statistic would be calculated using the mean DMFT, the standard deviation of DMFT, and the number of subjects in each exposure group. The formula for the t-statistic is found in Box 14-11. In this case, the t-statistic = 8.55. One can then use the t-statistic to look up the probability of this result, given that the null hypothesis is true on a t-table. Similar to the chi-square distribution table, the probability

associated with a given t-statistic depends on the degrees of freedom. For the t-test, the degrees of freedom would equal the sum of the number of subjects in each of the groups − 2; in this case, it would be (547 + 237 − 2) = 782. As there are increasingly greater degrees of freedom, the critical cutoff values for a given probability under the null change less and less. For example, consulting the selection of critical values shown in Box 14-11, you can see that the α = 5% critical value for DF = 60 is 1.980, whereas the 5% critical value for infinite DF is 1.9600. To be more conservative, in this case, we will look at the critical values for DF = 100. Because our t-statistic of 8.55 exceeds the 5% and 1% critical values, we conclude that we can reject the null hypothesis. There is a statistically significant difference between the mean DMFTs of children exposed and not exposed to the preventive program.

If one wishes to compare the mean of a normally distributed continuous variable across levels of a categorical variable with more than two levels, one needs to use **analysis of variance** (**ANOVA**) and the accompanying F-test. The F-test is a generalization of the t-test; they are equivalent when comparing two means. As an example, return to the hypothetical analysis of three programs: no prevention, a preventive program consisting only of educational materials being sent home to the parents, and a full preventive program. Suppose that we now wish to compare the mean DMFT among the three groups. We will abbreviate the mean DMFT in the full prevention program as μ_{FP}, in the education alone as μ_E, and in the no prevention group as μ_{NP}. Table 14-10 shows the hypothetical mean DMFTs and standard deviations for the three groups. The null hypothesis would be that the mean DMFT is the same in all three groups; H_0: $\mu_{FP} = \mu_E = \mu_{NP}$. The alternative hypothesis is that not all of the means are equal.

The appropriate statistical procedure in this situation is ANOVA and the F-test. Using ANOVA, we separate the data variability into two parts: between-group variability and within-group variability. Between-group variability is the variation between each group mean and the overall mean

BOX 14-11 The t-Test

When you want to test whether two independent groups have the same mean of a normally distributed continuous variable, use the two-sample unpaired t-test. Here, the numbers of subjects, means, and standard deviations of each group are referred to as: n_a and n_b, μ_a and μ_b, and s_a and s_b, respectively.

1. Stating the null hypothesis. The null hypothesis, when conducting a t-test, is that the mean of group a is equal to the mean of group b. Thus, the null may be stated as $H_0: \mu_a = \mu_b$, and the alternative may be stated as $H_A: \mu_a \neq \mu_b$.
2. Calculating the t-statistic. To perform the t-test, we assume that the samples came from populations in which the continuous variable is normally distributed with means μ_a and μ_b, respectively, and a common unknown variance. Under these assumptions, the sample variance of the difference in sample means is given by the pooled variance:

$$(s_{\bar{x}_a - \bar{x}_b})^2 = \left(\frac{1}{n_a} + \frac{1}{n_b} \right) \left(\frac{(n_a - 1)s_a^2 + (n_b - 1)s_b^2}{(n_a + n_b - 2)} \right)$$

The test statistic t is calculated by dividing the difference in sample means by the standard deviation of their difference. Recall that the standard deviation is the square root of the variance.

$$t = \frac{\bar{x}_a - \bar{x}_b}{\sqrt{(s_{\bar{x}_a - \bar{x}_b}^2)^2}} = \frac{\bar{x}_a - \bar{x}_b}{s_{\bar{x}_a - \bar{x}_b}}$$

3. Two-tailed t-distribution. When you have calculated the t-statistic, you can identify the corresponding probability under the null by consulting the appropriate degrees of freedom row of the t-table. The degrees of freedom can be determined by subtracting 2 from the total number of subjects in both groups, $(n_a + n_b - 2)$. Below you will find the 5 and 1% critical values for the two-tailed t-distribution.

DEGREES OF FREEDOM (DF)	5% CRITICAL VALUE	1% CRITICAL VALUE	DEGREES OF FREEDOM (DF)	5% CRITICAL VALUE	1% CRITICAL VALUE
1	12.7062	63.6567	16	2.1199	2.9208
2	4.3027	9.9248	17	2.1098	2.8982
3	3.1824	5.8409	18	2.1009	2.8784
4	2.7764	4.6041	19	2.0930	2.8609
5	2.5706	4.0321	20	2.0860	2.8453
6	2.4469	3.7074	30	2.0423	2.7500
7	2.3646	3.4995	40	2.0211	2.7045
8	2.3060	3.3554	50	2.0086	2.6778
9	2.2622	3.2498	60	2.0003	2.6603
10	2.2281	3.1693	70	1.9944	2.6479
11	2.2010	3.1058	80	1.9901	2.6387
12	2.1788	3.0545	90	1.9867	2.6316
13	2.1604	3.0123	100	1.9840	2.6259
14	2.1448	2.9768	Infinite	1.9600	2.5759
15	2.1314	2.9467			

TABLE 14-10 MEAN ± SD DMFT IN THE THREE LEVELS OF PREVENTION EXPOSURE IN A HYPOTHETICAL STUDY

	N	MEAN DMFT (SD)
Full preventive program	547	1.52 (2.03)
Education-only program	443	2.75 (2.07)
No preventive program	237	3.07 (2.91)

for all groups; within-group variability is the variation between each subject and their group mean. If the between-group variability far exceeds the within-group variability, there are likely to be differences in group means. The F-ratio quantitatively summarizes this by dividing the between-group variance by the within-group variance. A detailed discussion of the calculation of the F-ratio is beyond the scope of this chapter. An F-ratio = 1 would occur if the between-group variability equals the within-group variability; the F-ratio increases as the between-group variance grows relative to the within-group variance. The F-test assesses whether the observed treatment group differences are statistically significant. Although not explicitly shown here, the general steps are the same as for the other statistical tests: calculating the F-ratio from the data set and referring to the tabulated value at the appropriate critical value for the corresponding degrees of freedom. In the F-test, there are two degrees of freedom: one corresponding to the between-groups and one to the within-groups. Thus, the critical value on the F-distribution depends upon the α error selected, as well as both degrees of freedom. In our example, the F-ratio was 55.93, with df = 2 and 1224. This exceeds the critical value for both α = 5% and 1%; therefore, we reject the null hypothesis that all of the exposure groups have the same mean DMFT. However, this does not explicitly reveal the differences among the three groups. This

significant ANOVA result may indicate that all three means differ from one another. Alternately, it may indicate that the mean DMFTs of the no prevention and the education groups differ from the mean DMFT of the full prevention program groups but not from each other. To get this information, we would have to run a posttest, which is beyond the scope of this chapter (Box 14-2).

Exact and Nonparametric Statistical Tests

The tests discussed rely on meeting various assumptions. Because it can be unreasonable to make these assumptions, approaches must be taken that are not dependent on them: exact and nonparametric statistical tests. This chapter does not review these tests in detail but simply introduces the circumstances in which they may be employed. When examining cross-tabulations, we can use the chi-square test only if there are sufficient numbers of subjects in each cell of the table. Usually, if there are not at least five subjects per cell, we must use Fisher's exact test. In correlation, if the variables are not normally distributed, the Spearman rank correlation should be used instead of the Pearson correlation. When comparing the distribution of a continuous variable between two groups, the Mann-Whitney μ test should be used instead of the t-test when the continuous variable is not normally distributed. If comparing the distribution of a continuous variable among three or more groups, the Kruskal-Wallis test should be used instead of ANOVA/F-test if the continuous variable is not normally distributed.

ASSOCIATION AND CAUSATION

Association between two variables does not necessarily indicate causation. In the example study (Box 14-1), there is a statistically significant association between exposure to the preventive program and a lower relative DMFT. This does not necessarily mean that the preventive program *caused* the lower DMFT. There are many other potential explanations for the observed association. Chance/random error (Type I error) is one explanation,

BOX 14-12 ANOVA and F-Test

Use ANOVA and the F-test to compare the means of a continuous, normally distributed outcome across three or more groups. You must also assume that the data from all treatment groups have the same variance. Here, assuming three groups, the numbers of subjects, means, and standard deviations of each group are referred to as: n_a, n_b, and n_c; μ_a, μ_b, and μ_c, and s_a, s_b, and s_c, respectively. The total number of groups (exposure levels) is referred to as K, and the total number of subjects in all groups is referred to as N.

1. Stating the null hypothesis. The null hypothesis is that all of the groups have the same mean. Therefore, the null and alternative may be stated as H_0: $\mu_a = \mu_b = \mu_c$, and H_A: not all μs are equal.
2. Calculating the F-ratio.

$$F = \frac{\text{Between-group variance}}{\text{Within-group variance}}$$

The details of the calculation of the F-ratio are beyond the scope of this chapter; however, you should know that as the F-ratio increases, evidence against the null hypothesis mounts.

3. F-Distribution
   Once you have calculated the F-ratio, you can identify whether it exceeds the critical value for your set α by consulting the appropriate cell of the F-distribution table. The appropriate cell is identified using the set α error, the degrees of freedom for the numerator of the F-ratio, and the degrees of freedom for the denominator of the F-ratio. The degrees of freedom for the numerator of the F-ratio is (number of groups − 1), (K-1). The degrees of freedom for the denominator of the F-ratio is (total number of subjects − total number of groups), (N-K).

but there are errors that are not attributable to chance—systematic errors.

This systematic error is called **bias.** Bias is a consistent, repeated divergence in the same direction of the sample estimate from the true population value. For example, when a thermometer always reports the temperature to be 5 degrees lower than it truly is, the temperatures that are recorded using this thermometer will be biased. Bias can occur in many forms.[6] To illustrate this point, we will discuss an example of information bias. Information bias can occur whenever there are errors in the measurement of variables. In our study, the investigators measured DMFT. Suppose that when they encountered a questionable carious lesion, they were more likely to classify it as a

lesion if the child had not been exposed to the preventive program. Thus, independent of any effect of the preventive program, the children not exposed to the preventive program would appear to have a higher mean DMFT than those exposed.

A frequently encountered type of bias is **confounding** bias. To illustrate this, consider what would happen if those children exposed to the preventive program were of higher social class than those children not exposed to the preventive program. Even if they were not exposed to the preventive program, children of higher social class, as a group, would likely have a lower DMFT. If this were the case, social class, rather than the preventive program, may be responsible for the observed differences in DMFT between the exposure groups. This would be an example of confounding. The effects of two variables (in this case, exposure to preventive program and social class) on an outcome (here, DMFT) are said to be confounded when they cannot be distinguished from one another. We would then call social class a confounder or a confounding factor. To be a confounding factor, a variable must possess certain characteristics: (1) it must be associated with the exposure; (2) even among the unexposed, it must be associated with the outcome; and (3) it must not be an intermediate step in the path between exposure and disease. These concepts are graphically illustrated in Box 14-13.

One can control for confounding bias in the design phase or the analysis phase of the study. Two approaches to confounding control in the design phase are restriction and randomization. With restriction, you limit the eligible subjects to those who are in one category of the confounding variable. Referring back to the example in the previous paragraph, if we were to enroll only subjects classified as upper social class, it would limit confounding by social class because it would break the necessary link between exposure and the confounding factor. Both children exposed and not exposed to the preventive program would be equally likely to be of upper social class because all subjects would be of upper social class. Another approach would be to randomize exposure. A randomized trial is an experimental study in which exposure is randomly assigned. In this way, given a sufficiently large number of subjects, the exposed and the nonexposed are likely to have the same characteristics. Additionally, randomization is the only way to control for known and *unknown* confounders.

In the analytic phase, you can control for known confounding factors, *provided that you collected data on these factors*. This chapter covers two approaches: stratification and regression. Stratification in the analysis phase is analogous to restriction in the design phase. To control for the confounding factor, we would examine the relationship between exposure and disease in strata,

BOX 14-13 Confounding

A confounding factor must possess three characteristics:

1. It must be associated with exposure.
2. It must be associated with disease, even among the unexposed.
3. It must not be an intermediate on the causal pathway between exposure and disease.

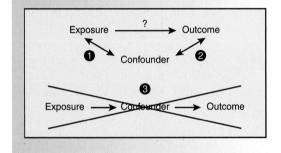

or levels, of this factor. In our example study (Box 14-1), the authors examined the relationship between exposure to the preventive program and presence of carious lesions in the permanent teeth (Table 14-4 and Table 14-11A). They found that the risk ratio between exposure and outcome was 0.74. Again, imagine that those exposed were more likely to be of upper social class and that social class is negatively associated with presence of carious lesions in the permanent teeth. In other words, social class is a confounder. To control for this confounding, we may stratify by social class. If social class had two levels, high/middle and low, we would create two 2×2 tables, as shown in Table 14-11 B–C.

You can see how the estimate of the risk ratio changes when we control for social status: exposure has a smaller effect. By controlling for confounding, we come closer to the true causal effect of the preventive program on the proportion of

TABLE 14-11 A–C OVERALL AND ADJUSTED (SOCIAL CLASS) RELATIONSHIP BETWEEN EXPOSURE TO THE PREVENTIVE PROGRAM AND PRESENCE OF CARIOUS LESIONS IN PERMANENT TEETH

A. Overall

	CARIOUS LESIONS IN PERMANENT TEETH	NO CARIOUS LESIONS IN PERMANENT TEETH	TOTAL
Exposed	289	258	547
Nonexposed	169	68	237
Total	458	326	

RR = 0.74

B. High/Middle Social Class

	CARIOUS LESIONS IN PERMANENT TEETH	NO CARIOUS LESIONS IN PERMANENT TEETH	TOTAL
Exposed	160	241	401
Nonexposed	81	101	182
Total	241	342	

RR = 0.9

C. Low Social Class:

	CARIOUS LESIONS IN PERMANENT TEETH	NO CARIOUS LESIONS IN PERMANENT TEETH	TOTAL
Exposed	82	54	136
Nonexposed	37	18	55
Total	119	72	

RR = 0.9

children with carious lesions in the permanent dentition. Stratification works well when you want to control only for a single confounding factor, but not when there are multiple confounding factors because you have to create a stratum for each

combination of factors. For example, if you have two binary confounding factors (e.g., gender and social status), you would have to consider four strata. Additionally, when the confounding factor is continuous, stratification would be impractical. In these cases, one relies on regression.

LINEAR AND LOGISTIC REGRESSION

There are several types of regression analyses. Here, we introduce linear and logistic regression, defined in Box 14-14. The subtleties of regression are beyond the scope of this chapter. For more detail, read *Fundamentals of Biostatistics* (Duxbury Press, 1995).[7] It is best to consult a biostatistician to assist you to perform regression.

Linear Regression

Linear regression assesses the relationship between a single, continuous outcome variable and one or more explanatory variables (e.g., exposures, confounding factors). The explanatory variables may take any form, continuous or categorical. The outcome variable is sometimes referred to as the dependent variable; the explanatory variables are referred to as independent variables. Several assumptions must be met to validly perform linear regression, which are beyond the scope of this book. Conducting linear regression results in the estimation of a linear equation relating the dependent to the independent variables. Let us first consider relating a single continuous outcome to a single exposure, returning to the hypothetical relationship between income and DMFT (Fig. 14-8). The equation resulting from this simple linear regression is in the familiar form of $y = mx + b$, where y is the value of the dependent variable, x is the value of the independent variable, m is the slope (also called the linear regression coefficient or β), and b is the intercept. In this case, the equation is DMFT $= -0.00014$ (income) $+ 7.94$. The intercept is the value of the dependent variable (y, DMFT in this case) when the independent variable (x, income in this case) is 0. Thus, the linear regression predicts that those with an income = 0

BOX 14-14 Linear and Logistic Regression

Simple linear regression: Used to evaluate the linear relationship between a *single continuous* dependent variable (outcome) and a *single* independent variable (exposure).

Multiple linear regression: Used to evaluate the linear relationship between a *single continuous* dependent variable (outcome) and *two or more* independent variables (e.g., exposures, confounding factors).

Simple logistic regression: Used to evaluate the relationship between a *single binary* dependent variable (outcome) and a *single* continuous or categorical independent variable (exposure).

Multiple logistic regression: Used to evaluate the relationship between a *single binary* dependent variable (outcome) and *two or more* independent variables (e.g., exposures, confounding factors).

would have a DMFT = 7.94. You interpret the linear regression coefficient as you would any slope: for every one-unit (dollar) increase in income, there is a 0.00014 decrease in DMFT. You may also conduct hypothesis testing on this coefficient. The null hypothesis is that the linear regression coefficient = 0. The alternative is that $\beta \neq 0$, in other words, that there is a linear relationship between income and DMFT. As with any hypothesis test, a p-value would result. In this case, the p-value associated with income is 0.022, which is below the threshold of $\alpha = 0.05$. In this way, we would reject the null hypothesis and conclude that there is a statistically significant, linear relationship between DMFT and income. Beyond determining the presence of a linear relationship, linear regression equations may be used to predict the value of the dependent variable, given the values of the independent variable(s). In our example, we would predict that someone with an income of $38,000 would have a DMFT of -0.00014 (38,000) + 7.94 = 2.62. To have a prediction model that included more than one independent variable or to control for confounding of an exposure–outcome relationship, you would use multiple linear regression. For example, suppose that we wanted to examine the relationship between income and DMFT, controlling for gender, because we suspect that gender may be a confounding factor. Let us say that we obtained the following equation: DMFT = -0.00019 (income) + 0.93 (gender) + 7.9. Focusing on the coefficient associated with income, we can see that *controlling for gender,* for every 1-unit increase in income, there is a 0.00019 decrease in DMFT. This is a different estimate than we obtained when we did not control for gender because we have removed the effects of confounding by gender. To fully interpret this equation, you would need to know that gender is coded as 0 for females and 1 for males. Thus, the interpretation of the coefficient associated with gender is that *controlling for income* males have a 0.93 higher DMFT than females.

Logistic Regression

Logistic regression examines the relationship between a single, binary outcome variable and one or more explanatory variables (e.g., exposures, confounding factors). As with linear regression, the explanatory variables may take any form; the terms *dependent variables* and *independent variables* refer to outcome and explanatory variables, respectively. Several assumptions, which are beyond the scope of this chapter, need to be met to validly perform logistic regression. Logistic regression results in odds ratio(s) describing the relationships between the outcome and explanatory variable(s). Here, we will focus on the interpretation of the odds ratio associated with a binary exposure. To illustrate, in our example study (Box 14-1), the authors first conducted a simple logistic regression analysis to examine the relationship between exposure to the preventive program and suffering from caries during the 7.5-year follow-up, both binary variables. They found an odds ratio of 0.42. Interpreting this as a risk ratio, those children exposed to the preventive program were 58% less likely to have experienced carious lesions during the follow-up period than those children who were not exposed. You may conduct hypothesis testing on this odds ratio to obtain a p-value. The null hypothesis would be that there is no relationship between exposure to the preventive program and experience of carious lesions 7.5 years after beginning the intervention; in other terms, the null hypothesis would be that the odds ratio = 1. The alternative hypothesis would be that OR ≠ 1. The authors conducted the test; the result was a p-value <0.0001, indicating that we can reject the null hypothesis. Next, the authors conducted multiple logistic regression; this allowed them to examine the relationship between exposure (prevention program) and outcome (one or more carious

lesions during the 7.5 years of follow-up), controlling for carious lesions at the beginning of the study, gender, malocclusion, presence of posterior cross-bite, and social class. Controlling for these factors, the odds ratio relating the preventive program to the experience of carious lesions was 0.40, almost identical to that obtained from the simple logistic regression.

GUIDELINES FOR INFERRING CAUSALITY

Researchers usually try to identify causation rather than just association. This certainly applies to the use of statistics to evaluate dental public health interventions; you want to be sure that any relationship you detect between an intervention and an outcome is a result of the intervention, rather than some other explanation. In 1965, Hill proposed a commonly referenced set of standards for evaluating causality.[8] Six of his criteria were strength, consistency, temporality, dose-response, plausibility, and experimental evidence. These criteria are assigned brief explanations in Box 14-15. Other than temporality, which is absolutely necessary to establish cause and effect, these criteria should not be viewed as rigid requirements; they are simply guidelines.

BOX 14-15 Six Standards for Causality

1. **Strength.** Stronger associations may be more likely to be causal than are weak associations.
2. **Consistency.** Consistent associations are those that are observed across various populations and circumstances. You should keep in mind, however, that some effects occur only in rare circumstances.
3. **Temporality.** A cause must precede an effect.
4. **Dose-Response.** As the "dose" of the cause increases, the likelihood of the effect occurring increases.
5. **Plausibility.** A causal relationship should be biologically plausible. Keep in mind, however, that the perception of plausibility may be limited by current understanding.
6. **Experimental evidence.** Experimental evidence provides a test of the causal hypothesis, but this is not always possible or ethical to obtain.

STATISTICAL VERSUS CLINICAL SIGNIFICANCE

Because a result is statistically significant, it does not mean that it is clinically significant. When a null hypothesis can be rejected (because the p-value is less than your cutoff α), there is good evidence that an effect is present; however, that effect may be so small as to be clinically meaningless. A small p-value, such as 0.0001, does not mean that there is a strong association; it simply means that there is strong evidence for some association. For example, suppose that the study described in Box 14-1 found a statistically significant association between exposure to the preventive program and mean DMFT, with a p-value of 0.04. We should ask the question: How large was the difference between the mean DMFTs? If those who received the preventive program had a mean DMFT of 1.0 and those who did not receive the preventive program had a mean DMFT of 5.0, the results would be more clinically important than if the children who did not receive the program had a mean DMFT of only 1.25. It is essential that you judge clinical significance on the basis of the magnitude of effect, rather than on p-value alone.

SUMMARY

The chapters in Module IV have given you a foundation in epidemiology and biostatistics. A basic understanding of these sciences is essential to the conduct of every stage of evidence-based public health practice: defining the problem, planning the initiative, implementing the initiative, and evaluating the program. Equally important, however, is the application of this knowledge to critically review published literature. This is the concern of Chapter 15.

RESOURCES

Moore DS. Statistics: Concepts and Controversies. New York, NY: W.H. Freeman, 1991.

Norman GR, Streiner DL. PDQ Statistics. Hamilton, ON, Canada: B.C. Decker, 1999.

Weintraub JA, Douglass CW, Gillings DB. Biostats: Data Analysis for Dental Health Care Professionals. Chapel Hill, NC: CAVCO, 1985.

Review Questions:

1. From the following selections (a-d), classify gender, race, and temperature in terms of type of variable.
   a. Binary nominal categorical
   b. Nominal categorical with >2 categories
   c. Ordinal categorical
   d. Continuous

2. What is the median of the following numbers: 12, 0, 5, 4, 10, 10, 8, 2, and 3?
   a. 5
   b. 10
   c. 6
   d. 4.5

3. What is the standard deviation of the series of numbers in Question 2?
   a. 15.3
   b. 16.3
   c. 3.9
   d. 6.2

4. Consider a standard normally distributed variable Z. Determine the probability that it will lie between -2 and -1.
   a. 13.6%
   b. 84.1%
   c. 15.9%
   d. 2.3%

5. A hypothetical cohort study was conducted on the relationship between current smoking and the presence of gingivitis or periodontal disease. The study yielded the following 2×2 table:

	GINGIVITIS OR PERIODONTAL DISEASE PRESENT	GINGIVITIS OR PERIODONTAL DISEASE ABSENT	TOTAL
Current Smoker	50	50	100
Not Current Smoker	50	100	150
Total	100	150	250

What is the risk ratio describing the relationship between current smoking and gingivitis and periodontal disease in the population?
a. 0.50
b. 0.33
c. 1.75
d. 1.52

6. A longitudinal study was conducted to determine the relationship between dmft (decayed, missing, or filled primary teeth) in first grade and DMFT in fifth grade. The scatter diagram of dmft versus DMFT looks like this:

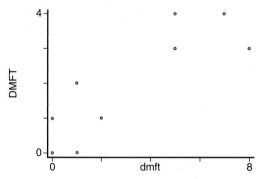

How would you describe the linear relationship between dmft and DMFT?
a. Positive
b. Negative
c. Nonexistent
d. Not enough information provided

7. A study was conducted to determine the relationship between flossing and the number of sites that bled on periodontal probing (BOP). Flossing was classified as daily, less than daily, and never. Assuming BOP was normally distributed, what statistical test would you use to formally assess the null hypothesis that daily flossers, less than daily flossers, and never flossers have the same mean BOP?
a. t-test
b. Correlation
c. Mann-Whitney μ test
d. ANOVA/F-test

8. A hypothetical cohort study was conducted on the relationship between presence of periodontal disease and subsequent development of coronary heart disease. Both variables were binary categorical. The authors calculated the risk ratio to be 1.5. What is your interpretation of the risk ratio?
a. 1.5 more people with periodontal disease developed coronary heart disease.
b. Those people with periodontal disease were 1.5 times more likely to develop coronary heart disease.
c. Those people with coronary heart disease were 1.5 times more likely to develop periodontal disease.
d. 1.5 more people with coronary heart disease developed periodontal disease.

9. Return to the example in Question 8. By conducting a statistical test, the authors found the p-value to be below the set α level of 0.05. What type of statistical error may you be concerned about?
a. None
b. β error
c. α error
d. Sampling error

10. Does statistical significance always imply clinical significance?
a. Yes
b. No

REFERENCES

1. American Dental Education Association. Competencies for entry into the profession of dental hygiene, Exhibit 7. J Dent Educ 2003;67(7):1–5. Available at: http://www.adea.org/cepr. Accessed February 2004.

2. Tapias MA, De Miguel G, Jimenez-Garcia R, Gonzalez A, Dominguez V. Incidence of caries in an infant population in Móstoles, Madrid. Evaluation of a preventive program after 7.5 years of follow-up. Int J Paediatr Dent 2001; 11:440–446.

3. Norman GR, Streiner DL. PDQ Statistics. Hamilton, Ontario: B.C. Decker, 1999.

4. Money Income in the United States: 1999. Washington, DC: U.S. Census Bureau, 2000.

5. Rothman KJ, Greenland S. Modern Epidemiology. Philadelphia, PA: Lippincott Williams and Wilkins, 1998.

6. Sackett DL. Bias in analytic research. J Chronic Dis 1979; 32:51–63.

7. Rosner B. Fundamentals of Biostatistics. Belmont, CA: Duxbury Press, 1995.

8. Hill AB. The environment and disease: association or causation? Proc Royal Soc Med 1965;58:295–300.

Scientific Communication

Objectives

After studying this chapter and completing the study questions and activities, the learner will be able to:

- Define evidence-based dentistry.
- Describe how scientific information is transferred to health professionals and the public.
- Access and assess the quality and applicability of information found in the scientific and public literature.
- List and describe sections of a scientific article.
- Describe different methods of communicating scientific information.
- Select an appropriate mode of communicating a new concept or information.
- Create and deliver a scientific presentation.

KEY TERMS

Abstract	MEDLINE	References
Critical review	Methodology	Results
Discussion	Oral presentation	Round table
Evidence-based care	Original source	Secondary source
Evidence-based dentistry	Peer-reviewed	Table clinic
Juried	Poster	Title
Literature review	PubMed	
Literature search	Refereed	

The American Dental Education Association competencies addressed in this chapter include[1]:

C.3:   Provide dental hygiene care to promote patient/client health and wellness using critical thinking and problem solving in the provision of evidence-based practice.

C.4:   Assume responsibility for dental hygiene actions and care based on accepted scientific theories and research, as well as the accepted standard of care.

C.8:   Communicate effectively with individuals and groups from diverse populations, both verbally and in writing.

CM.4:   Facilitate client access to oral health services by influencing individuals and/or organizations for the provision of oral health care.

HP.1:   Promote the values of oral and general health and wellness to the public and organizations within and outside the profession.

Introduction

It is the responsibility of scientists and innovators in a particular discipline to relate information, ideas, and results in a clear and concise manner. This facilitates the transfer of information from the point of discovery to potential users, including health professionals and the public at large. It is also of vital importance in the grant writing process in order to promote a new idea or concept to open the avenues of discovery. A clear and concise statement of purpose and plan for a research study increase the chance for funding a study to obtain new knowledge. There are several key ways scientists may effectively transmit findings and ideas, including professional journals and scientific presentations, such as poster sessions, table clinics, round tables, or oral presentations at professional meetings. Continuing-education courses are another mode of relaying information to user groups. Most states require professionals to stay current in their discipline in this way. In many cases, the media may also be a useful and effective tool for disseminating information. Internet-based information, including professional journals, government Web sites, professional listserves, and consumer information, is a rapidly growing form of information dissemination.

It is the responsibility of the dental public health practitioner to be able to evaluate the quality of new information from all of these sources using cultivated skills in critical thinking to determine the usefulness and applicability of the information to the practice setting. Staying abreast of current information contributes to the pursuit of lifelong learning and allows one to respond effectively and accurately to inquiries from patients and the public. In addition, this enables the practitioner to provide the most current, appropriate care for their patient population, based on the latest scientific evidence. This is referred to as **evidence–based care.**

EVIDENCE–BASED DENTISTRY

Chapter 2 stated that the goal of evidence-based practice is to facilitate timely translation of research findings into clinical and community practices that result in improved oral health. **Evidence-based dentistry** (EBD) is an approach to oral health care that requires the judicious integration of systematic assessments of clinically relevant scientific evidence relating to the patient's oral and medical condition and history, with the provider's clinical expertise and the patient's treatment needs and preferences.[2] The American Dental Association has defined EBD as a process that includes four components (Box 15-1):

1. Defining clinically relevant question(s).
2. Systematically conducting searches for all studies and databases, published or unpublished, that may help answer the question.

BOX 15-1 Evidence–Based Dentistry

Four components of evidence-based dentistry:

1. Defining clinically relevant question(s).
2. Systematically conducting searches for all studies and databases, published or unpublished, that may help to answer the question.
3. Translating the findings from systematic reviews for use by practitioners.
4. Assessing the health care outcomes that result from following the EBD process.

From: American Dental Association Policy on Evidence-Based Dentistry. Available at: http//www.ada.org/prof/prac/issues/statements/evidencebased.html#definition. Accessed May 9, 2003.[2]

3. Translating the findings from systematic reviews for use by practitioners.
4. Assessing the health care outcomes that result from following the EBD process.[1]

It behooves the dental public health practitioner to apply EBD methods to aid in program planning and clinical care. Applying these methods helps ensure quality care and programs. Several professional organizations and government entities worldwide have developed centers for evidence-based practice. Among these resources are the Cochrane Oral Health Group, the University of York National Health Service Centre for Review and Dissemination, and the Center for Evidence-Based Dentistry at the Institute of Health Sciences at Oxford University. These sites also provide valuable links to other information on evidence-based practice. The resource section at the end of the chapter contains a list of useful sites.

DIFFUSION OF INNOVATIONS

Chapter 9 introduced the Diffusion of Innovations theory (Table 9-2; Box 9-6). Health educators not only use the principles of this theory to select strategies for health education programs, but also for describing transfer of information from scientists or innovators at the point of discovery to the potential users of the information. A critical factor in the speed at which the diffusion of innovations (Fig. 15-1) or information occurs is the scientist's ability to disseminate the information quickly and efficiently and the professional's vigilance in staying abreast of new evidence, ideas, and treatment modalities.

Scientists, researchers, and industry are primary sources of new information. The role of these entities is to investigate new technologies, modes of care delivery, techniques, and materials in terms of safety, effectiveness, and quality. In ad-

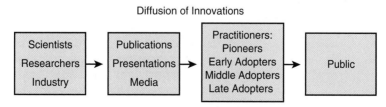

Diffusion of Innovations

FIGURE 15-1 Diffusion of Innovations. (Source: Becker MH. Factors affecting diffusion of innovations among health professionals. Am J Public Health 1970; 60(2):294–304.)[3]

dition, they may evaluate current methodologies to determine continued effectiveness in light of new information. It is also their role to initiate the dissemination of the information through effective channels of scientific communication. In most cases, the information is first made available to professional practitioners in the field.

The time lag that occurs between the disclosure of new knowledge and the use of this knowledge by health care professionals can deprive many citizens of the benefits of the information, sometimes for many years. Currently, more and more companies with a product to market are targeting the public directly through the use of the media in hopes that the public will receive the information sooner and will prompt providers to consider the product sooner. Although this is a marketing strategy, it also may shorten the time of diffusion (Fig. 15-2). In addition, it applies greater pressure to practitioners to stay abreast of new information. Because the media does not always portray health information accurately, providers should be prepared to educate their patients.

As described in Chapter 9, not all adopters of innovation are created equal. Not all providers adopt or embrace new procedures, technology, or materials at the same rate. Adopters can be pioneers (innovators), early adopters, middle adopters (majority), or late adopters (laggards).[2] Pioneers and early adopters are the first to hear of new innovations and the first to adopt them into practice. As a result, they become opinion leaders in the communication network in their respective field and, as such, are often looked on as highly credible sources of information. Middle and late adopters may rely on these opinion leaders for information or seek it out in other ways but, for various reasons, are not as quick to adopt the innovation into their

practices. When the information is disseminated and available to practitioners, it becomes the role of the practitioner to *access* and *assess* the information. Although the Internet now provides much quicker and broader access to information for all levels of adopters and may speed up the diffusion of new ideas, it also adds new challenges in assessing the quality of available information.

ACCESSING INFORMATION

To provide evidence-based programs, it is important to be able to locate the latest information. Most students and public health practitioners are familiar with seeking out resources through a library catalog to obtain information on a topic of choice. Many health science libraries have reference librarians who can assist in locating information or generating a computer literature search for you. If the library does not have the journal or book in their collection, they can assist in requesting the information from another library. This may be time consuming and costly and not feasible for the provider who needs it quickly. However, this method is becoming dated with the accessibility of online resources.

Many sources of information are available at the touch of a finger. Certain sources and advantages and disadvantages of each are detailed in Table 15-1. With access to the Internet, a **literature search** of the medical, dental, and other literature databases worldwide can be quickly performed. An example is **MEDLINE** or **PubMed,** an English language bibliographic database that allows free Internet access through the National Library of Medicine. A perfect example of the diffusion of innovations is that new search engines and databases are appearing constantly and many

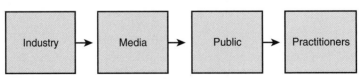

FIGURE 15-2 **New Path for Diffusion of Innovations.**

TABLE 15-1 ADVANTAGES AND DISADVANTAGES OF SOURCES OF INFORMATION

SOURCE	ADVANTAGE/DISADVANTAGE
Newsletters	Current; not scientific
Journals	Current information; rigor and objectivity varies
Books	Foundational knowledge; dated information
Published empirical reports	Current information; rigor and objectivity varies
Advertisements	Biased information
Newspapers	Clue to public interest; subject to interpretation and bias
Popular magazines	Readable; subject to interpretation and bias
Internet	Accessible; no control over validity of information
Professional meetings	Current information; rigor and objectivity varies

professional journals are becoming available on-line for immediate downloading without the delay of sending away for reprints from the author, publisher, or the nearest health sciences library.

In addition to professional journals and publications, the Internet provides access to a multitude of other sources of information, including funding agencies, foundations, census figures and immigration statistics, and oral health programs. In addition, information from most government agencies can be accessed, many of which have information and specific data about national efforts in your area of interest. These may include the Surgeon General's Report on Oral Health,[4] Healthy People 2010 Objectives for the Nation,[5] the National Center for Health Statistics—FastStats,[6] the National Oral Health Surveillance System,[7] the Centers for Disease Control and Prevention,[8] or the World Health Organization.[9]

Many listserves can be found on the Internet where professionals dialogue on topics pertinent to their practice. These listserves allow professionals to ask questions of colleagues and experts about sources of information, successful programs, and funding opportunities. It also can provide the opportunity for partnering to build alliances for oral health promotion. A well-established professional listserves in dental public health is listed in the resource section.

The Internet facilitates accessing an overwhelming amount of information but, unfortunately, does not assess the quality of information available. That process still remains with the user.

ASSESSING INFORMATION

Evaluating the quality of information involves the ability to discriminate between high-quality, valid information and information that is not predicated on sound scientific principles. Learning to critically review information may take time and practice to develop, but it is essential to the practice of public health. Scientific information and the number of journals are compounding at alarming rates, making it virtually impossible for professionals to stay abreast of new information without strong skills in critical review. Professional education and competence includes the ability to evaluate the quality of information. How does a health care professional decide which information is useful, pertinent, valid, or of high quality? How does one go beyond textbooks to make those decisions on their own?

Textbooks provide strong foundational knowledge in a specific field. However, the nature of the publishing process can render much cutting-edge information obsolete by the time of publication. The time line for publishing a text can be 2 to 3 years, and the information may be several years old at submission. Professional journals may bring information to the reader sooner because they are published more frequently. Even so, the process of publishing the paper may take 6 months to 1 year before it is available (Fig. 15-3). Presentations at scientific meetings may be made soon after results of a study or evaluation of a program take place, making this a more rapid form of information diffusion. Attendance at these meetings is an important part of being a professional and pursuing lifelong learning.

Assessing Written Information

Obviously, the source of information is an important factor in determining the quality of information. Textbooks and quality journals undergo a process of **peer review.** This means the information has been reviewed, **juried,** or **refereed** by other scientists or experts in the field before it is accepted for publication. This is usually achieved by an anonymous method carried out by the publisher or editor and ensures the quality of the publication and the reputation of the journal and/or the professional society sponsoring the journal. This is a several step process, which explains the delay in the information being available to the public (Fig. 15-3). However, that is a necessary trade-off to assure the quality of the information disseminated. Although textbooks lend themselves well to the educational process, journals are a more common source of information for practicing professionals.

Journals are not all created equally. Not all journals are peer-reviewed or published with the goal of strong scientific integrity. To determine if a journal is peer-reviewed, check for a listing of the editorial board and read through the journal's author instructions. Does it mention a review process or ask that multiple copies of an article be submitted? Contacting the editor directly can also be useful. Journals may be sponsored by a learned society or scientific publisher, a professional organization, or a commercial publisher.[10] Learned societies are formed for the purpose of disseminating scientific findings, and they maintain a

strong emphasis on scientific rigor. Advertising is rarely included in the publications. Reputable scientific publishers also place a premium on scientific rigor. Journals from professional organizations are peer-reviewed in some manner; however, there may be bias toward the views of the organization and considerable advertising may be included to offset the cost of publishing. This may not compromise the quality of the information, but it is important to consider in the evaluation of the content. Many more commercial publishers, including dental-related industries, are producing journals for practitioners. A review process, if present, is not nearly as scientifically rigorous and frequently handled in-house. Articles may be solicited or written by staff writers. It is important to consider the level of quality of the information in the article before deciding how to use the information in practice (Box 15-2).

When a health care practitioner is experienced in a field of interest and becomes familiar with the available journals, the quality of a journal can be quickly determined. If the publication is determined to be a reputable source of information, a more specific review can be applied to the article of interest. Are the authors well known in their field? Are they affiliated with a research or academic institution? Was the study funded by a federal agency or well-respected foundation or by a commercial enterprise?

Next, the **abstract** is critiqued for an overview of the content. Does the **title** reflect the content of the article? Does the content offer new information or concepts that would be useful to your program? What information is presented and how well is it supported by other literature or studies and by the results presented in the article? It is important to determine how this new information expands knowledge, is congruent or incongruent with what is known, and whether or not the conclusions presented are supported by the evidence. Keep in mind, causation cannot be determined by a single study, but must be developed over time, with multiple studies indicating a particular cause and effect. Claims of cause and effect must be considered with caution.

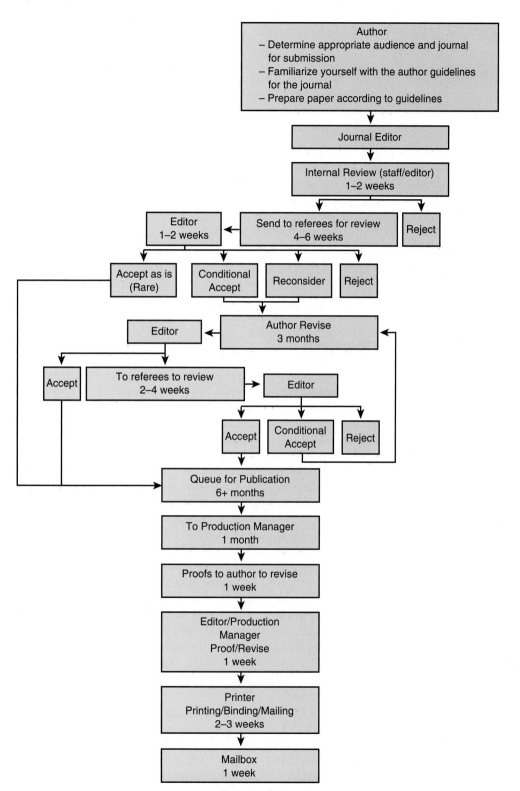

FIGURE 15-3 Steps to Publishing a Scientific Article. (Recognition to: Tomar S., ed., J Public Health Dent, for providing the information used for this timeline.)

BOX 15-2 Quality of Scientific Information

Quality of Information from highest to lowest:

- Experimental studies or clinical trials
- Rigorously-controlled cohort and case-control studies
- Clinical trials without concurrent control groups
- Retrospective cross-sectional studies without controls
- Descriptive surveys
- Case reports
- Personal opinion, subjective opinion, anecdotal accounts

Adapted from: Burt BA, Eklund SA. Dentistry, Dental Practice, and the Community. 5th Ed. Philadelphia, PA: WB Saunders, 1999, p 153.[10]

When the reader is satisfied that the source is reputable and the content of the article is of interest, it is time to read the entire article. Some practitioners prefer to read the **methodology** section first to determine if the methods employed are valid and reliable. Are there dental indices, survey instruments, or measurement tools presented that have not been previously used or tested? Are flaws in the sampling process evident? Are there flaws in the chosen research design that may influence the validity of the results? Research method and design have been addressed in earlier chapters.

If the methodology is acceptable and appropriate, the reader may continue with other sections. The **literature review** or introduction should clearly identify the problem and provide an unbiased presentation of background information about the topic. The **references,** therefore, should be current and represent both sides of the issue.

In the **results** section, any statistical tests should be described and be appropriate for the data collected. This was also addressed in more depth in Chapter 14. Are the results statistically significant or clinically significant? Could they be applied to any similar practice situation and to what extent? Is more information needed to assess the value of the results in relation to another practice?

When reviewing the **discussion** section, determine if the conclusions presented are supported by the results. Are the authors forthcoming about any potential limitations to the study? Can the results be generalized to other practice settings? Are there possible explanations for the stated outcomes other than those suggested by the authors? See Box 15-3 for a summary of items to consider when consulting written information.

A **critical review** of an article is not solely for the purpose of being critical of the research or the authors. It is to assess the level of quality of the information and how it may be used appropriately, if at all, in practice. Often, when first learning to review the literature, learners are focused so heavily on finding fault and criticizing that they neglect to consider how the information may provide some positive growth in the knowledge base of the field. Eventually, the pendulum swings back to a more neutral unbiased review. An unbiased critical review looks at both the positive and negative aspects of the information.

Assessing Internet Information

Techniques for assessing written scientific information have been available for some time, and each person may adapt them to their own personal

BOX 15-3 Assessing Written Information Sources

Publication Quality
- Peer-review process, editorial board
- Professional organization, learned society, commercial publisher
- Current
- Authors well respected, affiliated with research or academic institution

Title and Abstract
- Title clear, reflects content, useful to your practice
- Abstract complete, concise, expands knowledge, conclusions supported, major findings reported

Introduction/Literature Review
- Problem clearly stated and developed
- Unbiased presentation of topic

Methodology
- Sample appropriate—size and selection
- Indices/measurement tool reliable, valid, sensitive, specific
- Research design
- Relevant or adaptable to your practice

Results
- Appropriate statistical analysis chosen
- Charts and graphs clear and described in text
- Statistically or clinically significant
- Applicable to practice

Discussion
- Conclusions warranted from results presented
- Limitations described
- Generalizable to other situations
- Other explanations for results

References
- Current
- Thorough
- Useful for further investigation
- Original source of information

style or preference. The explosion of Internet information and the type and amount of information available for both scientists and the lay public through that source requires some additional evaluation. Guides are now being developed for review of Web sites and Internet material. Dalhousie University in Canada[11] has developed a list of six criteria for evaluating health information on the Internet: (1) credibility, (2) content, (3) disclosure, (4) links, (5) design, and (6) interactivity

(Box 15-4). In addition to the criteria already mentioned for assessing written information, these criteria are useful for Web sites in particular.

Assessing credibility includes considering the source of the information and its currency and relevance and whether it is subject to a review process. The content should be accurate, complete, and provide a disclaimer. It is also important that users are informed about collection of any information about them and how that information will be used. Links are provided for additional high-quality sources for information on that topic, and the design should provide for easy navigation of the Web site. The Web site should also provide a way for users to interact and provide feedback and comments.

COMMUNICATING YOUR MESSAGE

It was mentioned that it is the role of the scientist to effectively communicate new information to other professionals or the public. What if you have a striking new idea or discovery about which you want to inform people? The best way to communicate the message may be in the form of a journal article or presenting at a professional meeting by means of a table clinic, poster session, oral presentation, or round table. You may want to provide a continuing-education course for a local dental or dental hygiene society or other interested group. How will the presentation be organized? What is the best forum for presenting the message? All of these are considerations when communicating a message. This section will explore the various methods of communicating new information. There are many resources available for a more in-depth discussion of writing a research paper. Certain resources are listed at the end of this chapter. An important step for any author or presenter is to have a colleague(s) read, review, or listen to a presentation and provide feedback on content, style, and readability. This may help avoid many pitfalls, including grammar and spelling, especially those mistakes spell-checker does not catch!

BOX 15-4 Assessing Health Information on the Internet

Credibility
- Source
- Currency
- Relevance
- Review Process

Content
- Accuracy
- Disclaimer
- Completeness

Disclosure
- Data Collection

Links
- External links provided

Design
- Navigation

Interactivity
- Feedback
- Questions

Reprinted with permission from: Evaluation of Health Information on the Internet. W.K. Kellogg Health Sciences Library. Dalhousie University, Halifax, Nova Scotia, Canada. Available at: http://www.library.dal.ca/kellogg/internet/evaluate.htm.[11]

Although this section focuses on a typical journal article, the principles are the same for submitting a case study, a review of the literature, or other informational article for publication.

Journal Articles

A standard journal article describing a new scientific development or program includes six sections, abstract, introduction or review of the literature, methodology, results, discussion, and references. This is not necessarily the order in which they are written, but the order in which they may appear in the published article. Preparing an article for publication has many similar considerations as the critical review of articles from other authors.

Before beginning the writing process, consider the audience that may be most appropriate for the information. What professional journals might reach that audience? What are the style requirements for the publication(s)? Most publications publish instructions to authors at least once a year. Locate these instructions and follow them during the construction of the article. It will save considerable time reformatting.

LITERATURE REVIEW

The literature review, usually the first section written, begins with a thorough search of the available literature on the topic. This section is a review, synthesis, and evaluation of the current scientific knowledge on the subject of the report. It also points out where there may be gaps in the scientific knowledge. This process requires a base list of references, including those from MEDLINE or PubMed and other sources such as books, government agencies, and other official documents. For each pertinent reference located, the complete reference citation, including journal, author(s), volume number, pages, publisher and publisher location, and date of publication, should be documented. For Web sites, include the uniform resource locator (URL) and the date accessed. Index cards are useful for this purpose. Each index card should include the complete citation and a short synopsis of the article. These can easily be sorted and arranged according to topic or format for the paper. In addition, there are several reference programs available for use with the computer. These programs allow sorting and storing of references and article information.

When the information to be included is located, it is time to use skills in assessing the quality of the information and organizing it into a logical order. A working outline of the paper should include an introductory paragraph that states the purpose of the paper, program, or study. Following this statement of purpose, the analysis and synthesis of the information is presented in a specific manner, such as chronologically, geographically, by magnitude of results, or information supporting or refuting the concept. Subheadings may be useful for clarification of information. When the information is presented, concluding comments can tie the information together and to the original premise of the study or program.

METHODOLOGY

Methodology describes the details of how the study was performed or how the program was administered. This section should answer the questions of who, what, where, how, and why. It also should be in enough detail to allow others to evaluate the study or program and be able to replicate it or adapt it for their needs. This section details the research design, including sampling technique, procedures performed, data collection instrument(s) and criteria, process of evaluation, and the rationale for the procedures used.

RESULTS

The results section describes the analyses of the data collected or outcome of the evaluation procedures, including the statistical tests performed. Data also may be presented in table or graph form, together with the text for clarification and emphasis of important findings. It is important at this point to refrain from interpreting the results and discussing the implications, as that is reserved for the discussion section of the paper.

DISCUSSION

The discussion section provides the reader with the author's thoughts on what the results mean and the significance of the results to the profession. It discusses findings that agree or disagree with the current literature, the interpretation of the findings, and the significance of the results.

Opinions can be expressed, if they can be supported by the results. Any limitations in the study or applicability or generalization of the results to other settings should be included. A concise summary with conclusions should highlight the major findings and their significance. Suggested areas of further study are also a beneficial addition.

REFERENCES

The reference section is a fluid portion of the paper. The list of references will grow as the paper or program develops, new information becomes available, and references are gleaned from information read while preparing the paper. From the beginning of the process, they should be complete and reflect the most current research in the field. They should be generated from the **original source** or author of the information. This means that the reference quoted should be the original study or article and not from a **secondary source** that has quoted the material in a later publication. Quoting the secondary source may not accurately reflect the intent of the original author and may result in inaccuracies if the original intent was taken out of context or misquoted by the second author.

To avoid plagiarism, credit is given to the original author for direct quotes, paraphrased ideas, factual statements, and information that is not common knowledge. Also avoid "selective referencing" in which only references that support a single opinion on a subject are included. An unbiased presentation of opposing views increases credibility of an author.

Placing the reference numbers in the text in a way that clarifies the source of the information and yet does not disrupt the flow of the paper for the reader is an important consideration. Too many references in the text become unreadable, whereas inappropriate location in the text makes it difficult for the reader to determine the source of the information. Check the style requirements for the publisher to whom the paper will be submitted and follow them closely. This includes material found both in written sources and on the Internet.

While constructing the paper, it is convenient to use the author's name and date of publication in parentheses in the text, rather than a number of a reference. This allows easier revision and reorganization or addition of references as the writing process develops. The final numbers in the text and a bibliographic list can be easily generated as a last step in the process.

ABSTRACT AND TITLE

The abstract is usually written last because it is a concise summary of the entire paper. Again, refer to the style requirements of the publisher for proper format of the abstract. An abstract is usually 200–300 words long and includes purpose, methodology, results, and conclusions. It is a vehicle for the reader to determine if the content of the paper is of relevance to their practice and whether or not to read the entire text. As such, clarity and brevity are the keys to getting the point across in a limited space.

You most likely used the abstracts and titles of other articles in your literature search to determine the usefulness of articles for your own paper.

The title will be indexed and used as a guide or screening tool by readers and other researchers. Use words that accurately reflect the nature of the information. Avoid using unnecessary words that add length and not clarity. Many publications have a limit on the number of characters allowed in the title.

Oral Presentations

An **oral presentation** is another forum for communicating a message. This forum works well for describing a program or presenting research findings. Most professional associations have annual meetings at which the diffusion of new information is a core expectation. A common method of disseminating the information is to have speakers present their work in an oral format, including lectures, symposiums, or panel discussions. Oral presentations often follow a format similar to scientific journal articles and should include a statement of the problem or purpose, a brief review of the literature, the methodology employed, results, and a discussion of the relevance of the findings. In this format, presentations must closely follow a time schedule. The length of time allowed for each presenter is designated by the meeting planner, commonly between 10 and 20 minutes, with a short question-and-answer period at the end. This format does not usually allow audience interaction.

This may be one of the most difficult delivery approaches because of the inflexibility in time, difficulty in determining audience characteristics, and performance in front of an audience. If some form of media is used, the size and layout of the room and familiarity with equipment available will determine appropriate use of audiovisuals. If a speaker is not experienced in presenting in front of an audience, then practicing in front of colleagues to get feedback on style, content, and pace is advised. If there is to be a question-and-answer period, it is important to anticipate what questions may be asked and to provide concise responses to allow several people to be able to participate. If one is unable to answer a question, do not attempt to make up an answer. Ask the participant to write the question and their contact information on a piece of paper. The information and response can be communicated later. Another member of the audience may have the information and wish to respond. The honesty of admitting you do not have the information and the offer to follow up is much more refreshing than an attempted response that, in its own way, clearly indicates you do not know.

Table Clinics

A **table clinic** is effective for demonstrating a new clinical technique or product. This is a visual format that allows hands-on demonstrations on a tabletop and open discussion with the viewer. A short presentation of the concept or procedure is followed by audience questions and interaction. The presentation is repeated frequently to allow several small groups to attend. Space may be

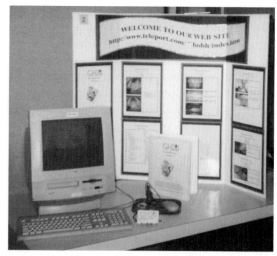

FIGURE 15-4 Outstanding Achievement in Community Dentistry. Dental Hygiene Student Merit Award [Honorable Mention]. Honolulu, HI: American Association of Public Health Dentistry, October 1999.

limited to six to eight people or the number who can easily gather around the table area. This format allows a great deal of interaction with the audience.

Attractiveness of the display is important in generating interest in your message. One may use video, slides, or computer-generated visuals. A brief handout or samples of the new product are often expected. Some organizations sponsor table clinic competitions in which the presentation is viewed by a group of judges and prizes are awarded (Fig. 15-4). Use techniques described in Chapter 10 for suggestions on how to create an attractive visual display.

Scientific or Programmatic Posters

A **poster** session format is becoming more popular at professional meetings, as it allows for a greater variety of information to be displayed in a smaller time frame and space. Usually lasting 2–3 hours, a poster session allows the participants to selectively view topics in which they are interested and allows open discussion with the presenter. This style of presentation promotes communication among professionals who may have similar interests. The presentation is visual in nature and may use photos, graphs, or bullet lists, but also should follow the format of abstract, methodology, results, summary, and conclusion. Again, follow suggestions in Chapter 10 for creating an effective visual effect.

Be prepared to answer questions on the topic of the presentation. A nice touch would be to offer a short handout or abstract that reinforces the material. Include contact information to allow viewers to contact the presenter later if they have other questions. This promotes collegiality with other professionals who may have similar interests and may lead to future projects, job opportunities, or grant proposals.

Again, some organizations sponsor poster competitions in which the presenter has a time limit to make a formal presentation to a group of judges and to respond to their questions (Fig. 15-5).

Round Table Discussions

A **round table** is yet another way to disseminate information and receive feedback on a topic, a study design, or new program. This is an interactive format and an excellent way to generate interest in a new theory, political agenda, or other topic in which you would like to brainstorm or build coalitions.

Skills in small group facilitation are extremely useful for this format to be productive. Conversations can easily divert to other subjects and decrease the effectiveness of this group process. Tips include having a set agenda with a preliminary introduction of all of the participants, a short presentation of the topic to center the discussion, and a handout with discussion points and contact information for all participants after the meeting for participants to continue the dialogue if they desire. This format is limited in attendance to the number of people who can be accommodated at the table, usually eight to ten people. Audiovisuals are only limited by the time frame allowed and room accommodations.

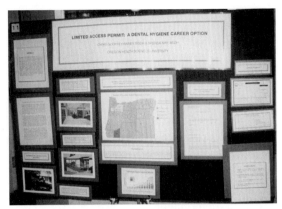

FIGURE 15-5 Limited Access Permit: A Dental Hygiene Career Option. San Diego, CA: American Dental Hygienists' Association Student Poster Competition [4th Place], June 1999.

SUMMARY

Scientific communication is a critical component of public health practice. Whether you are the grant writer for the development of a new idea, a scientist, a program administrator imparting information about a program or discovery, or the practicing professional trying to stay abreast of new information pertinent to your practice, the dissemination of information is important. Accessing and assessing the information pertinent to the practice of public health is a skill that requires practice, diligence, and a desire to be a continual learner. There are many ways to access information. However, the Internet is fast becoming the preferred mode because of its efficiency and the amount of information available. Efficiently assessing the quality and usefulness of that information is an invaluable skill. Being able to express your ideas, opinions, and concepts in a concise, clear manner using any one of many different formats is another skill that takes creativity and practice.

RESOURCES

AAPHD listserve for professionals in dental public health. Available at: http://www.aaphd.org. (Internet discussion group related to dental

Learning Activities

1. Locate form and style recommendations from various journals and compare and contrast them.
2. Create a poster, table clinic, or round table discussion format centered on a topic of interest (group or individual).
3. Write a scientific paper based on your own research or community project (group or individual).
4. Perform an Internet- or Web-based literature search on a topic of choice (individual).
5. Choose an article to critically review and share with the class (group or individual).
6. Write a review of the literature on a topic of choice, comparing and contrasting several articles, assessing quality, and deriving conclu-

sions based on what you read (individual or group).
7. Establish a weekly journal review group, rotating leadership of the discussion, to develop small group facilitation and leadership skills.
8. Visit a dental consumer Web site and evaluate the quality of information based on credibility, content, disclosure, links, design, and interactivity.
9. Select an evidence-based dentistry Web site and evaluate the site based on credibility, content, disclosure, links, design, and interactivity.
10. Identify a public health issue in the popular media and evaluate the content and appropriateness of the information.

public health topics. Access AAPHD Web site to join the listserve)

ADHA. Writing Research Papers. J Dent Hyg 1996;70(1):10–13.

Alley M. The Craft of Scientific Presentations: Critical Steps to Succeed and Critical Errors to Avoid. New York: Springler-Verlag, Dec. 13, 2002.

American Association of Public Health Dentistry (AAPHD). Available at: http://www.aaphd.org.

Briscoe MH. Preparing Scientific Illustrations: A Guide to Better Posters, Presentations, and Publications. 2nd Ed. New York: Springer-Verlag, 1996.

Center for Evidence-Based Dentistry, Institute of Health Sciences, Oxford University. Available at: http://www.ihs.ox.ac.uk/cebd/index.htm.

Cochrane Oral Health Group. Available at: http://www.cochrane-oral.man.ac.uk.

University of York, National Health Service Centre for Reviews and Dissemination (CRD). Available at: http://www.york.ac.uk/inst/crd/centre.htm.

Fourth National Research Conference: An evidence-based approach in dental hygiene practice, education, and research. J Dent Hyg (Online Suppl), Spring 2001. Available at: http://www.adha.org/publications/nrc.

Lester JD. Writing Research Papers: A Complete Guide. MLA Update. 10th Ed. New York, NY: Longman Publishing, 2003.

National Library of Medicine. Available at: www.ncbi.nlm.nih.gov/PubMed/.

Agency for Healthcare Research and Quality. Available at: http://www.ahrq.gov.

Review Questions

1. Which method of scientific communication would be MOST appropriate for demonstrating a new method of fluoride application?
   a. Oral presentation
   b. Round table discussion

c. Poster presentation

d. Table clinic

e. Journal article

2. Which of the following is NOT one of four components of evidence-based dentistry as defined by the American Dental Association?

a. Systematic literature review

b. Defining a question

c. Translating findings for use

d. Assessing health outcomes

e. Presenting findings at a professional meeting

3. Opinion leaders in the diffusion of innovations theory are most likely:

a. early adopters.

b. middle adopters.

c. late adopters.

d. nonadopters.

e. the general public.

4. The most current source of valid and reliable scientific information is most likely found:

a. in a textbook.

b. in a journal article.

c. at a professional meeting.

d. on the Internet.

e. in an advertisement.

5. The highest quality of scientific information is based on:

a. case reports.

b. retrospective cross-sectional studies without controls.

c. anecdotal accounts.

d. clinical trials with control groups.

e. clinical trials without control groups.

REFERENCES

1. American Dental Education Association. Competencies for entry into the profession of dental hygiene, Exhibit 7. J Dent Educ 2003 July;67(7):1–5. Available at: http://www.adea.org/cepr. Accessed January 2004.

2. American Dental Association Policy on Evidence-Based Dentistry. Available at: http://www.ada.org/prof/resources/positions/statements/evidencebased.asp. Accessed July 2004.

3. Becker MH. Factors affecting diffusion of innovations among health professionals. AJPH 1970;60(2):294–304.

4. Oral Health in America: A Report of the Surgeon General. Rockville, MD: U.S. Department of Health and Human Services, National Institute of Dental and Craniofacial Research, National Institutes of Health, 2000.

5. U.S. Department of Health and Human Services. Healthy People 2010. Washington, DC: January 2000. Available at: www.health.gov/healthypeople.

6. National Center for Health Statistics–FastStats. Available at: http://www.cdc.gov/nchs/fastats.

7. National Oral Health Surveillance System. Available at: http://www.cdc.gov/nohss.

8. Centers for Disease Control. Available at: http://www.cdc.gov.

9. World Health Organization. Available at: http://www.who.int.

10. Burt BA, Eklund, SA. Dentistry, Dental Practice, and the Community. 5th Ed. Philadelphia, PA: WB Saunders, 1999.

11. Evaluation of Health Information on the Internet. W.K. Kellogg Health Sciences Library. Dalhousie University, Halifax, Nova Scotia, Canada. Available at: http://www.library.dal.ca/kellogg/internet/evaluate.htm.

ETHICS AND THE LAW IN PUBLIC HEALTH PRACTICE

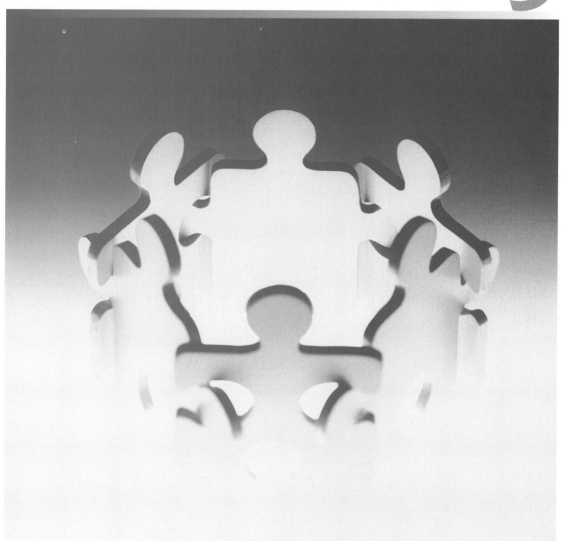

Ethical Principles

16

Objectives

After studying this chapter and completing the study questions and activities, the learner will be able to:
- Describe the characteristics of a profession.
- Identify responsibilities that contribute to professional behavior and attitude.
- Identify clinical professional responsibilities, focusing on patient care and patient–operator interactions.
- Understand the underlying ethical theories that are the foundation of ethical principles.
- Identify and describe the ethical principles guiding ethical behavior and decision-making.
- Identify the purpose of a professional code of ethics.
- Describe the concept of the common good.
- Describe the concepts of cultural competence, cultural sensitivity, and cultural knowledge.
- Define an ethical dilemma.
- Describe the steps outlined in the ethical dilemma resolution framework.
- Apply the ethical dilemma resolution framework model to ethical dilemmas encountered in community settings.

KEY TERMS

Autonomy	Deontological ethics	Professional responsibilities
Beneficence	Ethical dilemma	Professionalism
Bioethics	Ethical decision framework	Social justice
Code of ethics	Ethics	Utilitarian ethics
Common good	Fidelity	Veracity
Confidentiality	Justice	Virtue ethics
Cultural competence	Moral values	
Cultural knowledge	Nonmaleficence	
Cultural sensitivity	Profession	

The American Dental Education Association competencies addressed in this chapter include[1]:

C.1:   Apply a professional code of ethics in all endeavors.

C.6:   Promote the profession through service activities and affiliations with professional organizations.

HP.2:   Respect the goals, values, beliefs, and preferences of the patient/client while promoting optimal oral and general health.

Introduction

Ethical principles are the core elements characteristic of dental professionals and professional behaviors. Professional and personal communications, actions, and decisions are guided by a profession's code of ethics. Codes of ethics encourage oral health providers to commit to contribute to the well-being of patients and the communities in which they practice and live. The specialized expertise and knowledge of an oral health care provider allows them to impact a community's oral health status and well-being. With the responsibility of contributing to attaining and maintaining the oral health of the citizens of a community, come challenges and dilemmas. It is useful to be familiar with an ethical decision-making framework that can address the ethical dilemmas encountered by practitioners in their many roles and responsibilities—in their practice, in their community, and in their professional associations.

PROFESSIONALISM AND PROFESSIONAL RESPONSIBILITY

A special relationship exists between a provider and patient. The patient trusts that the provider will demonstrate professional judgment and behavior. Dental hygienists are members of a profession. A **profession** is an occupation with a specific set of characteristics; one that is self-regulated through systematic training and collegial discipline, with a foundation in technical, specialized knowledge requiring advanced education and

skill. Additional characteristics are a service focus and code of ethics. **Professionalism** is defined as a set of values, attitudes, and behaviors that place the client's self-interest before the self-interest of the professional.

A dental hygienist is required to enroll in a rigorous academic program that assesses skills, knowledge, critical thinking, and judgment. In addition to the academic program required, the dental hygienist must successfully complete specific written and clinical examinations. There is a unique scope of practice for the dental hygienist. When a license has been granted, the dental hygienist joins a profession that demonstrates an attitude and set of behaviors that places patients' interest and well-being as a priority. A **code of ethics,** which is drafted and approved by peers in the American Dental Hygienists' Association (ADHA), provides a framework for the dental hygienist's actions and decision-making.

An individual who identifies himself or herself as a professional must also satisfy certain **professional responsibilities.** A critical professional responsibility is to remain current in scientific and clinical knowledge that will assist the practitioner in making evidence-based decisions. This responsibility is encompassed in the concept of being a lifelong learner and seeking to continue one's professional education throughout the professional career. There is also a responsibility to demonstrate a commitment to professional ethics and ethics-based decision-making, which is based on the expectation that professionals place patient well-being as a priority. The oral health care of patients by dental hygienists also serves the needs of society. Oral health and its relationship to general health, individual comfort, and personal self-worth and aesthetics is important to society. A society in poor oral health is unhealthy and unable to contribute.

Each element of professionalism reinforces and supports the others. There are also clinical elements to professionalism. The following traits can be considered clinical aspects of professionalism and professional responsibility:

- **Suspension of self-interest:** The patient's welfare and the welfare of the community takes priority.
- **Honesty and integrity:** These qualities are important in the provider–patient relationship because of the trust required when sharing health information. These qualities are also fundamental in relationships with dental colleagues, third-party payers, other health and allied health professionals, and students.
- **Technical competence:** Patients must be assured that the provider meets high standards of care. Members of the dental or medical team must be confident that the dental hygiene professional is committed to excellence in all aspects of assessment, treatment, and evaluation.
- **Accountability:** A licensed professional is responsible to apply certain skills and knowledge, according to certain standards dictated by state laws and dental practice acts. The authority to provide specific services carries with it a responsibility to be accountable to patients, employers, government agencies, insurers, and society. This refers to the ability to answer for one's actions.
- **Communication:** Clear communication skills, which demonstrate cultural sensitivity and competence, are necessary to appropriately interact with patients. All patients must be treated with respect and dignity. Effective listening enhances respect and communication. A dental provider must be attentive, seek understanding, and show respect.
- **Tolerance:** This responsibility addresses the acceptance of all individuals and the qualities and characteristics they bring to the workplace or the provider–patient relationship.

PRINCIPLES OF ETHICS

A hallmark of a health profession is its use of ethical principles to guide decisions about patient interactions and care. All oral health care providers make clinical decisions using evidence-based information. In oral health care situations, the dental provider and patient have similar goals, to either attain or maintain optimum oral health. The provider uses knowledge, experience, and judgment and considers the needs of the patient in making treatment recommendations. Together with the patient, treatment decisions are made and implemented by the provider. **Ethics** concerns the standard of behavior and the concept of right and wrong. **Bioethics** is the discipline related to the ethical implications of biologic research methods and results.

Practitioners are faced with dilemmas in their daily interactions with patients and colleagues, whether in the small business climate of a private practice or in more complex organizations, such as a public health clinic or community-based health program. The resolution of a dilemma is guided by ethical principles, professional responsibilities, and moral values. **Moral values,** influenced by family, religion, culture, and society, contribute to ethical conduct. Health professionals must not rely on their own value system however; instead, they should use ethical principles and professional codes to assist them.

A brief review of ethical theories and principles provides the foundation necessary to assist the practitioner in resolving frequently encountered issues and dilemmas. Ethical principles frequently cited in health care settings are based on ethical theory. Ethical theory attempts to provide a general set of considerations for moral behavior. Three major ethical theories are described. The first is **Utilitarian ethics,** proposed by John Stuart Mill, a nineteenth century English philosopher, which suggests that the rightness of an act is measured by the outcome. What makes an action correct or incorrect is the good or evil that results, not the act alone. Utilitarian ethics suggests that the end justifies the means. Utilitarian ethics approaches an issue with a belief that the action or actions should produce the greatest good for the greatest number. Community water fluoridation, in addition to being a significant public health measure, is an example of utilitarianism in dental public health. This action, which reduces caries rates, is available to all members of a community at a low cost. Access to community water fluoridation satisfies the utilitarian's requirement to produce benefits for the largest number.

A second ethical theory, **Deontological ethics,** was proposed by Immanuel Kant, an eighteenth century German philosopher. Deontology is derived from the Greek word *deon,* meaning duty. A deontologist suggests that an action is right when it satisfies an obligation or duty. A decision is not viewed based on the potential consequences, but rather a sense of duty. A dental hygienist, who is required by law to report suspected cases of child abuse, fulfills that decision because of a sense of duty. If the dental hygienist is aware that a child is at risk, the duty overrides any personal concern about losing a friend, colleague, or patient when the duty is fulfilled. Deontologists also suggest that performance of acts in the past creates obligations in the present. For example, if one has a contractual promise, one is bound by the terms of the contract.

A third ethical theory is **Virtue ethics.** Aristotle and Plato, fourth century BC Greek philosophers, were proponents of virtue ethics. This theory is based on the concept of the moral, virtuous, health care provider striving for excellence. This theory is viewed in terms of personal qualities, such as honesty, fidelity, wisdom, and self-restraint.

Ethics in Health Care

Ethical principles important to the health care environment are as follows:

- Beneficence
- Autonomy
- Veracity
- Justice
- Nonmaleficence
- Fidelity
- Confidentiality

These principles are a guide to conduct. Each principle can be applied to the professional interactions of the dental hygienist with patients, dental colleagues, health care providers, and community members.

Beneficence advocates providing benefits, preventing harm or evil, and promoting good. This suggests that the health care professional must, through their actions and reactions, seek to "do good" for the patient. The dental provider who develops and implements a smoking cessation program at a local church or community center is promoting good oral health. Educating clients about tobacco and tobacco cessation strategies uses the skills and knowledge of the dental hygienist.

Autonomy flows from the concept of respect for individuals. All individuals have the right to self-determination, allowing that individual to decide on a course of action as it relates to their health care. A health care provider demonstrates respect for a patient's autonomy in all interactions with the individual. An oral health care provider keeps the patient informed during assessment, diagnosis, treatment planning, and treatment. Informing a patient of the outcomes allows the patient to make informed decisions. Obtaining informed consent from a patient prior to providing treatment is a structured method of providing information about their status in a comprehensive and understandable manner. The informed consent process allows the practitioner to explain a procedure, the need for the procedure, alternatives, and risks. This process also allows the patient to ask questions and have their questions answered. Each step in the process contributes to a patient's understanding and their ability to make a decision about their health status.

Veracity is telling the truth, honesty, and integrity. This principle is important in many aspects of oral health care, primarily in the area of written and oral communication. Health care providers are expected to be truthful in their interactions with patients. If harm or an unanticipated, untoward incident occurs, the provider should communicate clearly and accurately to the patient or the person responsible for the patient. Dental professionals must also demonstrate integrity in the business aspect of oral health care delivery. Altering records, committing insurance fraud, or purposefully failing to correctly document in a patient record are examples of dishonesty.

Justice focuses on fairness and equality. Individuals are treated justly when they are given what they are owed, deserve, or can legitimately claim. It can also be described as fair equality of opportunity. All patients should be treated fairly and equally. Justice issues are important in oral health care delivery on many levels. All patients receive the same quality of care, whether as a privately insured patient or a subsidized patient. Justice also impacts decisions about community-based programs and the distribution of services. Dental professionals whose interests are in serving the needs of a community seek to ensure that services, preventive therapies, oral health education, and other efforts are equitably distributed to all those individuals who would benefit. **Social justice** also describes the concept of fairness in distribution of resources. Social justice, in view of health care and oral health care, suggests addressing unmet needs and taking actions to improve and increase access to services to meet those needs.

Nonmaleficence requires the oral health care provider to avoid harming the patient; "above all, do no harm." Dental professionals consistently take steps to prevent patient harm. Sterilization of instruments, disinfection of a unit, and the use of universal precautions are examples of a provider taking steps to prevent patient harm. By their actions, dental providers are "doing good." The operators, using their skill and knowledge, strive to never inflict harm, to prevent harm if able, and to remove or reduce opportunities for harm (e.g., the accurate recording of a patient's health history). An up-to-date, accurate health history, for example, assists the provider from inflicting harm by

identifying a local anesthetic allergy or preventing the incorrect anesthesia from being administered.

Fidelity is the requirement to keep implied or explicit promises. It is faithfulness to duty and obligation. The dental provider who promises to assist a local high school district in educating the students about the value of mouth guard use during athletic activities is expected to keep that promise. There are other responsibilities inherent in fidelity; fidelity includes a broader range of responsibilities than keeping a promise: (1) The responsibility to maintain confidentiality, which is implied by the relationship between the provider and patient when a health history is recorded. The patient assumes the provider will keep the information confidential unless appropriate steps are taken to acquire the patient's permission to share the information. (2) The responsibility of professional competence. If specific services are provided, the dental provider must have a certain level of knowledge, judgment, and skills that meet acceptable practice standards. The principle of fidelity supports the provider–patient relationship. Other responsibilities include keeping contractual agreements and never abandoning the patient prior to completion of treatment.

Confidentiality obligates the provider to keep all information about a patient private and to not share the information with a third party without consent. Confidentiality has its foundation in trust. The importance of confidentiality is identified in the Hippocratic oath, which states, "What I may see or hear in or outside the course of treatment . . . which on no account may be spread abroad, I will keep to my self, holding such things shameful to speak about." This principle of confidentiality respects the patient's privacy. Thus, information about patients is not discussed with family members or friends. Permission must be granted prior to sharing health information with another party. There are exceptions to maintaining patient confidentiality. For example, there are legal requirements in certain situations to report specific infectious diseases, such as sexually transmitted diseases. In this instance, the individual's right to privacy is balanced against the need to protect the public good.

Code of Ethics

Oral health care providers are guided in their decisions by their personal values. These values are influenced by education, personal and professional experiences, and religious and cultural background. A code of ethics is important to all health professions. A code of ethics is a formalized description of principles that govern the behavior of a profession's members and provide a framework for decision-making. The ADHA Code of Ethics provides guidance to its members for appropriate behaviors in various situations and assists in monitoring the profession. As new issues emerge that must be addressed, the codes are edited or expanded to assist practitioners to address current issues. The codes of ethics for dental professionals highlight common themes. The codes define the ethical principles that serve as a foundation for all health care providers. The ADHA code describes the importance of oral health and the role of the dental hygienist in preventing and treating oral diseases. Advocating for patients is an important aspect of the code. The principles are described in a manner that applies to patients and clinicians. In addition, there are statements that address competence and personal well-being and that encourage teamwork and collaboration in the work environment. The importance of respect for colleagues and patients is also highlighted. A code of ethics, such as ADHA's Code of Ethics, also encourages practitioners to contribute to their professional organizations and research- and community-based efforts. The ADHA code specifically addresses the ethical obligation that dental hygienists have to their communities. The ADHA Code of Ethics supports an approach called a hierarchy of duties. The hierarchy suggests that professionals have obligations to society, employers, patients/clients, colleagues, and professional organizations.

CONTRIBUTING TO THE COMMON GOOD

Dental professionals are citizens of various "communities," including the local area where they reside or are employed. A population with a specific socioeconomic status, ethnic and religious affiliation, or other unique qualities may characterize this local community. The professional communities to which a dental hygienist belongs is defined by many factors, including education, credentials, experiences, and interests. A dental hygienist may belong to the ADHA and a state and local dental hygiene component. The membership in this professional community is dictated by the state and city where the dental hygienist resides. In addition, because of personal or professional interests, the dental hygienist may also hold memberships in other professional or service organizations. For example, a dental hygienist interested in oral cancer prevention and education may be an active member of the local American Cancer Society. An oral health care provider interested in dental public health may join a professional organization such as the American Association of Public Health Dentistry or the Association of State and Territorial Dental Directors. Each organization has a specific mission and assists the member by being a source of information on current trends, professional publications, and research. Dental professionals are also members of a scientific community. To be a skilled professional, it is imperative to maintain a current knowledge level. Dental professionals use scientific publications, professional meetings and seminars, and continuing-education resources to keep current in dental and related sciences. Decisions about patient care, oral health recommendations to patients and community groups, and approaches to resolving oral health problems must be based on sound scientific evidence. These reasons link dental professionals to the scientific community.

The participation in various communities, in conjunction with the professional education and credentials of an oral health care provider, includes a social responsibility. This social responsibility arises from the provider's ethical responsibilities of nonmaleficence and justice. The social responsibility is to take a specific action or set of actions to address the oral health needs of a society, using the skills and knowledge of the professional. A professional may work independently to address needs or work in tangent with a larger group of professionals. There is a broad range of commitment to the social responsibility aspect of being a professional; for example, a dental hygienist in private practice who contributes twice a year to an oral cancer screening activity at a local retail mall. Other dental professionals may join the U.S. Public Health Service to provide services to many different groups, including Native Americans. In each instance, there is a commitment to improve the well-being of individuals and contribute to a better society.

The U.S. Surgeon General's Report highlighted that the distribution of oral diseases is disproportionate among the U.S. population. The report emphasized that certain ethnic and racial minorities and the elderly, disabled, and medically compromised have a disproportionate amount of oral disease as compared with the rest of the population. This report triggered a series of initiatives focusing on oral health, educational and preventive strategies, and collaborative efforts between government agencies, educational institutions, and community groups. Oral health professionals can effect the changes needed to maintain and improve the oral health status of all citizens. A National Call to Action to Promote Oral Health outlines specific actions that could be taken, including:

- Change perceptions regarding oral health and disease, so that oral health becomes an accepted component of general health.
- Accelerate building the scientific and evidence base and apply science effectively to improve oral health.
- Build an effective infrastructure at the local, state, and national levels.

- Strengthen and expand oral health research and educational capacity.
- Remove known barriers between people and oral health services.
- Use public–private partnerships and build on common goals to improve oral health.

These action steps direct providers to work toward the **common good.** The common good is defined as working in a manner that benefits all people. Dental professionals easily understand the philosophy of striving to take steps to benefit the larger community. Dental professionals recognize individual rights. However, as members of a community, it is also the obligation of all members of the dental team to collaborate to benefit all citizens. Ethical oral health care providers put the interests and needs of the patients and communities before their own interests.

Oral health care professionals, especially those with a career in community-based service, contribute to the common good. Activities such as screening, preventive education, treatment, and referral are examples of actions that impact the well-being of a community. Fluoridation of community water supplies enhances the capacity to reduce caries in an area, benefiting many. Many dental hygiene and dental education programs have students provide oral health services to underserved or special needs populations in their communities. This community outreach experience for students is an example of contributing to the common good. When they graduate, students who participate in community outreach activities are enriched by their experiences and sensitized to their obligation to contribute to the well-being of people of all communities. The community benefits because the student-provided care allows access to services that may otherwise be unavailable. Licensed dental practitioners staffing community-based clinics, mobile dental van clinics, or other dental public health service sites are enhancing access to care and contributing to the common good. The members of the dental professions who use their skills to provide dental care in the community are contributing to a common purpose—to assist citizens within a community to attain and maintain oral health.

Communities are defined by geography; socioeconomic status; and cultural, religious, and ethnic characteristics. In addition to considering the oral health status and needs of a specific community, the dental provider should demonstrate cultural competence and sensitivity. **Cultural competence** is described as having a defined set of values and principles that allow a provider to demonstrate behaviors and attitudes that enable them to work effectively cross-culturally. **Cultural sensitivity** is awareness that cultural differences and similarities exist, without assigning values (i.e., better or worse, right or wrong) to those cultural differences. **Cultural knowledge** is familiarization with the selected cultural characteristics, history, values, belief systems, and behaviors of members of another ethnic group. Awareness of religious or cultural beliefs that impact health beliefs and practices are critical on all levels. Culturally sensitive oral health care is a delivery system that is accessible and respects the beliefs, attitudes, and cultural lifestyles of the provider and the patient. The provider must be aware that different cultures view the aspect of health and illness in different ways; for example, an illness may be caused by a specific virus for one patient, whereas another patient may attribute the same illness to a spiritual imbalance. The provider caring for patients in a clinic that provides care to a Hispanic population understands the importance of autonomy and the need for the patient to understand their oral health status as they make decisions about treatment. The clinic may have health history questionnaires, patient information brochures, and informed consent forms written in Spanish to assure that patients are correctly comprehending and responding to inquiries about their health.

Communication is important in providing culturally competent care. The provider–patient interview is an opportunity to determine important features of the patient, including family dynamics, beliefs about health and illness, and specific concerns about oral and general health care. In other instances, cultural beliefs or practices may influence provider–patient interactions during treatment. Patients who traditionally may not complain about discomfort or pain will not share that information with the provider. The provider, seeking to do no harm or prevent harm, must determine whether a patient is comfortable by relying on nonverbal responses or reactions.

When a dental professional is providing services in a community with cultural or religious practices different from his or her own, it is recommended that the provider take steps to become familiar with the culture, religion, and other characteristics of the patient population. Information can be solicited from colleagues, community or religious leaders, local community centers, focused research, and certain Web sites. A practice, clinic, or center may have written or other resources available to all employees. Actions taken to treat patients with respect and understanding support all ethical principles, but particularly those of autonomy, justice, and nonmaleficence.

ETHICAL DILEMMAS

The oral health care provider is frequently challenged by situations in which there is difficulty determining the ethically correct action, one in which there is not a simple solution. An **ethical dilemma** occurs when one duty or obligation is in conflict with another. For example, as part of the discussion with a dental provider at a dental clinic, a 28-year-old patient indicates that she wants all her teeth extracted. She explains that this is based on her limited financial resources, her family history of everyone "losing their teeth," and her lack of interest to return to the clinic for multiple appointments. The dental provider understands that patient autonomy and respecting the patient's right to determine his or her care is a necessary component of the patient–provider relationship. However, the provider also knows that extracting all of this patient's teeth may create a potential for "harm." Two ethical principles are in conflict: autonomy versus nonmaleficence.

Conflicts or dilemmas arise in community settings for other reasons. In public health settings or community sites where oral health services are provided, there are also instances in which professional values may be in conflict with community values. A simple example is the nursing home setting. The nursing home "community" includes health care professionals, licensed and nonlicensed staff, and patients. A dental professional, following a needs assessment, may determine that specific services are needed for every resident. The nursing and nursing support staff may not agree, believing the priorities are staff education and in-service presentations, with limited oral health care services. Conflicts arise between the two groups; however, each group is basing their beliefs and recommendations on ethical principles. The dental professionals are interested in promoting good, thus supporting beneficence. The staff, knowing that education assists the staff to screen for cancer, provides better preventive care, and prevents harm, is contributing to nonmaleficence. Both sides are advocating with an ethical principle as a foundation for their interest. A conflict may arise if there is a limited budget for the nursing home and a decision has to be made. Which recommendation will get funded? How might one make that decision? An ethical decision-making model is a framework that provides a strategy to resolve issues.

Ethical Dilemma Resolution Framework

Individuals and dental teams are apt to face ethical dilemmas during their professional experiences. An **ethical decision framework** is recommended to give the provider a mechanism to address issues, individually or as part of a team. Ethical dilemmas cannot always be resolved by a code of ethics alone. It is useful to have a framework with which to analyze and make ethical decisions. The following framework suggests a method that can be used by providers in community or public health settings. The model recognizes the value of making a decision or choice and considers the profession's viewpoint, as well as other stakeholders. The dilemmas encountered in community settings can involve provider–patient interactions, staff relationships, community networks and expectations, and professional organization and political issues. The model encourages an approach to resolving the dilemma through the identification of multiple alternatives that are carefully evaluated. The individual or individuals responsible for solving the dilemma are required to gather information from multiple sources to allow for an informed decision. Each alternative is evaluated, using legal, ethical, and policy guides for anticipated outcomes. When an alternative is chosen, the model emphasizes which action should occur and which consequences should be evaluated.

1. Define the problem. A problem or dilemma occurs when ethical principles or obligations are in conflict.
2. Identify the stakeholders. Stakeholders include licensed and nonlicensed personnel, patients, the surrounding community, dental and interdisciplinary health colleagues, and professional associations and licensing agencies.
3. Identify available alternatives to the problem. In considering alternatives to resolve the dilemma, the individual using the decision-making framework must consider all alternatives. The purpose of the model is to encourage broad thinking. Frequently, in attempting to resolve ethical dilemmas, there is a tendency to think of one or two solutions, limiting possible alternatives. A few narrow choices reduce the possibility for a solution that would satisfy ethical and legal obligations.
4. Gather information to assist in evaluating the alternatives. Prior to evaluating the alternatives, investigating information that is important to better understand the dynamics of the current dilemma. The type of information gathered is influenced by the dilemma presented. In instances in which a patient care dilemma is evident, reviewing the patient's chart may provide

all the information necessary to assist in evaluating possible alternatives to resolve a dilemma. If a dilemma is evident because of a pattern of behavior by a provider or employee, more information may be necessary, including information about individual policies and procedures. Examples of information to consider include:

- Data: including history, current health status, trends, and practices. Depending on the dilemma, the data sought can be for a patient, group of patients, or target population within a community, such as senior citizens.
- Personnel: licensed and nonlicensed individuals, credentials, experience, and skill levels
- Cultural, ethnic, religious, and socioeconomic factors
- Rules and regulations: policies and procedures in a particular employment setting, standards of care, licensing, and other regulatory requirements
- Philosophical: the approach to oral health care
- Historical: previous practices, annual reports, or meeting minutes.

5. Evaluate the identified alternatives using the following filters. As each alternative is reviewed, consider the following:
- Review relevant ethical principles and codes.
- Compare consistency with policies, procedures and guidelines.
- Keep alternatives acceptable within applicable laws and regulations.

6. Rank the alternatives:
- List the results each alternative will achieve.
- List the consequences of each chosen alternative.

7. Make a decision.
8. Act on the decision.
9. Evaluate the decision.

Use of the Ethical Dilemma Resolution Framework

The following scenario is provided, followed by an analysis using an ethical dilemma resolution framework.

Scenario: Substandard Care Provided. The city health department is located in a former major hospital near the downtown area. Most patients are residents of the metropolitan area and have dental care paid through the Medicaid program or assistance from other public organizations willing to pay for dental care. The dental clinic clearly informs the patients that it provides "cleanings, fillings, and extractions." No prosthodontic care is provided, although dentures are occasionally repaired because the staff dentist is willing to help out. There are two part-time dentists and one full-time dental hygienist. The dental hygienist is completing a second year of employment at the clinic.

The dental hygienist is concerned about the quality of care provided by one dentist. At maintenance visit appointments, the dental hygienist repeatedly observes caries in teeth that have been restored by the dentist. The patients are unaware of the problem and happy that they have their "fillings." The dental hygienist has observed that the same dentist is consistently responsible for not removing caries. She has discussed her concerns with the clinic manager who, although somewhat sympathetic, emphasizes how difficult it is to get dentists to work in the clinic. The clinic manager points out that the clinic has gone for months without a dentist on staff; she is just happy that there are two dentists willing to treat patients.

As part of the annual evaluation of the clinic and its services, the health department is conducting volunteer staff interviews to obtain feedback about the health department and its clinics and personnel. The announcement about the volunteer interviews indicated that all attempts would be made to keep all interview discussions confidential. The dental hygienist is interested in discussing her observations and concerns, but unsure about what to do. The scenario is discussed using the ethical dilemma resolution framework.

1. **Define the problem.** There are several conflicts presented in this scenario. The dental hygienist is aware that harm is occurring; the patients are not receiving optimal care; and the

ethical principle of beneficence, do no harm, is compromised. The failure to remove all caries places the inadequately treated patient at risk for future dental problems. An opportunity exists for the dental hygienist to provide information about poor quality care so that steps to correct the problem can be implemented. The information could result in the dentist's employment being terminated; however, if the dental hygienist does not inform someone about the compromised care, her integrity and honesty, or veracity, is compromised. Justice is also a concern. The patients treated by the dentist should receive the same quality of care as the patients whose treatment is provided by the other dentist on staff. All dentists providing care should meet the technical standard for removing all caries from a tooth.

2. **Identify the stakeholders.** The stakeholders are primarily those patients in the community who rely on the dental clinic to provide dental services. Additional stakeholders include the public health clinic (as the employer) and the dental hygienist who works with the dentist and the dental community.

3. **Identify possible alternatives to the problem.** Possible alternatives include:
   a. The dental hygienist can speak with the dentist and use radiographs to assist in identifying the caries removal problem.
   b. The dental hygienist could speak to the other dentist in the clinic, share the radiographs, and suggest the dentist discuss the issue with the dental colleague.
   c. The dental hygienist could notify the individual conducting the quality assurance assessment of the trends observed in patient care and recommend that a peer review evaluation be conducted by a dentist.
   d. The dental hygienist could contact the professional association state peer review board.
   e. The dental hygienist could ignore the situation.

4. **Gather information to assist you in evaluating the alternatives.** In preparation for pri-

oritizing the alternatives, the dental hygienist can take several steps:
   a. Determine the length of employment and years of practice for the dentist.
   b. Contact the state board of dentistry to determine if issues of lack of competence for that particular dentist are documented and on record.
   c. Conduct a chart review so that a sample of patients treated by that dentist could be reviewed to determine if poor caries removal is a consistent or long-term problem. The chart review could be conducted by the other dentist on staff, to assess each patient's oral health status, number of visits, cooperation level, and preventive practices.
   d. The dental hygienist could also determine how appointment scheduling occurs and if adequate time is allotted for patient care.
   e. The dental hygienist may be aware of the dentist's philosophy of care from working together in the same clinic.
   f. Determine if a peer review process or staff evaluation occurs as part of the policies of the clinic. There may be evaluation mechanisms in place that could be used to make the appropriate supervisors aware of the situation.

5. **Evaluate the identified alternatives.** The dental hygienist should evaluate each alternative using different resources. The ADHA code of ethics encourages dental hygienists to act as patient advocates. In this instance, the dental patient is unaware of the quality of care that is provided. The ethical principles of beneficence, doing good and nonmaleficence, and do no harm are important to the facts. The dentist is providing care that is substandard. The patient is at risk for future problems. The dental hygienist is aware of this and, to be fair, must let someone know the truth. Each ethical principle can be applied to this scenario and used to evaluate each alternative. Within the health department, policies and procedures for communicating issues or concerns may be available,

including quality assurance reporting mechanisms, patient advocates, specific feedback forms, or other mechanisms, to assist the dental hygienist. Patient treatment guidelines or standards may also exist that are used by the dental clinic for peer evaluation. Professional association peer review protocols need to be evaluated to see if they exist and to learn the mechanism for reporting members.

6. **Rank the alternatives.** Each alternative has advantages and disadvantages for the dental hygienist, the dentist involved, and the patients treated by the dentist. The dental hygienist must consider the anticipated outcome of each chosen alternative. The ranking must be based on sound ethical and legal principles. The dental hygienist should consider the impact of each alternative on the work environment and the interpersonal relationships within the office. The patient's interests are paramount in the ranking because of the ethical obligations of preventing harm and promoting good. Reviewing each alternative and ranking them from worst to best forces the dental hygienist to consider all aspects of the issue. However, because there are multiple factors involved, there is a possibility that, although the first ranked alternative is the best choice, it is the second ranked alternative that will be chosen by the dental hygienist. In all instances, the dental hygienist is most likely guided by the principle of doing the right thing, even it if means the decision will jeopardize the relationship with the dentist. The dental hygienist is interested in protecting the health and well-being of the patients who trust the health department to provide optimum care.

7. **Make a decision.** The dental hygienist, or any provider faced with a dilemma, must make a decision to resolve the dilemma. This decision is based on a thorough analysis of the situation, the options available, and the potential outcomes for each alternative. It is important that a decision be made that allows resolution of the issue.

8. **Act on the decision.** This particular step may appear to be an understood aspect of the decision-making framework. The dental provider must follow through on the alternative chosen, taking the steps to complete the process. Delaying or avoiding a resolution to the problem creates additional dilemmas and, depending on the circumstances, may lead to violation of legal obligations.

9. **Evaluate the decision.** The evaluation process begins when the decision is acted on. The consequences may be immediate. For example, if the dental hygienist chose to report the dentist to the quality assurance representative, the dentist may resign from the position on notification of the allegation. Or, in some circumstances, because the dental hygienist notified the appropriate personnel, the dental hygienist's employment may be terminated. Each alternative must be weighed for personal and professional consequences. Yet, each dental provider is obligated by their code of ethics to fulfill the obligations suggested by each ethical principle.

Cases With Ethical Dilemmas

Use the ethical decision-making model to resolve the issues presented in Cases 1–6 or use them to discuss the concepts presented in the chapter.

CASE 1: PROFESSIONAL VERSUS COMMUNITY VALUES

It's My Money and My Child! The dental provider is noticing a trend in the patients visiting the dental clinic located in the local health department. Many teenage clients are requesting stainless steel crowns for their anterior teeth. A popular musician wears the stainless steel crowns during concerts, and his young audience wants to look like him. The teenagers' crowns are not covered by dental insurance or other subsidies. In most cases, however, the parents are finding the financial resources to pay for the care. The dental provider is concerned because the trend is increasing. However, the patients, although requesting the crowns for healthy teeth, are declining preventive care, including maintenance visits and needed restorative work. The parents claim they want their financial resources to go toward the crowns, not the other dental care. The parents all indicate that they should get what they ask for because, after all, "it's my money and my child!" *What should the provider do to resolve the conflict?*

CASE 2: ALLOCATION OF RESOURCES

Who Receives the Grant? The dental provider in charge of the dental portion of a health clinic located in the Hispanic community recently received notification that a grant application was successful. A local foundation agreed to provide $500,000 to support a preventive dentistry program coordinated by the dental clinic. Following consultation with other members of the interdisciplinary health team, two primary groups were identified that could benefit from the funds. The first group is the significant number of teenage parents within the community. An oral health education program is needed that focuses on infant oral health, preventive strategies, and diet and nutrition. Educating the teenage parents about oral health, tobacco use, and the role of diet and nutrition on oral health should be addressed. At the same time, the clinic staff also identified the number of elderly in the community, many without teeth and needing dentures. The physician in charge of the health clinic decided to let the dental provider choose which target group should benefit from the funds. The dental provider is now faced with a dilemma. *What should be done?*

CASE 3: PROVIDING SERVICES BEYOND THE SCOPE OF PRACTICE

It's Our Secret! A dental hygienist recently joined the staff of a dental clinic located in an isolated, rural area of the state. The clinic had been seeking to employ a licensed dental hygienist for a long time. Because of a spousal relocation, the dental hygienist was happy to find employment. One dentist and a full-time dental assistant staffed the dental clinic. The dental assistant was a long-time employee who lived in the community. For the first 6 months, the new dental hygienist enjoyed the work environment, collegiality, and patients. On a few occasions, while passing one of the dentist's operatories, she noticed the dental assistant performing root planing or scaling the teeth and, sometimes, polishing. The law in the state where the dental clinic was located did not allow dental assistants to perform those procedures. The dental hygienist knew that dental assistants could not practice like a dental hygienist because, prior to getting a license, she had to take the state's jurisprudence test—the law is clear. The dental hygienist decided to approach the dentist to determine if the observations were correct. The response of the dentist surprised the dental hygienist. He indicated that because it had been difficult to employ a dental hygienist, a decision was made to allow the dental assistant to perform as a dental hygienist when required by the circumstances. The dentist assured the dental hygienist that the assistant was skilled because he had "trained" her. The assistant had read a few of his textbooks and had attended a continuing-education course for dental hygienists. The dentist assured the dental hygienist that it was in the community's best interest to have two employees providing dental hygiene services to "meet the needs of the community." He also emphasized that the patients did not know the difference between a dental assistant and dental hygienist. He ended the conversation by reminding the dental hygienist that no one would find out if no one shared the "secret." *What should the dental hygienist do?*

CASE 4: FAILURE TO FOLLOW APPROPRIATE LEGAL MANDATES

It's the Mayor! The dentist's office scheduled the mayor's 8-year-old daughter for prophylaxis, radiographs, fluoride treatment, and examination.

During the intraoral examination, the dental hygienist noted some bruising on the child's soft palate and frenum. The little girl was wearing a turtleneck with long sleeves, which was unusual in the warm and humid July weather. During the head and neck examination, the dental hygienist also noticed some bruising along the back of the neck. The girl was cooperative and responded to all the requests made by the provider during the treatment phase. The provider waited until the end of the appointment, when the girl appeared a little more comfortable, to ask about the bruises in her mouth and on her neck. The little girl became quiet and pensive. The dental hygienist tried a few more times to elicit responses, but the child indicated she wanted to see her mother. The dental hygienist left the operatory to talk with the dentist prior to the dentist examining the child. The dentist listened and then went to the operatory to complete the examination. He dismissed the child. At the end of the day, he indicated that he wanted to speak with the dental hygienist. The dental hygienist assumed that they would discuss a concern about potential child abuse that, under state law, must be reported. Instead, the dentist chastised the dental hygienist for even suggesting abuse had occurred. After all, she's the mayor's daughter! *What should the dental hygienist do?*

CASE 5: SUBSTANDARD CARE AND INSURANCE FRAUD

We're Doing Them a Favor! During an office staff meeting, the dental hygienist was pleased to hear that the office was going to begin scheduling Medicaid patients for treatment. The community where the practice was located was near a section of the city that was popular with immigrants settling in the area. Many immigrants qualified for Medicaid and other social service benefits. The office manager indicated that the component dental society was putting "pressure" on dentists in the community to provide access to care to the underserved members of the community. The day following the meeting, the dental hygienist and office

manager had a private conversation prior to the first patient's arrival. The office manager indicated that all Medicaid patients would be allowed 30 minutes with the dental hygienist. The office manager indicated that the dental hygienist should perform a "rubber cup prophy" for all children and adults, give them a toothbrush with some fluoridated toothpaste, and dismiss them. However, the dental hygienist's records would indicate more treatment than occurred. For adult patients, root planing and scaling, radiographs, examination, and patient education would be recorded. For child patients, prophylaxis, fluoride treatment, and radiographs would be recorded. The office manager indicated that Medicaid reimbursement was not adequate. The dentist had decided to provide some treatment but would bill for as much as possible to "cover the costs." The office manager commented that, at least, the patients were receiving some treatment. *What should the dental hygienist do?*

CASE 6: POLITICS VERSUS PROFESSIONAL OBLIGATIONS

Supervision Required. The dental hygienist was employed by the state public health division to provide care in isolated clinics throughout the state. The service has a mobile dental van that traveled from community to community, providing treatment. Local dentists were asked to volunteer their time and provide restorative care; however, the assigned dentists were frequently not available or chose not to staff the mobile van.

One dentist in the state was a strong advocate of expanded duties for dental hygienists who chose to be employed in community-based settings. His recommendation included training public health dental hygienists to do preventive resin restorations (PRR). His argument was that many children seen in the clinics or mobile vans returned year after year for prophylaxes but, because of a lack of dental providers, had little or no restorative work provided. Each year, the caries in the children became more serious and resulted, for many children, in toothaches and, ultimately, extractions. Allowing public health dental hygienists to do PRR would begin to address the significant needs of the children.

The dentist was active in the local dental society and had made his views known at local and state meetings. Recently, however, rumors had started about his past. Apparently, the dentist, while battling a substance abuse problem, had gotten into trouble with the law. A few people knew about his past, including one of the dental hygienists staffing the dental van. A public hearing was going to be held at the state board level to discuss the proposed change to the state law that would allow dental hygienists to do certain expanded duties. The dental hygienist had been approached by a number of dentists, through e-mail and telephone calls, to talk about the advocate dentist's past. Certain dentists in the state wanted to harm his reputation, so that state board members and other influential dentists questioned his credibility. At least one dentist had indicated that if the dental hygienist did not cooperate, funding for the mobile van might disappear. *What should the dental hygienist do?*

SUMMARY

All members of the dental team are obligated to practice using ethical principles and codes of ethics for guidance. The dental hygienist involved in community service, provision of care, or education is expected to demonstrate professional behavior. In addition, the dental hygienist is required to fulfill professional responsibilities, including competency; sensitivity to cultural, ethnic, and religious characteristics; written and oral communication skills; and contributing to the well-being of the community. In situations in which the dental hygienist encounters an ethical dilemma, the use of an ethical decision-making framework provides a structured assessment and resolution of the problem. The framework can be used for patient–provider, colleague-to-colleague, and provider-to-community dilemmas. Dental hygienists and all health care providers recognize the importance of ethics and ethical decision-making as a core aspect of the profession.

RESOURCES

Access to Care [Position Paper]. American Dental Hygienists' Association, 2001. Available at: http://www.adha.org/profissues/access_to_care.htm. Accessed Fall 2002.

American Dental Association. Available at: http://www.ada.org.

American Dental Education Association. Available at: http://www.adea.org.

American Dental Hygienists' Association. Available at: http://www.adha.org.

A National Call to Action to Promote Oral Health. Rockville, MD: U.S. Department of Health and Human Services (USDHHS), Public Health Service, Centers for Disease Control and Prevention, National Institutes of Health, National Institute of Dental and Craniofacial Research. NIH Publication No. 03-5303, May 2003.

Code of Ethics for Dental Hygienists, 1998–1999. American Dental Hygienists' Association.

Haden NK. Improving the oral health status of all Americans: roles and responsibilities of academic dental institutions. Report of the ADEA's President's Commission. American Dental Education Association, March 2003.

Hasegawa T, Welie J. Role of code of ethics in oral healthcare. J Amer Coll Dent 2000;63:5–8.

Health and Health Disparities. Available at: http://ncmhd.nih.gov/.

International Dental Ethics and Law Society: IDEALS. Available at: http://www.ideals.ac.

Mutha S, Allen C, Welch M. Toward culturally competent care: a toolbox for teaching communication strategies. center for health professions. UCSF. Available at: http://futurehealth.ucsf.edu/cnetwork/resources/curricula/diversity.html.

O'Neil EH. Pew Health Professions Commission. Recreating health professional practice for a new century: the fourth report of the Pew

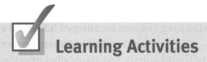

Learning Activities

1. Develop a code of ethics. Divide a class into small groups and assign the task of drafting a class code of ethics. The code can address relationships with student colleagues, faculty, and staff, as well as a student code of conduct. Each group can report their suggestions. Compile the consistent themes and adopt the code as a guiding framework to be used during the enrollment in the program.

2. Obtain a copy of the American Dental Association's Code of Professional Responsibility and Ethics and the American Dental Hygienists' Association Code of Ethics. Review both codes. Identify common themes and principles. Identify how and where obligations to society and community are identified in each code.

3. Identify actions that a dental professional can take to contribute to the "common good" of their local community. Begin by identifying the action and what steps would be needed for the action to be implemented. Identify the target group, anticipated outcomes, potential collaborators within and outside the dental profession, and possible sources of funding.

4. Think about ethical dilemmas that you have experienced as a student, employee, or employer. Summarize the dilemma, in writing or in a group, and identify which ethical principles were violated. Use the ethical decision-making model to "solve" the dilemma, allowing classmates or colleagues to present alternatives. Discuss if the dilemma was resolved and what approach was taken to resolve it. What were the consequences of the resolution?

5. Using the cases presented in this chapter, or other individually reported cases, role play a conversation between the dental provider faced with the dilemma and a key figure in the dilemma.

6. Invite local dental public health practitioners to discuss ethical issues and or specific cases with students. Distribute the issues or cases prior to the class meeting, divide the class into small groups, and assign practitioners to each group. If the practitioners are unable to visit a class, assign students to interview individuals by visiting community sites.

7. Research a particular ethnic or cultural group and their health beliefs and practices. Discuss how the knowledge gained would influence the interaction between a dental provider and patient.

Health Professions Commission. San Francisco, CA: Pew Health Professions Commission, December 1998.

Oral Health In America: A Report of the Surgeon General—Executive Summary. Rockville, MD: USDHHS, National Institute of Dental and Craniofacial Research, National Institutes of Health, 2000. Available at: http://www.surgeongeneral.gov/library/oralhealth/.

Ozar DT, Sokol DJ. Dental Ethics Chairside. 2nd Ed. Washington, DC: Georgetown University Press, 2002.

Principles of Ethics and Code of Professional Conduct with Official Advisory Opinions. Chicago, IL: American Dental Association. Revised January 2003.

Professional Ethics in Dentistry Network: PED-NET. Available at: http://www.luc.edu/depts/ethics/dental_ethics.htm.

Purtilo R. Ethical Dimensions in the Health Professions. 3rd Ed. Philadelphia, PA: WB Saunders, 1999.

USDHHS. Office of Minority Health. National Standards for Culturally and Linguistically

Appropriate Services. Rockville, MD: USD-HHS, March 2001. Available at: http://www.omhrc.gov/clas/.

Review Questions

1. The local health department is interested in purchasing a mobile dental van that would allow access to care for regions of the city that do not have dental practitioners. A health department dental hygienist wants to collect data about oral health status from elementary school children and begins visiting the schools and evaluating the children, using an oral hygiene index. She fails to obtain consent from the children's parents for the evaluation. Which of the following ethical principles did the dental hygienist violate?
   a. Autonomy
   b. Beneficence
   c. Justice
   d. Veracity
   e. Fidelity

2. The clinic dentist is running late and is noticeably flustered. She quickly reviews the chart and proceeds to begin the extraction. The dental assistant is surprised to see that instead of extracting tooth #3, as treatment planned, the dentist is extracting #4. The dental assistant discreetly points to tooth #3 and the treatment plan sitting on the counter. The dentist, realizing her mistake, replaces #4 in the extraction site, extracts #3, and sutures the patient. She provides postoperative instructions and reminds the patient to make an appointment to have the extraction site checked. The dentist says nothing to the patient about the wrong tooth being extracted. Which of the following ethical violations did the dentist violate?
   a. Autonomy
   b. Beneficence
   c. Justice
   d. Veracity
   e. Fidelity

3. A small dental clinic is the recipient of grant funding. There are no specific stipulations about how the funds should be used, only that they should contribute to the improvement of oral health in the community. The dental hygienist charged with using the funds decides she wants use the money in a way that would benefit a significant portion of the community, in this case, the senior citizens residing in the town. Which of the following ethical theories do this dental hygienist's actions support?
   a. Deontological ethics
   b. Utilitarian ethics
   c. Virtue ethics
   d. Professional ethics
   e. Antifraud ethics

4. Which of the following are characteristics of a profession?
   (1) Adherence to a code of ethics; (2) Specialized and rigorous academic training; (3) Monitoring by colleagues; (4) Professional association membership requiring dues; and (5) Service orientation
   a. 1, 2, and 3
   b. 1, 2, 3, and 4
   c. 2, 3, and 4
   d. 1, 2, 4, and 5
   e. 1, 3, and 5

5. A dental hygienist is employed on a Native American Reservation. The hygienist is working with local tribal leaders to address certain oral health problems evident in the community. The dental hygienist seeks out the advice and input of the member of the tribe that has traditionally provided medical advice and care to the tribe's members. The dental hygienist is interested to learn how oral health problems, including caries and periodontal disease, have been addressed by the tribal members. Which of the following is the dental hygienist attempting to improve?
   a. Cultural competence
   b. Cultural sensitivity
   c. Cultural knowledge
   d. Cultural domain
   e. Cultural practices

6. A dental hygiene program allows its students to provide care in an outreach clinic located in a part of town where there has been an influx of Spanish speaking immigrants. The dental hygiene program makes a curriculum change, requiring all students to enroll in a conversational Spanish class so that students and patients can communicate clearly and accurately. Which of the following National Call to Action steps is the dental hygiene program addressing?
   a. Changing perceptions regarding oral health and disease, so that oral health becomes an accepted component of general health.
   b. Building an effective infrastructure at the local, state, and national levels.
   c. Removing known barriers between people and oral health services.
   d. Using public–private partnerships and building on common goals to improve oral health.

Questions 7–10. Use the following scenario as a basis to respond to Questions 7–10.

A dental hygienist, a recent graduate, is the newest staff member of a progressive clinic. The quality that attracted the dental hygienist to the position was the apparent commitment of the office to treating all patients from the surrounding community. She has been seeing various patients; some self-pay, others have their care paid for by state Medicaid funds. Today's patient is covered by Medicaid. During the intraoral examination, the dental hygienist notes a lesion that may require biopsy. The dental hygienist brings the lesion to the attention of the supervising dentist, who indicates that it is not "anything to worry about." The dental hygienist is surprised that the dentist did not make a recommendation for an evaluation of the lesion. Later in the day, the dentist comments that "he didn't make the recommendation because most people like her patient don't follow through on recommendations." The dental hygienist is concerned at the dentist's philosophy of care. More significantly,

the dental hygienist is concerned about the patient's well-being.

7. The dentist's failure to refer the patient for a biopsy violates which of the following ethical principles?
   a. Autonomy
   b. Beneficence
   c. Veracity
   d. Fidelity
   e. Competence

8. The dental hygienist decides to use the ethical dilemma resolution framework to resolve the situation. Which of the following is NOT an ethically based alternative to consider?
   a. Reappoint the patient and have another dentist on staff examine the lesion.
   b. Talk with the dentist about the dental hygienist's concern about the patient and reappoint the patient so that the dentist can reexamine the lesion.
   c. Reappoint the patient and ask a dental hygiene colleague to conduct an examination.
   d. Wait until the patient returns for a maintenance visit in 6 months and see how the lesion appears.
   e. Call the patient and encourage them to get a second opinion.

9. Prior to considering all the alternatives recommended, the dental hygienist gathers information that would be useful. Which of the following is the type of information that should be obtained?
   a. A careful review of the patient's chart and previous intra- and extra-oral findings
   b. Review an oral pathology book specifically related to oral lesions similar to the one observed
   c. The referral policies and protocol followed by the office
   d. a and c only
   e. a, b, and c

10. The dental hygienist chooses to confront the dentist, based on a belief that all patients in

an office should receive the same treatment. Which of the following ethical principles influenced the dental hygienist in her reasoning?

a. Autonomy
b. Veracity
c. Justice
d. Confidentiality
e. Beneficence

REFERENCE

1. American Dental Education Association. Competencies for entry into the profession of dental hygiene, Exhibit 7. J Dent Educ 2003;67(7):1–5. Available at: http://www.adea.org/cepr. Accessed February 2004.

Legal Principles

17

Objectives

After studying this chapter and completing the study questions and activities, the learner will be able to:

- Identify common sources of law.
- Describe contract principles and associated duties for providers and patients.
- Identify intentional torts that a dental provider may be at risk for committing.
- Describe the intentional tort of negligence and the elements necessary to prove a provider negligent.
- Describe the necessary criteria to obtain informed consent.
- Describe the necessary criteria to obtain an informed refusal.
- List common exceptions to obtaining informed consent.
- Describe the concept of standard of care and related duties to meet the standard for dental hygienists.
- Describe recommended risk management techniques.
- Describe the purpose of a state dental practice act.
- Describe the steps involved for a proposed bill to become a law.
- Describe federal laws that prevent discriminatory practices by employers and protect the safety and health of employees and wage and employment benefits.

KEY TERMS

Abandonment	Contract law	False imprisonment
Administrative law	Damages	Fraud
Assault	Deceit	General supervision
Assignment	Defamation of character	Implied contract
Battery	Defendant	Implied duties
Beyond a reasonable doubt	Dental practice act	Indirect supervision
Case law	Direct supervision	Informed consent
Civil law	Employment discrimination laws	Informed refusal
Collaborative practice	Duty	Intentional tort
Consideration	Expressed contract	Laws

Libel

Negligence

Plaintiff

Preponderance of evidence

Punitive damages

Slander

Standard of care

Statute of limitations

Technical battery

Tort law

Trespass

Unintentional tort

Unsupervised practice

The American Dental Education Association competencies addressed in this chapter include[1]:

C.2:   Adhere to state and federal laws, recommendations, and regulations in the provision of dental hygiene care.

C.5:   Assume responsibility for dental hygiene actions and care based on accepted scientific theories and research, as well as the accepted standard of care.

C.10:   Provide accurate, consistent, and complete documentation for assessment, diagnosis, planning, implementation, and evaluation of dental hygiene services.

CM.4:   Facilitate client access to oral health services by influencing individuals and/or organizations for the provision of oral health care.

HP.2:   Respect the goals, values, beliefs, and preferences of the patient/client while promoting optimal oral and general health.

HP.3:   Refer patients/clients who may have a physiologic, psychological, and/or social problem for comprehensive patient/client evaluation.

PC.1:   Systematically collect, analyze, and record data on the general, oral, and psychological health status of a variety of patients/clients using methods consistent with medicolegal principles.

PC.3:   Collaborate with the patient/client and/or other health professionals to formulate a comprehensive dental hygiene care plan that is patient/client-centered and based on current scientific evidence.

PC.5:   Evaluate the effectiveness of the implemented clinical, preventive, and educational services and modify as needed.

Introduction

All members of the dental team, as part of their professional responsibility, attempt to comply with the laws that regulate the practice of their profession. Each dental professional makes decisions or provides treatment with the goal of fulfilling their legal obligations as a health care provider. However, dental hygienists and other members of the dental team live and practice within a litigious society. Allegations resulting in a lawsuit can occur on many levels. Patients may sue oral health care providers or an employee may sue an employer. The oral health care provider must be aware of legal principles—to guide their actions, written and verbal communication, and personal and professional relationships. In addition, dental hygienists employed in community-based settings may also be negotiating contracts, conducting research, lobbying, and advocating for a particular target group or change in legislation and need a foundational knowledge about the legal system as a tool they can use in their many roles.

THE PURPOSE OF LAWS

Laws are developed to protect the public. The drafting and implementing of a specific law is a codification of rules with specific consequences. Law is a rule of conduct or action prescribed or formally recognized as binding or enforced by a controlled authority. The purpose of laws is to regulate the behavior of citizens and protect the public's oral health and well-being. Laws are described as the minimum standard required to keep a society functioning. Issues and concerns in society influence the development of specific laws. A new law is drafted and instituted because of changing patterns of behavior and values, technology, advancements in science, and other influences on lifestyle. With the increased use of computers, for example, privacy laws have been updated to include protection from identity theft or purchase fraud. Laws are developed to contribute to a civilized society, one in which people conform to certain behaviors to prevent harm.

OVERVIEW OF THE LEGAL SYSTEM

The United States' legal system has one federal legal system and fifty separate state systems. The federal government administers the U. S. Tax Court, while state government administers traffic or small claim courts. The state government also administers dental and dental hygiene licensing acts.

There are multiple sources of law. Constitutional law includes laws derived through both the U. S. Constitution and the constitutions of individual states. The Constitution, however, only addresses the relationship between individuals and the government. An additional source of law is when elected officials in governing bodies, such as the U. S. Congress or a state legislature, enact a law to become effective at a specific date. The Congress and state legislatures enact statutory and legislative laws. Lower jurisdictions, such as a city government, may enact codes or municipal ordinances. Laws passed by Congress impact the entire United States, whereas state law or local law is specific to an individual state or city. Another source of law is common law or case law. English Common Law is based on principles, including justice, reason, and common sense. When these principles are applied to a specific situation, as during a trial, they become case law. **Case law** is developed when a court explains or interprets other sources of law (e.g., when a case interprets the meaning of a particular statute). In addition to interpreting other sources of law, common law may define other legal rights and obligations. For example, a dentist's obligation to use reasonable care in treating a patient is a legal obligation from a series of court cases. If the case is decided in federal court, it has a wider impact. Cases decided on by an appellate or state court are state specific.

Laws are classified as public and private. Public law includes criminal, administrative, constitutional, and international law. Private laws or civil laws include tort, contract, property, inheritance, family and corporate law. Health care providers need to know about two specific areas in civil law, tort and contract law.

Civil Law

Civil law focuses on the relationships between individuals or between individuals and the government. Two areas of civil law are **tort law** and **contract law.** Tort law includes acts that result in harm against another person. The acts are classified as intentional or unintentional. Contract law is a violation of an agreement or promise between two persons to do or not to do something. The two parties in a lawsuit are the **plaintiff,** the individual bringing charges in the lawsuit, and the **defendant,** the individual or party against whom criminal or civil charges are brought in a lawsuit. In a civil law trial, the jury is asked to listen to the evidence presented by the plaintiff and the defendant and make a decision of guilt or innocence. The standard used by the jury to make a decision in a civil trial for a determination of guilt or innocence is **preponderance of evidence.** Preponderance of evidence means that one side of the case must demonstrate a greater weight of evidence than the other side. The plaintiff must provide, that it is more likely than not, that a dentist or dental hygienist caused the injury. The evidence may include dental records, scientific publications, and oral testimony by expert witnesses. In a criminal trial, the level of proof required is **beyond a reasonable doubt.**

Contract law addresses a breach or neglect of a legally binding agreement. A breach of contract may be alleged if either individual or party involved fails to comply with the terms of the legally valid contract. The agreement is referred to as a contract, which is a voluntary agreement between two parties in which specific promises are made for consideration. **Consideration** is a legal term meaning something of value is bargained. In dentistry, the consideration for the extraction of a tooth is a specific fee. There is an agreement between two parties because the oral surgeon offers to extract the tooth and the patient accepts. A contract is only valid if both parties are competent. Competence indicates that the individual is mentally competent and not mentally ill or incapacitated or making the agreement under the influence of drugs or alcohol.

For purposes of a contractual agreement, minors lack competence, although there are special situations when a minor can legally consent. In most situations, a minor, an individual below the age of 18 (or in some states 21), cannot consent to treatment. Only a parent or legal guardian is able to consent for a minor in nonemergency situations. There are exceptions, including the mature minor, an individual younger than age 18 who is mature enough to understand a physician's instructions and obtain medical care for treatment of drug, alcohol abuse, contraception, venereal disease, or pregnancy. Some state laws clearly define those rights. An emancipated minor is an individual between the ages of 15 and 18 who is self-supporting and not living with or financially reliant on a parent and who may have children, be married, or be in the military. Parental consent is not required. Proof of the emancipation should be kept in the dental record (e.g., marriage certificate).

Two types of contracts exist: expressed and implied contracts. An **expressed contract** is an agreement that is explicitly stated, either orally or in writing. For example, a written treatment plan that describes the procedures to be performed and the costs of the procedures may be viewed as an expressed contract. To be legally valid in some states, some contracts must be in writing. In some states, the Statute of Frauds indicates which contracts must be in writing. In those states, the contract that is frequently impacted is the third-party payer contract. This contract is a written agreement signed by a party other than the patient who promises to pay the bill. If, for example, a grandmother agrees to pay a visiting grandson's dental bill for an emergency root canal, the dental office may ask the grandmother to sign a third-party payer contract. An **implied contract** is an agreement that is shown by inference through signs, inaction, or silence. Therefore, it is the conduct of the parties that created the contract, not specific or expressed words. A patient with an appointment in a dental office is examined by the dentist and treated by the dental hygienist. There is no statement of offer or acceptance or discussion of consideration. However, the patient's actions imply a promise to pay for the services. The action of the patient and the dental provider implies an agreement.

Dental providers do not always state an agreement in writing, or explicitly, using words. The terms of the contract are not listed or outlined. However, the courts have determined that there are many terms implied because of the provider–patient relationship, referred to as **implied duties.** There are implied duties owed by the provider to the patient and implied duties owed by the patient:

- Exercise reasonable skill, care, and judgment in the assessment, diagnosis, and treatment of patients.
- Have proper license and registration, comply with all laws, and practice within the scope of practice dictated by state law.

- Use standard drugs, materials, and techniques; refrain from experimental procedures.
- Never abandon the patient; arrange for care during absences.
- Charge reasonable fees based on community standards.
- Complete procedures within a reasonable time.
- Inform the patient of progress and of any untoward incidents.
- Obtain informed consent.
- Refer unusual cases to specialists.
- Maintain patient privacy and confidentiality.
- Keep accurate records.
- Maintain a current level of knowledge.
- Practice in a manner consistent with a code of ethics for the profession.

There are also duties owed by the patient to the provider, which include:

- Follow home oral health care instructions.
- Keep appointments and notify a provider if an appointment cannot be kept.
- Pay fees for services in a reasonable time.
- Cooperate with the provider.
- Give honest answers to information requested.
- Notify a dental provider if a patient's health status has changed or if there are changes in medications.

When a provider has agreed, either in writing or by action, to have a professional relationship with a patient, the contract relationship cannot be terminated improperly. A relationship between a provider and patient can terminate if, for example, the patient moves to another location or the provider is a specialist and the treatment required is completed. However, if a dental provider fails to provide formal notice of the ending of a relationship, they may be accused of **abandonment.** Abandonment is the discontinuation of an established patient–provider relationship. A dental office or clinic should inform the patient in writing that the relationship is ended for protection from accusations of abandonment. The letter can indicate a notice that the relationship is being termi-nated with or without a reason, which should be presented using professional, nonsubjective, or accusatory language. The letter may identify a reason for termination including:

- Failure to schedule maintenance appointments
- Failure to resolve an unpaid balance or pay for a service
- Missed appointments
- Failure to follow instructions
- Disagreement about treatment philosophy
- A written or oral statement from the patient that they are seeking the care of another dentist (e.g., their insurance coverage has changed).

The letter also should include a specific date that the relationship is terminated and an offer to provide emergency care during that period. The letter should encourage the patient to seek another provider and indicate that dental records will be forwarded to another provider, for a reasonable fee, upon receiving a signed request from the patient.

Tort Law

Tort law is a civil violation in which an individual harms another's person (body), privacy, or property because of negligent or intentional actions. To sue for a tort, a patient or employee must have suffered mental or physical injury. When an individual is found to have harmed another, the injured person is allowed by law to seek a remedy, **damages,** in a civil lawsuit. Damages are monetary compensation. If the conduct is considered malicious or fraudulent, then another category of damages, **punitive damages,** can be granted. Punitive damages are damages over and above the award to compensate for harm.

There are two categories of torts—intentional and unintentional. An **intentional tort** is a deliberate and purposeful act that has a substantial certainty of untoward consequences from the act. Intentional torts include assault, battery, deceit, defamation of character, false imprisonment, fraud, trespass, or invasion of privacy. Dental professionals, like all citizens, can be subject to allegations of an intentional tort. **Battery** is any bodily contact without permission, also described as unlawful touching without consent. **Technical battery** is when a dental provider, in the course of treatment, exceeds the consent provided by a patient. Although no wrongful intent is present and there was a sincere interest to treat the patient, there still may be damages awarded. If the patient does gain some benefit, nominal damages may be awarded. If a restraint device is used on a child without parental permission and harm occurs, a battery may be alleged. If a dentist is given consent to extract tooth #30 and proceeds to extract #31 and no patient consent occurred, a technical battery may be alleged. **Assault** is threat of bodily harm. There does not have to be any physical contact for an assault to occur. Threatening to harm a patient with specific actions, resulting in apprehension, is a form of assault. A dental provider threatening to "hurt" someone if the "patient does not cooperate" may cause apprehension, especially if the statements are made in a harsh, loud manner. Dental professionals may also be accused of **deceit**—a false statement or deceptive practice with intent to injure someone. **Defamation of character** is the wrongful act of injuring someone's reputation by making false statements in writing (**libel**) or verbally (**slander**). **False imprisonment** or false arrest is unlawful restraint. **Fraud** is described as dishonest or deceitful practices in depriving or attempting to deprive another of his or her rights. An individual that misappropriates funds that were designated to pay for dental care is depriving a population of their right to access to dental services. **Trespass** is injury or interference with the property of another. Invasion of privacy is interference with a person's freedom from intrusion.

The **unintentional tort** is **negligence.** Unlike intentional torts, there is no intent to cause harm. Negligence is an unintentional tort alleged when one may have performed or failed to perform an act that a reasonable person would have done in similar circumstances. The following elements must be present to determine that a dental provider is guilty of negligence:

- A duty or legally recognized obligation exists.
- A breach of duty occurred. This can be an act of commission or omission.
- The breach of duty was a direct cause of the patient's injury.
- There is a legally recognizable injury.

The burden to prove the defendant guilty is on the plaintiff. An important question to consider is duty. **Duty** is defined as an action or conduct based on a legal obligation. A dental hygienist is required to meet various duties based on the accepted scope of practice allowed in a particular state. Dental hygienists conduct assessment, determine dental hygiene diagnoses, make a treatment plan, provide treatment, and evaluate outcomes. One cannot list a specific set of duties; however, some examples are to competently and appropriately treat, refer to dental specialists or physicians for consultations, provide patient education, and clearly communicate to allow for informed consent or refusal.

Dental hygienists must meet the **standard of care** in all settings where care is provided. Standard of care is the level of care expected of a reasonable and prudent practitioner in the same or similar circumstances. Dental hygienists are educated and expected to complete certain procedures during the various phases of dental hygiene care. Any compromise of care resulting in harm to a patient could be interpreted as failure to meet a duty. The dental hygienist that inadequately completes a health history may not identify a health condition requiring premedication. The dental hygienist has a duty to carefully review the health history, ask appropriate follow-up questions and, if necessary, obtain a medical consult. A dental hygienist has a duty to thoroughly scale and root plane a periodontally involved patient to control disease. Failure to adequately sterilize and sharpen instruments, treat disease, educate the patient, and provide postcare instructions are all examples of dental hygiene obligations that, if not done prudently and reasonably, may result in patient harm. The resulting harm may include infection, trauma, and periodontal disease advancing to a more serious state. The patient needs to allege the negligence and provide proof of the direct relationship between what the dental hygienist did or did not do (an act of commission or omission) during the appointment that led to harm.

Informed Consent and Refusal

One important duty that is based both on ethical and legal principles is the need to obtain **informed consent** from the patient for treatment they receive. Informed consent is the act of providing information and assuring that the patient understands the treatment risks and advantages, options available, and the nature of the disease or problem. The act of obtaining an informed consent recognizes the patient's autonomy and their right to determine what treatment they do or do not receive. The elements of informed consent require the dental provider to explain the following, using understandable language:

- The proposed treatment for the identified disease or diagnosis
- Reason(s) the treatment is necessary
- The advantages and risks of the proposed treatment
- Available alternatives to the proposed treatment
- The advantages and risks of the alternative treatments discussed
- Potential outcome(s) of treatment
- Risks involved if treatment is refused
- An opportunity for the patient to ask questions and receive answers.

It is difficult to completely inform the patient of all potential risks. However, there should be a reasonable attempt made on the part of the provider so that the patient can make an informed decision. The informed consent is for only those procedures to which the patient consented. This principle comes from a medical case that occurred in the early 20th century. A woman consented to have an operation on her diseased right ear. While under anesthesia, the physician determined the left ear was more seriously diseased than the right and operated without consent. The operation was successful. However, the patient was never awakened and permission never granted. The plaintiff sued for battery and won. (*Mohr v Williams,* 104 N.W. 12, [Minn. 1905]). This medical malpractice case highlights the importance that dental providers should only complete procedures consented to by the patient. A dental hygienist that received consent to place sealants on specific teeth cannot choose to provide the treatment on teeth for which the parent did not consent. Informed consent should be documented, either by using a form that lists the elements described or documenting consent in the progress notes. It is advised that the patient sign and date the informed consent, as should a witness. Written documentation, such as a signed informed consent, documents information that is useful if a lawsuit occurs. The informed consent provides a source of reference and assists the dental provider in proving that a duty to obtain informed consent was met.

There are exceptions to obtaining informed consent unique to each state. The more general exceptions include:

- Emergency treatment.
- Not informing the patient about commonly known risks. One should be cautious because what is "known" to the dental professional is not necessarily the patient's understanding.
- The risk is too minor or remote.
- The disclosure of risks may be more detrimental to the patient's well-being, sometimes referred to as therapeutic privilege.
- The risk not known to the profession.
- The patient indicates they are waiving their right to know. The provider should be cautious and obtain informed refusal if the patient indicates they do not want an explanation of the procedure, risks, and alternatives.

- Regular explanation of a procedure. If a regular explanation is always used, such as the reason for root planing and scaling or use of an ultrasonic scaler, it is advisable to have the explanation documented in an office or clinic manual. Caution is advised against relying on the "regular" explanation for failing to obtain consent because informed consents are tailored to the patient's situation.

A consent form should comply with state law. Handing the form to the patient is not advised; rather orally discussing the information and obtaining a written consent is recommended. If a preprinted form is used, notations should be made on the form to show topics or aspects of informed consent were discussed. The notation can be initials of the patient or provider, handwritten explanations or additions, checkmarks, words added or a line drawn through words. In most jurisdictions, only a dentist can obtain informed consent. Concurrently, in some states, dental hygienists are allowed to treat patients of record without a dentist on the premises. Dental hygienists provide treatment that may include administration of local anesthetic and periodontal and ultrasonic instrumentation. There are treatment justifications and benefits for all procedures. There are also risks with each procedure. Risks for anesthesia can be sensitivity, temporary or permanent paresthesia, or an allergic reaction. The risks for periodontal treatment can include failure of the treatment, infection, periodontal abscess, and sensitivity.

If state law does not allow the dental hygienist or dental assistant to obtain consent, the dental hygienist may want to develop a protocol in which the information included in an informed consent is reviewed and discussed with the patient. A notation in the chart could indicate the content of the discussion and record that the patient understood what was to occur during the appointment. The provider could also record questions posed by the patient, as well as responses. The information can

be documented in a precise manner; however, it should be clearly recorded that the patient was informed of the planned treatment and accepted. Dental hygienists treating compromised patients, including the mentally impaired or elderly patients with compromised ability, must strive with other members of the dental team to obtain consent. For those patients with compromised ability, the patient record should clearly document who can provide consent—a legal guardian, a spouse, a divorced parent, or an adult child. If an individual indicates legal right to give consent for another's treatment, such as a biologic parent in the case of a child of divorced parents, it is advisable to request a copy of documentation, stating who is legally allowed to consent to treatment. Frequently, a grandparent, indicating they have responsibility for a child, accompanies children scheduled for an appointment. The child cannot give consent because of minor status; the provider should request documentation to confirm the relationship of the grandparent and determine if the grandparent has legal rights. A frequent dilemma is the minor child that is left alone for a scheduled appointment by a parent or guardian. The dental provider, seeking to obtain consent, finds the parent unavailable. Dental services, especially those with potential risks involved, should not be provided without consent. One may consider telephone consent, with the increasing number of cell phones available, or if the parent is at work. However, if telephone consent is obtained, it is suggested that a second person "witness" the consent by also speaking to the person granting the consent. The circumstances for obtaining consent by phone should be recorded, including the date, time, and witness. Other instances in which consent by telephone occurs may be when a child has been brought to a dental clinic by a caregiver, teacher, or friend. If a patient is mentally compromised but legally allowed to consent to treatment, the provider should attempt to explain the procedures in a language the patient understands, allow the patient to repeat what they comprehend, and record the interaction.

The dental provider must evaluate the necessary procedures and the risk of harm.

Challenges occur for dental hygienists in all practice settings. An employer or a supervising dentist may request that a dental hygienist compromise assessment or treatment protocol. An employer dentist may request that the dental hygienist spend less time with a patient whose oral health care is paid for by a state welfare agency because the compensation level is considered (by the dentist) to be below usual, customary, and reasonable fees. The dental hygienist may provide substandard care, not appropriately root planing or educating the patient and, therefore, not fulfilling a standard of care.

A dental hygienist faces other challenges in certain work settings. Parents or guardians are not always committed to optimum oral health care and may be uncooperative in getting the patient to an appointment, reinforcing preventive care, or agreeing to treatment. In a situation in which either the patient or the patient's parent or guardian refuses recommended treatment, the dental provider should get a signed **informed refusal.**

An informed refusal is documentation that the recommended treatment is refused. This type of written documentation protects the provider from subsequent allegations of negligence. Informed refusal is an outgrowth of informed consent. A dental hygienist conducts an intraoral examination and identifies a lesion that the dentist agrees needs to be referred. The patient refuses to go for the biopsy and later develops oral cancer and subsequently dies. The dentist could be sued for failing to inform the patient of the consequences of refusal for a biopsy. An informed refusal form or documentation is similar to informed consent. The informed refusal should document the recommended procedure (e.g., referral to a periodontist because of advanced periodontitis). The general and oral health risks to the procedure being refused should be documented. The refusal should document any patient questions and the responses made and include dated signatures of the dentist,

the patient, and a witness. Another form of informed refusal is a patient statement in the chart, indicating refusal of a recommendation. For example:

> *I, Connor Burton, refuse to have a complete set of radiographs (x-rays) taken by the dentist/dental hygienist. Dr. Alex has informed me that by refusing the x-rays I am not allowing her to appropriately evaluate my oral health status and plan my dental treatment. I understand the risks are that Dr. Alex will not be able to determine if I have cavities, gum disease, or other problems, such as cancer in my mouth. I also understand that she may not be able to treat my disease, resulting in my condition becoming worse. I refuse the x-rays, understanding the risks to my oral and general health.*
> *Signed,*
> *Connor Burton*
> *March 21, 2005*

A written statement, such as the one presented, either typewritten or in the patient's handwriting, is clear documentation that the patient refused a recommendation and is aware of the risks of the refusal. In certain situations, when patients are asked to sign such a statement, they change their decision and cooperate. Another term used for informed refusal is "against dental advice," or similar language. The purpose of informed consent and refusal documentation is to maintain a record that shows the provider attempted to meet their duty to inform and that the patient either consented or refused.

Risk Management

A basic understanding of civil law related to contract and tort law is important to all dental professionals. The legal principles assist in guiding the dental team in developing protocols for patient care, working as a team, and preventing the potential for litigation. In addition to understanding the concepts to reduce the risks for allegations of negligence, risk management techniques can be incorporated in daily activities and as part of an approach to the management of a clinic. Risk management includes assessing licensed and unlicensed office personnel, office protocols, record keeping and storage, facilities, and personal interactions to determine if there are at-risk practices. If there are activities or actions that place the office at risk for a potential lawsuit or allegation of failing to comply with a state or local ordinance or regulation, steps should be taken to remedy the risk. Depending on the identified risk, the actions could be as simple as updating an outdated health history or more difficult, such as terminating the employment of an unprofessional or incompetent employee. Additional risk management techniques important to dental providers in community-based clinical settings are:

- Clear, concise, and accurate documentation. An office manual should outline a framework for documenting treatment notes, patient cancellations, informed consent, informed refusal, and telephone conversations with patients or other health professionals. The recommended documentation should comply with state law requirements. If acronyms are used, such as WNL (within normal limits) or S/RP (scaling and root planing), office manual descriptions should provide a definition. This is critical in multistaff employment environments, ensuring that all providers can understand the records and what has occurred. Staff in-service and reviews of record keeping protocols are also recommended on a regular basis.
- Personnel should be currently licensed and credentialing checks should occur at initial employment and throughout the term of employment, including requests for educational credentials, CPR certification, specialty board certification, current licensure documentation, and evidence of continuing-education activities. If appropriate, peer review can allow opportunities for consistency in skill and treatment protocols.

- Clear written and oral communication. The setting for the provision of dental care may include a diverse staff and patient population. Sensitivity to cultural differences, language, health beliefs, and practices is important. If a particular ethnic patient population is represented in a practice, health history forms, informed consent and refusal forms, postoperative forms, and other patient-focused forms should be translated. Bilingual staff is also recommended.
- Awareness of state practice acts, state statutes, public health codes and local ordinances that impact facilities, records, supervision requirements, and reporting requirements (for infectious diseases) is important. It is critical that all members of the dental team are familiar with the scope of practice allowed by the state dental practice act. Copies of pertinent materials can be on file or a listing of Web sites where information can be obtained should be provided in an area accessed by all personnel.
- Knowledge of federal and state laws impacting record keeping and patient confidentiality and patient safety, including OSHA and HIPAA regulations.

Administrative Law

Administrative law is a body of law created by administrative agencies in the form of rules, regulations, orders and decisions. State governments are responsible for protecting the health, safety, and welfare of their citizens. In most states, the legislative branch of government enacts the state's **dental practice act.** The state dental practice act can be a single law or compilation of laws that regulate the practice of dentistry and dental hygiene. Other laws may exist in a state within public health law, child protection laws, elder rights and protections, occupational safety, informed consent, health care fraud, and education and training requirements for relicensure. For example, the dental practice act may indicate a minimum number of clock hours for license renewal, whereas a public health law requires all health care professionals to participate in domestic and child abuse training. Dental providers must be aware of the scope of the laws that impact their ability to practice and interact with patients. In certain states, the ability for a dental hygienist to practice in a clinic or health care delivery setting without a dentist on the premises required special laws to be promulgated. The language allowing specific practice rights may not appear in the dental practice act but in other legislation, such as a state senate bill. The type of supervision required to practice dental hygiene varies from state to state, by definition of dental hygiene scope of practice and, in some instances, the location of the practice. The definitions are state specific and, although similar terms are used, the descriptions may also vary (i.e., direct supervision may mean slightly different practices in different states). Specific types of supervision requirements are found in most states.

Direct supervision usually requires examination and diagnosis by a licensed dentist, for a patient of record. The dentist may delegate or authorize the dental hygienist to complete the procedure. The dentist needs to be on the premises and may be required to examine the patient before and after the procedure. Direct supervision requirements also apply to many tasks performed by a dental assistant.

The terms *assignment, indirect,* and *general supervision* are also used to describe supervision requirements. It is imperative that the dental hygienist read state law carefully to determine the requirements. In one state, indirect supervision is defined as requiring a diagnosis of a patient's condition and authorization by a dentist to complete a procedure, with the dentist on the premises. In another state, this same description may be defined as general supervision. Assignment, or a similar term, is used in some states to describe a type of supervision in which the dental hygienist is allowed to treat a patient of record without the dentist on the premises. However, a patient of record is defined as someone who has been examined and diagnosed by a licensed dentist and whose treatment the dentist has planned. The dentist then assigns the care to the dental hygienist to complete.

To increase access to care for underserved populations, some states allow **unsupervised practice,** including Colorado, Connecticut, and New Mexico. The practice status allows an individual to root plane and scale, perform curettage, apply preventive measures such as fluorides, assess the patient, record patient data, and administer topical anesthetic. Under Colorado regulations, unsupervised practice can be provided by a licensed dentist or dental hygienist without the supervision of a licensed dentist.

Collaborative practice is an emerging practice model in which dental hygienists strive to prevent and treat oral disease through the provision of educational, assessment, preventive, clinical, and other therapeutic services. In this model, practiced by certain dental hygienists in New Mexico, the dental hygienist works in collaboration with the dentist but without general supervision, as defined by New Mexico law. Dental hygienists choosing to practice in traditional and nontraditional settings should be familiar with the law and their rights and responsibilities.

For the implementation of a law to occur, the executive branch of the government is responsible. Within the executive branch are departments and agencies of the state government, including the Department of Consumer and Industry Services and the Secretary of State. To implement statutory law, specific requirements are developed (rules). Dental hygiene is regulated by a governing body (e.g., the Board of Dentistry or State Dental Commission). The rule-making body allows a public forum and process to get input and make changes in the rules for a profession. State boards of dentistry have responsibilities that may include definitions of supervisory requirements and categories, such as direct or general supervision of dental hygienists; issuing, renewing, and revoking licenses; protocol for disciplinary allegations; and outlining of scope of practice for dental assistants, expanded duties assistants, and dental hygienists.

The dental practice act, or other legislation, may promote or deter the role of the dental hygienists in providing services to populations in need. Certain states, for example, have strict rules governing the supervision of dental hygienists by a licensed dentist on site at all times. This may limit access to care in geographic locations where there are not enough dentists in practice or in locations where dentists prefer not to practice. If a dental hygienist chooses to provide care without appropriate supervision, the dental hygienist would be violating the state practice act and may be subject to disciplinary actions. The challenge of unmet dental need is a frequently encountered scenario. Many state dental hygiene associations have taken measures to try to change laws to permit dental hygienists to practice in public or dental health clinics to provide access to preventive services for underserved populations. The success to change the laws in different states has varied. Dental hygienists have collaborated with other health professionals, public health agencies, and consumer groups to promote changes in state regulations. This has required knowledge about how an idea for change becomes a change or addition to the law. Knowledge about the legislative process is an important skill for dental hygienists and others interested in making changes to improve access to care and address other issues related to community service and education.

CREATION OF LAWS

Dental hygienists active in community-based education or service frequently take on the additional role of a change agent. A dental hygienist, or group of dental or other professionals, determines that a law needs to be introduced or changed. This new law or change in law may be to expand the roles and responsibilities of a dental hygienist, such as allowing the administration of local anesthesia. Or, the change may be in reallocation of funds for dental reimbursement by modifying Medicaid requirements. The federal and state process for the introduction of a bill to become a law is similar, although there are variations state by state. States may vary as to the roles of the state assembly or legislature, but the process follows a core of basic steps.

The bill is introduced, or started, on either the house/assembly or senate side of the state legislature. Any legislator in the senate or house/assembly can introduce a bill. In some states, dental hygienists have worked with a supportive senator or representative to have a specific bill introduced. After each bill is introduced, it is sent to an appropriate committee. Four things can occur—the committee reviewing the bill:

1. Agrees with it in its original form and, if it was proposed on the house/assembly side, it is sent to the senate side.
2. Modifies the bill after listening to public comment and/or expert testimony.
3. Allows the bill to "die" in committee. It is then returned to the author. The individual who proposed the bill can either rewrite and reintroduce the bill or drop it.
4. Can "pigeonhole" the bill if it appears extreme —it will remain there until it is reconsidered.

If the committee has rewritten or modified the bill, it will come back to the house/assembly floor where all members of the house/assembly listen to the bill be read, sometimes line-by-line. The house/assembly members present the pros and cons and debate the bill. Each house/assembly member is asked to vote. If the bill passes the house/assembly side of the state legislature, it goes to the senate where the same process occurs. In certain states, the legislation must "age" for a short period (e.g., 3 days) prior to being sent to the other legislative body. If it successfully passes senate debate and discussion, it is forwarded to the governor. If the governor signs a bill, it is law. If the governor vetoes the bill, it returns to either the house/assembly or senate to be voted on again. Usually, it must receive a 2–3 majority vote in both houses to become law and override a veto. The U. S. Congress would follow a similar pattern for a bill introduction, such as prescription drug coverage or campaign finance reform. If the U.S. President signs a proposed bill, it becomes public law.

Public Law

Public or federal laws impact dental professionals personally and professionally. Public or federal laws protect individuals as employees, offer guidance to employers, and guarantee certain rights to groups of individuals. Dental hygienists have roles of both employee and employer. The federal laws may only apply to situations in which a minimum number of individuals are employed.

The employment relationship is one of two types: (1) at will, with indefinite duration; or (2) contractual, with definite duration. The employment at will concept governs the employment relationship, meaning the employment takes place at the will of either the employer or employee. The employment can be terminated at any time for no reason. Similarly, the employee can quit at any time. Many dental professionals have an at will employment situation. The exception is when there is a specific employment contract between the employer and employee that outlines the duration and terms of employment. The protocol or reasons for termination are outlined in the contract. Unfortunately, termination for certain individuals is based on a particular status or characteristics. Federal legislation was initiated and passed to protect certain classes of individuals.

The following are brief descriptions of laws important to dental providers for individual protection against discrimination or loss of federally mandated rights.

1. **Employment Discrimination Laws**
   - Title VII of the Civil Rights Act of 1964 prohibits discrimination in hiring and discharge and in employment compensation, terms, conditions, and privileges because of an individual's race, color, religion, sex, or national origin. Title VII covers employers of 15 or more employees, working at least 20 weeks of the year. Title VII created the U.S. Equal Employment Opportunity Commis-

sion (EEOC). The EEOC enforces Title VII provisions. A prerequisite of a court action under Title VII is filing a complaint with the EEOC within 180 days or, in a deferral state, 300 days. Title VI of the Civil Rights Act of 1964 forbids discrimination in all aspects of patient care in institutions that receive federal financial assistance, such as Medicare and Medicaid. Title VII also makes sexual harassment a form of unwelcome sexual discrimination.

   - Age Discrimination in Employment Act of 1967 (ADEA) prohibits discrimination based on age against any employee or applicant for employment that is at least 40 years of age and applies to employment settings with 20 or more employees.

   - Rehabilitation Act of 1973 applies to employers with federal contracts of $2500 or greater. It prohibits discrimination in employment practices based on physical or mental disabilities. The act also requires federal contractors to implement an affirmative action plan in hiring and promoting disabled employees.

   - Americans with Disabilities Act of 1990 (ADA) impacts employers with 15 or more employees working at least 20 hours a week. Titles I and II ban discrimination against disabled persons in the workplace, mandate equal access for the disabled to certain public facilities, and require commercial firms to make existing facilities and grounds accessible to the disabled. Patients are also protected under this statute. Title III of the act prohibits discrimination based on disability and indicates patients should receive all goods, services, facilities, and accommodations of any privately owned place of public accommodation, including hospitals and professional offices. Three categories of persons are considered disabled under this law:

   a. A person who has a physical or mental impairment that substantially limits one or more of the major activities of that person.

    b. A person who has a record of such an impairment.

    c. A person who, although not actually being disabled is regarded as disabled.

- 1976 Pregnancy Discrimination Act is an amendment to Title VII of the Civil Rights Act that makes it illegal to fire an employee based on pregnancy, childbirth, or related medical conditions. An employer cannot force a woman to quit her job because she is pregnant and a woman cannot lose her job because she had an abortion. Pregnancy must be covered in employer's medical plans similar to any other medical condition.

2. Employee Safety and Health

- The Occupational Safety and Health Administration (OSHA) act of 1970 protects worker safety and prohibits firing an employee for reporting workplace safety hazards or violations. OSHA regulations preempt all state and local regulations regarding employee safety and health. In 1991, OSHA developed rules to protect health care workers from bloodborne disease, called the OSHA Occupational Exposure to Bloodborne Pathogens Standards. There are significant penalties if an employer violates the standards.

- Consolidated Omnibus Budget Reconciliation Act (COBRA) requires that an employer with 20 or more employees must provide extended health care insurance for as long as 18 months following termination of employment usually, but not always at the expense of the employer.

- Drug Free Workplace Act of 1988 requires an employer contracting to provide goods or services to the federal government to certify that they maintain a drug-free workplace.

3. Wage and Benefits

- Equal Pay Act (EPA) of 1963 is an amendment to the Fair Labor Standard Act that requires equal pay for men and women doing equal work. Equal work is work that requires equal skill, responsibility, and effort under the same or similar working conditions.

- Family and Medical Leave Act (FMLA) of 1981 applies to public and private employers with 50 or more employees. This act allows employees to take an unpaid leave for up to 12 weeks if they have been employed for more than 1 year and worked for at least 1250 hours. Leave is allowed for maternity, adoption, or for caring for ill family members. Individuals may be allowed leave to provide:

    a. care for ill and injured children younger than 18.

    b. care for adult children who cannot take care of themselves because of physical or mental disability.

    c. care for a son or daughter, including biologic, adopted, or foster children; stepchildren; or legal wards.

    d. for personal health problems (physical or psychological) that affect employee, spouse, or parents (in-laws are not included in the definition of parents and unmarried partners are excluded).

Federal laws do not only focus on employment protection and discrimination. The Health Care Quality Improvement Act of 1986 was a federal statute passed to improve the quality of medical care nationwide. One provision that came from this act was the National Data Practitioner Bank, a repository of all payments made on behalf of physicians and dentists in connection with malpractice settlements or judgments and adverse peer review actions against licenses. The law requires that medical malpractice information must be reported so that the information is available to state licensure boards and certain professional societies. The purpose was to improve the quality of health care by encouraging licensing boards to identify and discipline practitioners who engage in unprofessional behavior and restrict the ability of incompetent providers to move from state to state without knowledge of previous history. The Health Insurance Portability and Accountability Act of 1996 (HIPAA) has three primary purposes:

(1) to help employees keep continuous health care coverage for themselves and their dependents if they leave one job for another; (2) to protect confidential medical information from unauthorized disclosure and/or use; and (3) help curb the rising cost of fraud and abuse through streamlining of codes and billing procedures.

State Law

State laws may be similar to federal laws and, in certain instances, stricter. A state law can never conflict with a federal or public law. State laws are also designed to protect the rights of employers and employees. State modified laws related to employment discrimination may add additional factors that cannot be used for discriminatory purposes, such as height, weight, marital status, or sexual orientation. A state law may broaden the definition as compared with federal law (e.g., the term disability would include a larger scope of conditions). State laws may define **the statute of limitations** for specific legal actions. The statute of limitations is the length of time during which a legal action must be taken and can be a state law or part of a statute. Limitations are put on the ability to collect, retention of medical records, medical or dental malpractice claims, and damages for child sexual abuse. The statute of limitations for filing a negligence suit against a health professional varies by state. The range of time may be from 1 to 6 years, with 2 years the most common. Some states define the start of the limitation period from the time the negligent act was alleged to occur; in some states, from the time it was discovered or should have been discovered or the date the provider–patient relationship ended. In addition, the statutory period in certain states is modified for minors or other categories of patients, such as the imprisoned or legally insane. Dental providers should be familiar with the laws in their state. State laws may also require specific continuing-education courses for health care providers. A state law may impose a requirement on a health care provider in a specific setting, such as an institution or hospital, to obtain testing for specific diseases, such as the tuberculin test. A state may also have language in a statute that forbids a health care provider to treat a relative or person with whom there is a personal relationship.

A TOOLBOX FOR THE ORAL HEALTH PROVIDER

An oral health provider who treats patients evaluates each patient's oral health status and plans the treatment specific to the patient's needs. The provider uses skills and knowledge acquired through education, both formal and lifelong learning; experience; and networking with colleagues. The provider picks which "tools" are needed to complete a task, whether a dental instrument, an oral hygiene index, or a consultation with a dental or health professional. The dental hygienist in a community setting may have various roles, including provider, manager, negotiator, change agent, advocate, researcher, record keeper, or quality controller. The dental hygienist or dental provider relies on the public health model or approach that includes assessment, analysis, prioritization, planning, implementation, and evaluation, with education and financial considerations a common aspect of all phases. There must be an understanding of the legal principles and local, state, and federal laws that apply to the circumstances in that individual's toolbox.

A dental hygienist should rely on a toolbox that includes knowledge and skills important to the provider to fulfill the roles and responsibilities of a particular position. The toolbox should include personal, professional, legal, and ethical tools that can be accessed and used when needed

The following are suggested tools to include in a dental public health provider's toolbox:

1. Personal
   - Ability to recognize deficiencies and seek assistance or opportunities to remedy skill or knowledge weaknesses. Example: cultural knowledge acquisition about a particular ethnic or religious population

- Negotiating skills
- Conflict resolution strategies and how to use them
- Commitment to lifelong learning
- Ability to access information about rules, regulations, practice acts, and other statutory information pertinent to public health settings, state or local agencies, federal agencies or groups, and oral health care providers. Sources may include libraries, telephone numbers, Web sites, professional associations, online archives, or educational institutions.

2. Professional
   - Awareness of local and state government priorities focused on oral health care, including access issues and financing mechanisms
   - A database of names and office locations and e-mail addresses for local and state politicians and their political agendas
   - Names and goals of state political actions groups (PACS) or other lobbying groups interested in relevant issues, including general health, oral health, citizen well-being, sports injury safety, and smoking cessation
   - Advocacy skills
   - Knowledge of potential allies or resources, including major health professional advocacy groups or associations in the city, state, or region (e.g., nursing and medical societies, visiting nurse associations, migrant services, ethnically or religiously based coalitions)
   - List of state colleges and universities with dental, dental hygiene, allied health, and health education programs
   - Knowledge of the local or state public health system, with an emphasis on the dental division or department and its agenda, personnel, budget, and annual or strategic plan
   - The names of individuals in the local and state dental and specialty dental societies responsible for community liaison, community service planning, grant funding, and political networking

- Copies of the latest public health codes and dental practice acts and/or Web sites for access
- Advocacy skills, including the ability to access information using listserv memberships, local publications, attendance at annual meetings of health professions groups, and subscriptions to online or mailed newsletters
- Contributions to political allies or volunteer time for political campaigns to develop a network for support

SUMMARY

Oral health providers practice within ethical and legal guidelines to protect themselves and the patients and communities they serve. A basic foundation in legal principles, including contract and tort law, will protect the dental provider in their day-to-day activities and decisions. Knowledge about state and federal laws that impact the employment settings and outline the rights and responsibilities of employers and employees contributes to a professional employment situation and reduces the risks of allegations of unprofessional conduct, discrimination, or harassment. The community-based dental provider must also be knowledgeable about changing the legal system to resolve issues impacting access to care. Awareness of the legislative process assists the dental hygienist and other members of the dental team to appropriately resolve issues in a professional, yet significant, manner. Dental providers should use the legal concepts and federal and state laws to protect their rights, and those of the patients and communities they serve, as providers and as citizens.

RESOURCES

Beemsterboer PL. Ethics and Law in Dental Hygiene. Philadelphia, PA: WB Saunders, 2001.

Council on Dental Insurance. Informed consent: a risk management view. J Amer Dent Assoc 1987;115:630–635.

✓ Learning Activities

1. Obtain a current copy of the dental practice act for the state where you received your education and also a copy of a dental practice act from another state. Compare and contrast the acts. What are the similarities? What are the differences?

2. Identify a patient situation in which it was apparent that there were irreconcilable differences between the provider and the patient regarding treatment. Draft a letter indicating that the relationship is ending, including the key elements to prevent allegations of abandonment.

3. Contact the state dental hygiene association or dental association. Invite the lobbyists to a student dental association or component meeting to discuss their role in advocating for oral health issues on the state level.

4. Review the list of contractual responsibilities that outlines the duties of the provider to the patient. Divide the students into two groups. Have one group give an example of how a violation of the responsibility could occur and have one group discuss strategies that could prevent the violation from occurring.

5. Individually, or as a group, identify a federal or state law or laws that you want additional information for or one that is unknown to you. Log on to the Web site that provides information about the law. Prepare a brief report for a presentation. Discuss how the law impacts dental hygiene practice. Compile each report into a packet and copy and distribute to all classmates to use as a future reference.

6. Identify procedures or treatments commonly provided for patients in clinical settings. Using the informed consent criteria, identify the procedure, possible risks and benefits, alternatives, and other information necessary to obtain an informed consent.

7. Identify a procedure, or procedures, that patients could refuse. Draft an informed refusal statement for the patient to sign. Or, role-play a situation in which a patient is declining a recommended treatment and the response of the provider.

8. Draft a dental hygiene office manual. As a group, identify a table of contents, including (but not limited to) topics such as employee rights and responsibilities; sexual harassment policy; termination notice guidelines; policies and procedures; dental hygiene record keeping guidelines; commonly used acronyms, with descriptions; sample termination letters; and other information that all dental hygiene team members should know. Assign portions to small groups within the class or component society. Review the drafts and compile.

9. Obtain a copy of state senate or house/assembly bill as a prototype. Draft a bill for submission to your state legislature. Identify a topic or issue that would impact on oral health status within your state. For example, a no-smoking policy in all restaurants or a mandatory bike helmet safety law. Divide the class into groups and then report the different "bills" that were proposed. If time allows, select certain students to present both sides of the bill (in favor and opposed) and listen to the arguments. Vote on the bill.

10. Obtain a copy of the Title VII of the Civil Rights Act of 1964 and the specific state law that protects civil rights. Compare and contrast the language found in the federal and state law. Is the state law stricter or more comprehensive and, if so, how?

Garner BA. Black's Law Dictionary. 7th Ed. St. Paul, MN: West, 1999.

Pollack BR. Law and Risk Management in Dental Practice. Chicago, IL: Quintessence, 2002.

Review Questions

A patient presenting to the clinic completes the health and dental history. Following a review of the data and radiographs and clinical examination, the dentist diagnoses the patient's condition and recommends two appointments of root planing and scaling. The patient nods his head in agreement and schedules an appointment with the dental hygienist. Answer Questions 1–3.

1. Which of the following relationships exist?
   a. A promise
   b. An expressed contract
   c. An implied contract
   d. An implied warranty
   e. An implied guarantee

2. On return for the recommended root planing and scaling, the dental hygienist informs the patient that she will be administering anesthesia as part of the procedure. The patient becomes upset and declines the anesthesia. Which of the following should be done?
   a. Treat the patient by root planing and scaling
   b. Obtain an informed refusal for the anesthesia
   c. Confirm that informed consent was obtained for the root planing and scaling by the dentist and obtain an informed refusal for the anesthesia
   d. Obtain informed consent for scaling and root planing
   e. Reappoint the patient

3. The patient tells the dental hygienist that she read about a new mouth rinse, developed by a local practitioner, that dissolves calculus. The dental hygienist indicates to the patient that she would not use the mouth rinse if the dental association did not approve of it. Which of the following contractual responsibilities is the dental hygienist fulfilling?
   a. Exercise reasonable skill, care, and judgment in the assessment, diagnosis, and treatment of patients
   b. Have a proper license and registration and comply with all laws and practice within the scope of practice dictated by law
   c. Use standard drugs, materials, and techniques; refrain from experimental procedures*
   d. Complete procedures within a reasonable time
   e. Keep the patient informed of progress

4. A dental hygienist is applying dental sealants to the posterior teeth of a 12-year-old child. The sealants were treatment planned a few months ago. The sealants treatment planned were for teeth 3, 14, 19, and 30. Informed consent was obtained for applying sealants on those teeth. Since the teeth were treatment planned, numbers 18 and 31 have completely erupted. The child is cooperative. The dental hygienist decides to apply sealants to numbers 18 and 31. Which of the following might the dental hygienist be accused of?
   a. Invasion of privacy
   b. Assault
   c. Technical assault
   d. Battery
   e. Technical battery

5. A dental hygienist is accused of negligence by a dental patient. Which of the following does the patient need to prove?
   a. The dental hygienist intended to harm the patient.
   b. The dental hygienist had a legally recognized duty or responsibility that the dental hygienist omitted.
   c. The harm that occurred is directly related to what the dental hygienist failed to do.

d. a, b, and c

e. b and c only

6. A state dental hygiene association seeks to change the dental practice act to allow a collaborative practice model for the state. The association determines that the governor needs to sign the law to make the change. Which of the following is the best approach to make the change occur?

a. Ask the dental association to work to change the law.

b. Petition the state board of dentistry to change the law.

c. Hire a lobbyist to talk with a state legislator to get the law changed.

d. Find a supporter or supporters in the state senate or assembly to sponsor the bill and offer to provide expert testimony.

e. Petition the governor to change the law.

7. A federal law that protects employees from discrimination in hiring and firing based on pregnancy, childbirth, or related conditions is the:

a. Americans With Disabilities Act.

b. Pregnancy Discrimination Act.

c. Title VII of the Civil Rights Act of 1964.

d. Family Medical Leave Act.

e. Rehabilitation Act of 1973.

8. Prior to beginning two quadrants of root planing and scaling, the dental hygienist wants to obtain informed consent (legal for dental hygienists in the state). The dental hygienist describes the periodontal status of the patient and then discusses other important information. Prior to outlining the possible outcomes of the procedure, the dental hygienist describes the benefits and anticipated outcomes of the treatment. The dental hygienist describes the possibility of infection, sensitivity, trauma, bleeding, shrinkage in gingiva, and redness. The dental hygienist also describes how the procedure may not succeed in stopping the progression of the disease that could lead to tooth loss. The dental hygienist then proceeds to explain the risks and benefits of administering local anesthesia during the procedure. The dental hygienist then proceeds to begin the treatment. Which of the following elements of informed consent were missing in the scenario?

a. Alternative treatments to root planing and scaling and the risks and benefits to the alternatives

b. The cost of the treatment

c. The patient's obligation to cooperate in care

d. An opportunity for the patient to ask and have questions answered

e. a and d

REFERENCE

1. American Dental Education Association. Competencies for entry into the profession of dental hygiene, Exhibit 7. J Dent Educ 2003;67(7):1–5. Available at: http://www.adea.org/cepr. Accessed February 2004.

NATIONAL BOARD PREPARATION

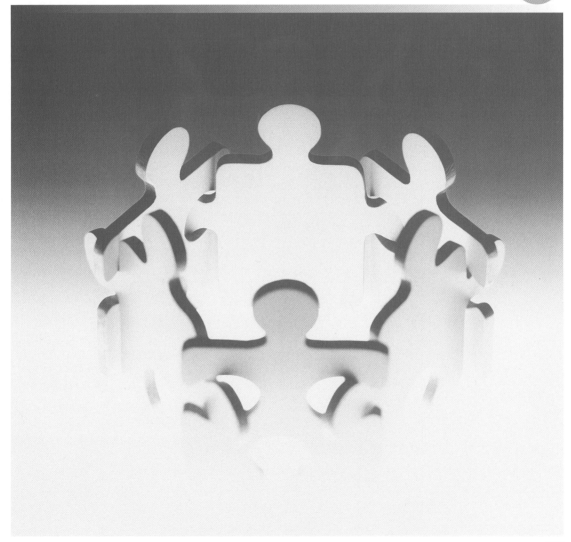

National Board Preparation

18

Objectives

After studying this chapter and completing the study questions and activities, the learner will be able to:
- Describe study skills helpful in preparation for the NBDHE.
- List test-taking strategies useful for the Community Dental Hygiene portion of the NBDHE.
- Identify personal preparation skills for the NBDHE.

KEY TERMS

Learning style   Study skills   Testlets

The American Dental Education Association competencies addressed in this chapter include[1]:

Community Involvement:

CM.1:   Assess the oral health needs of the community and the quality and availability of resources and services.

CM.2:   Provide screening, referral, and educational services that allow clients to access the resources of the health care system.

CM.3:   Provide community oral health services in a variety of settings.

CM.4:   Facilitate client access to oral health services by influencing individuals and/or organizations for the provision of oral health care.

CM.5:   Evaluate reimbursement mechanisms and their impact on the patient's/client's access to oral health care.

CM.6:   Evaluate the outcomes of community-based programs and plan for future activities.

Health Promotion and Disease Prevention:

HP.1: Promote the values of oral and general health and wellness to the public and organizations within and outside the profession.

HP.2: Respect the goals, values, beliefs, and preferences of the patient/client while promoting optimal oral and general health.

HP.4: Identify individual and population risk factors and develop strategies that promote health related quality of life.

HP.5: Evaluate factors that can be used to promote patient/client adherence to disease prevention and/or health maintenance strategies.

Introduction

Preparation and success in the Community Dental Hygiene portion of the National Board Dental Hygiene Examination (NBDHE) will be enhanced through understanding and implementing personal preparation, **study skills,** and test-taking strategies. Not only must the candidates possess knowledge of community dental hygiene concepts, they must also develop the skills necessary to identify the key issues factored into each examination question and the ability to respond appropriately.

THE NATIONAL BOARD DENTAL HYGIENE EXAMINATION (NBDHE)

The NBDHE is administered by the Joint Commission on National Dental Examinations. The purpose is to assist state boards in determining the professional competency of applicants who seek licensure to practice dental hygiene. The examination assesses the ability of the candidate to understand, recall, analyze, and apply important information from basic biomedical, dental, and dental hygiene sciences in a problem-solving context. The NBDHE is composed of approximately 350 multiple-choice questions. The examination is delivered in two sessions, with the morning session (component A) allowing 3 hours and 30 minutes and answering 200 traditionally styled, stand-alone test items. The remaining 150 questions are based on 12–15 dental hygiene case scenarios (component B). Component A includes the Community Health/Research Principles portion of the examination, with 20 questions, which are distributed within the following categories:

1. Promoting health and preventing disease within groups (including media and communication resources) (20%)
2. Participating in community programs (40%)
   - Assessing populations and defining objectives
   - Designing, implementing, and evaluating programs
3. Analyzing scientific literature, understanding statistical concepts, and applying research results (40%)

Note: The distribution of questions may change at the discretion of the NBDHE Joint Commission. It is recommended that candidates visit the American Dental Association Web site for the most current guidelines.

The Community Dental Hygiene section test format is presented as **testlets.** A testlet is a short descriptive scenario of a problem, situation, or event. Each scenario is followed by five or more situation-related multiple-choice questions for which there is only one correct or "best choice" answer. The Community Dental Hygiene section differs from traditional stand-alone, factoid, or case-based questions because the testlet format requires analysis and application of problem-solving skills, rather than memorization.

EXAMINATION PREPARATION

There are many resources available to help the candidate prepare for the NBDHE (see Resources). In addition to reviewing the material, the candidate will find it beneficial to incorporate personal preparation strategies to aid in their success.

General Preparation

1. Allow plenty of time. Nothing boosts confidence like advanced preparation. It is prudent to begin the review process at least 4 months prior to the examination. Plan small blocks of uninterrupted time for review. In this way, it will be possible to complete a structured sequence of review without excessive pressure.

2. Become familiar with the examination format by obtaining a recent release of the National Board Dental Hygiene Examination. Many dental hygiene schools have these examinations on file or you may obtain a copy for a fee from the Commission (National Board of Dental Hygiene Pilot Examination, 211 East Chicago Avenue, 6th Floor, Chicago, Illinois 60611).

Use this examination to test yourself on a day without potential interruptions. Identify areas of strength and weakness. Use this information to plan and organize your sequence of review in the coming months. Include all areas you marked incorrectly on the examination, as well as areas that were questionable in your review plan (even if you guessed correctly).

3. It is advisable to obtain a review text to aid in your study. Many comprehensive dental hygiene review texts are available and are listed in the resource section. Additionally, textbooks used in your program of study should be reviewed. Although the Commission states that National Board test items are not based on specific textbooks, it has published a list of reference texts used by the test construction committee. Those texts having significance in Community Dental Hygiene are listed in Box 18-1. The most current list is available online.

4. Schedule study time. Plan on approximately 4 hours per week to review for the examination. Designate a specific day and time to devote to this preparation. Study the most difficult material when you are most alert. Without a

---

BOX 18-1 Reference Textbooks Used for NBDHE

The ADA test construction committees have used the latest editions of the following textbooks as references for the Community Dental Hygiene testlets:

Burt BA, Eklund SA. Dentistry, Dental Practice, and the Community. Philadelphia, PA: WB Saunders.

Darby M. Mosby's Comprehensive Review of Dental Hygiene. St. Louis, MO: C.V. Mosby.

Darby ML, Walsh MM. Dental Hygiene Theory and Practice. Philadelphia, PA: WB Saunders.

Geurink K. Community Oral Health Practice for the Dental Hygienist. Philadelphia, PA: WB Saunders.

Gluck GM, Morganstein WM. Jong's Community Dental Health. St. Louis, MO: C.V. Mosby.

Harris NO, Garcia-Godoy F. Primary Preventive Dentistry. Upper Saddle River, NJ: Prentice Hall.

McKelvey ND. Saunders Review of Dental Hygiene. Philadelphia, PA: WB Saunders.

Wilkins EM. Clinical Practice of the Dental Hygienist. Baltimore, MD: Lippincott Williams & Wilkins.

Woodall IR. Comprehensive Dental Hygiene Care. St. Louis, MO: C.V. Mosby.

plan, best intentions are often put aside to focus on the immediate task or school assignment. If you find your plan is not working, reassess and reorganize to allow adequate time for preparation.

5. Read and understand the format and design of the examination. A printable version of the *Candidate's Guide for the National Board Dental Hygiene Examination* is available online.

6. Many comprehensive Board review courses are available. Many of these are marketed directly to dental hygiene programs. Information may be available through your school or program director. If you desire to take a course, thoroughly investigate the content and reputation of the course. They can be expensive and require travel, but can also reduce anxiety about the examination.

Study Skills and Learning Styles

It is important to identify your **learning style** to maximize your study strategy. Learning styles are traits that reflect how an individual approaches learning new material or tasks. Various recognized self-scoring inventories include the Kolb Learning Style Inventory[2] and the Myers-Briggs Type Indicator.[3] Various learning styles include reflective or active, sensing or intuitive, visual or verbal, and global or sequential. Most individuals are a combination of the various learning styles, with a preference for one aspect over another.[4]

There are many opportunities to discover your preferred learning style. A college testing center can help, many books are written on the subject, and several Web sites are available to obtain a free inventory. North Carolina University[4] offers an index of learning styles questionnaires that are automatically scored to aid individuals who wish to determine their own learning style preference. Knowing your preferred learning style can help you plan a more efficient and effective method of study. Table 18-1 provides a brief overview of learning styles and suggestions about how to maximize study strategies based on learning preferences.

Test-Taking Strategies

It is advantageous to employ general test-taking strategies during the examination. These strategies will help the candidate focus on pertinent details and eliminate any distracters within the testlet or multiple-choice answers.

1. Approach the examination with confidence. View the examination as an opportunity to show how much you have learned.

2. Listen and carefully read all instructions. Mark spaces on the answer sheet clearly, avoiding marks that extend outside the answer box.

3. Read the stem of the question completely and carefully to determine what the question is asking. Identify and underline key words and information.

4. Try to formulate an answer before looking at the options presented.

5. Read all answers carefully to determine if the response to the question is complete and appropriate. Look for the best answer that generally applies in *most* situations to conditions presented in the question.

6. Eliminate all obviously incorrect answers immediately to narrow the choices.

7. Make an educated guess if the correct answer is still in doubt after the choices have been narrowed as much as possible. There is no penalty for a wrong answer.

8. Skip a question if you "go blank" and move on. Make a light mark on the answer sheet by the number of the question you skipped. Be careful to mark the next answer in the appropriate box. (Erase the light mark when you go back and answer the question).

9. Be alert for grammatical clues. If a question indicates a plural response, all options in singular format may be an indication of an incorrect answer.

10. Be alert to any answer that contains the words: *always, never, none, all,* or *every.* Absolutes are seldom appropriate for health conditions and are usually incorrect answers.

TABLE 18-1 LEARNING STYLES AND STUDY STRATEGIES

LEARNING STYLE	CHARACTERISTICS	TO MAXIMIZE STUDY STRATEGY
Sensing	• Likes learning facts and solving problems • Detail oriented • Practical • Likes connections to real world • Dislikes complications and/or surprises	• Identify specific examples of concepts • Relate information to real world situations
Intuitive	• Innovative • Likes discovering possibilities • Tends to work faster • Dislikes memorization and routine calculations	• Find theoretic connections and apply to facts • Slow down to avoid mistakes due to lack of attention to detail
Visual	• Tends to remember what they see • Likes pictures, charts, and diagrams • Dislikes strictly reading text	• Create concept maps to represent visual connections • Find pictures, charts, and diagrams to aid memory of information
Verbal	• Tends to remember words (written and spoken)	• Write outlines or rewrite information in your own words • Working in groups may be helpful as you hear others verbalize information
Sequential	• Tends to understand in linear steps • Follows a logical path in problem solving • Dislikes skipping steps or jumping from topic to topic	• Outline material in a logical order • Study in the order of the textbook, handouts, or as the information was presented in class • Create inventories
Global	• Tends to gather information somewhat randomly, often without initially identifying the connections. • Frequently experiences the "Ah ha" moment of suddenly understanding a concept.	• Identify the "big picture" of a topic before trying to master the details • Review the objectives and skim the entire chapter to get an overview prior to focusing on details • Try to relate the topic to things already known • Rather than planning to study several topics in an evening, try to set aside larger blocks of study time for individual subjects
Active	• Tends to retain and understand information best by doing something active. This may include explaining or discussing material with others.	• Study in a group to facilitate an active relay of information on the topic • Create games or role plays to review information • Brainstorm with a peer • Participate in active discussion
Reflective	• Tends to think about information • Often prefers to work alone	• Pause while studying new material to review the reading • Pause to think of possible applications or questions about the information presented • Write a simple summary of the information to help retain the material

(Adapted from: Felder R, Soloman B. Learning styles and strategies. Available at: http://www.ncsu.edu/felder-public/ILSdir/styles.htm. Accessed December 2003.)[4]

11. Be alert for the words *except, not,* and *least* in the question. Errors are made by overlooking these key words. If a question does not make sense, read the question carefully and underline these key words to aid in formulating the answer.
12. Be alert to answers revealed within the examination itself. Sometimes clues or answers may be found in other questions. As you read the questions, jot down brief notes in the margins of the booklet, indicating ideas you may use later in your answers.
13. Do not change answers unless you are sure of the correction. Remember, your first answer is usually correct.
14. Be comfortable but alert. Change positions periodically to help you relax; however, maintain an upright posture in your seat to avoid unwanted fatigue.
15. Mark your answer on the answer sheet immediately, rather than waiting until finishing the examination and transferring all answers at one time. You may run out of time and be prevented from entering your answers. Additionally, errors are often made when transferring several answers at one time.
16. Review the answer sheet periodically to confirm you are marking the corresponding answer. One mark placed in the wrong space can throw off an entire portion of the exam. A quick review will help prevent a mistake from going too far before realizing you have made an error.
17. Reserve approximately 10% of your test time for review. Resist the urge to leave as soon as all the items are completed. Don't panic when other candidates start handing in their answer sheets. There's no advantage to being the first to complete the examination.
18. Make sure you have answered all questions; do not leave blanks. Remember, there is no penalty for guessing.

Personal and Physical Preparation

To prevent test anxiety, it is recommended to take care of personal and physical needs prior to the ex-amination. The guidelines in Box 18-2 will help ensure that the candidate arrives at the test site calm and ready to tackle the examination.

CONSIDERATIONS FOR DIVERSE LEARNERS

Candidates With Disabilities

Special arrangements may be granted to enable candidates with a qualifying disability to be examined. To be considered for special arrangements, the candidate must submit a written request well in advance of the testing date. Refer to the guidelines outlined under the National Board Dental Hygiene Examination Testing Services available from the American Dental Association for qualifying disabilities and application deadlines.

Candidates With English as a Second Language (ESL)

The Joint Commission states that translators will not be allowed in the testing area. Applicants with English as a second language may encounter unique problems when studying for the National Board Dental Hygiene Examination. ESL candidates may enhance their learning and test-taking skills by employing one or more of the following strategies:

- Reading and then writing the information when reviewing.
- Monitoring comprehension by summarizing information.
- Seeking visual aids to support verbal explanations.
- Working in groups to promote the sharing of information.

EXAMINING A TESTLET

The questions in the NBDHE have been written with specific intent and, as much as possible, extraneous information has been eliminated. Only one option is clearly the best answer for each question. Other possible options are designed to distract the attention of a candidate who lacks

BOX 18-2 Guidelines for Personal Preparation

The week before:

- Review the examination procedure posted from the ADA testing services.
- Avoid cramming; maintain your regular study schedule; review the most difficult areas.
- Plan your route to the examination site and determine travel time. Be generous in your estimate of travel time.
- Exercise; however, this is not the time to begin a rigorous new exercise program.
- Eat healthy foods, drink lots of water, and avoid alcohol.
- Get plenty of rest.
- Do not panic; panic decreases effectiveness. Assume there will be questions on unfamiliar content.
- Think positive. Relax. Envision yourself passing the examination. Taking the test with the attitude that one is prepared and capable of success is imperative. Having a clear and relaxed frame of mind is essential to the success of the candidate.

The night before:

- Do something fun.
- Eat healthy.
- Get a good night's sleep. (Do NOT take a sleep aid if you are unfamiliar with the effects it may have on you.)
- Avoid alcohol.
- Plan a relaxing evening. Avoid studying the night before the examination.
- Do not talk to other students about the examination. Anxiety is contagious!
- Set out all needed material (e.g., several pencils and erasers, watch, admission card, identification, magnifying glass, and water bottle).
- Lay out clothing for the morning. Dress for comfort. Layer clothing in case the room temperature is too hot or cold.
- Set your alarm; give yourself plenty of time to get ready and travel.
- Think positive. Envision yourself passing the examination.

That morning:

- Give yourself plenty of time.
- Eat a healthy breakfast before the examination: protein for endurance and carbohydrates that easily convert to energy on demand. Avoid caffeine and sugar as these often have a let-down effect.
- Arrive early; allow plenty of time for traffic, parking, and bad weather.
- Come prepared. Bring all needed materials (e.g., several pencils, erasers, watch, admission card, identification, magnifying glass, lunch). Leave all study materials at home. Note: mechanical pencils, eating, and drinking are not permitted in the testing room.
- Stay calm. A little anxiety is normal. Take regular deep breaths. Maintain a positive attitude and reaffirm that you will pass.

sufficient knowledge of the material; therefore, it is imperative the candidate understands the information the question was designed to seek.

The following scenario is an example of a testlet. To demonstrate test-taking strategies, key factors in the scenario have been identified.

Example Testlet: You are employed by a local health department. The department just received a small federal grant to provide smoking cessation services to a local middle school. Your job is to ascertain tobacco use and manage the development of the project. You create a student questionnaire to determine the current level of smoking behavior and the awareness of the dangers of smoking. After the program, you will reassess the population with the same questionnaire to determine if the program had an effect on the population.

Key identifiers for this question include: (1) The population: middle school students; (2) The types of assessment needed: tobacco use and dangers of smoking; and (3) How the assessments will be gathered: questionnaire.

1. Discussion of which of the following smoking related issues would MOST appeal to this population?
   a. Halitosis
   b. Tooth loss
   c. Heart disease
   d. Emphysema
   e. Low-birth-weight babies

Answer: a. Halitosis is a smoking related issue that would appeal the most to the middle school population. The other issues would be of relatively low interest as they occur much later in life and would not be perceived as imminent problems.

2. Any combination of preventive, educational, organizational, economic, and environmental supports for behavior conducive to health describes:
   a. health education.
   b. dental public health.
   c. health promotion.
   d. educational theory.
   e. community assessment.

Answer: c. Health promotion. Health education is related to educational or learning activities designed to increase knowledge.

3. Students who participate in a presentation of the dangers of smoking will decrease their use of cigarettes. This statement is an example of a (an):
   a. instruction.
   b. observation.
   c. objective.
   d. hypothesis.
   e. null hypothesis.

Answer: d. Hypothesis is the statement of expected outcomes of a study, whereas a null hypothesis states no difference will be found.

4. All of the following areas need to be examined when performing a needs assessment EXCEPT:
   a. demographics.
   b. behavioral characteristics.
   c. hereditary characteristics.
   d. health status.
   e. availability of providers.

Answer: c. Hereditary characteristics are not significant in determining the oral health needs of a community group.

ADDITIONAL SAMPLE TESTLETS

Testlet #1

A dental hygienist has recently taken a position with the Indian Health Service. His responsibility is oral health promotion for the Native American community. The community water system is not fluoridated. Data from the Surgeon General's Report suggest a usage of spit tobacco as high as 40% in junior high and high school children within the Native American population. To develop appropriate health promotion strategies, the dental hygienist wants to determine the oral health status and cumulative dental experience of the teachers and students in the local school.

1. What are the BEST indices to evaluate the oral health status of the teachers in the school?
   a. OHI-S, dmfs
   b. PII, TSIF
   c. PDI, CPI
   d. GI, DMFT
   e. CPI, DMFS

Answer: e. Teachers, as adults, would best be assessed by the CPI and DMFS (permanent teeth).

2. Based on the Surgeon General's Report, which of the following would be appropriate topics to discuss with the elementary school classes and teachers?
   a. Oral hygiene instructions
   b. Careers in the dental field
   c. How to respond to peer pressure regarding risky behaviors
   d. Risks of tobacco product use
   e. C and D

Answer: e. Students need education about the risks of tobacco use and the skills to counter peer pressure.

3. Which of the following would be the MOST cost-effective method to increase fluoride exposure in this community?
   a. Encourage parents to purchase toothpaste products with fluoride.
   b. Encourage local physicians to write prescriptions for fluoride supplements.
   c. Implement a program for annual professional fluoride treatments for all appropriately aged schoolchildren.
   d. Implement a fluoride tablet program in the school for appropriately aged children.
   e. Work with the city council and local leaders to implement community water fluoridation.

Answer: e. Community water fluoridation is the most cost-effective and socially equitable way to deliver fluoride to a community.

4. The dental hygienist wishes to assess the oral health status of the students. Because of time constraints, he samples grades K, 3, and 6 to determine student oral health status. Which oral health indices would be the BEST to use?
   a. GI, PI
   b. DMFS, dfs
   c. OHI-S, dmf
   d. TSIF, CPI
   e. CPI, DMFS

Answer: b. For children with a mixed dentition, both DMFS and/or dfs may need to be used. Other indices evaluating plaque, fluorosis, or periodontal disease would not provide useful information for this age-group.

5. There have been 18 new cases of squamous cell carcinoma this year in the elder population of this community. This is an example of:
   a. rate.
   b. incidence.
   c. prevalence.
   d. proportion.
   e. average.

Answer: b. Incidence is the number of new cases of a disease in a population.

Testlet #2

Residents in a low socioeconomic West Coast community have an average annual income of $15,000. Public facilities include two local medical clinics, a skilled nursing facility, home health services, and dental clinics. The nearest medical center is more than 30 miles north. There are three elementary schools, one middle school, and one high school. A local community college is in the neighboring city, 10 miles west of the community.

There is no fluoride in the public water supply. Several legislative attempts have been made to institute water fluoridation, but none have passed. The local elementary schools participate in a weekly fluoride mouth rinse program. Local dentists and pediatricians typically prescribe fluoride supplements; however, compliance is low. A study to determine the caries status of children is being planned. The age-groups to be studied are listed in the following table:

AGE OF STUDENTS IN STUDY

AGE	NUMBER
6–8	473
9–11	428
12–14	417
15–18	398

1. Which sampling method would best accomplish the task of determining caries status?
   a. Random
   b. Stratified
   c. Validated
   d. Convenience
   e. Systemic

Answer: b. Stratified: randomly selects a specific number of residents from each age-group listed, allowing a representative sample of the actual population to be included. Random would not guarantee proportional representation of each age-group. A convenience sample would be the least representative of the age-groups.

2. Which epidemiologic index would be the BEST choice for evaluating caries prevalence of this population?
   a. GI
   b. CPI
   c. RCI
   d. PDI
   e. DMFS

Answer: e. DMFS. RCI is a root caries index (most often seen in the elderly), CPI and PDI assess periodontal needs, and GI assesses the gingival condition.

3. What is the recommended dosage of supplemental fluoride for a 6-year-old at risk of caries in this community?
   a. 1.5 mg/day
   b. 1.0 mg/day
   c. 0.5 mg/day
   d. 0.25 mg/day
   e. No supplemental fluoride is needed.

Answer: b. 1.0 mg is the recommended dosage of supplemental fluoride for a 6-year-old in a nonfluoridated community.

4. If a sealant program is implemented in the elementary school, measuring sealant retention rates of the program is an example of what kind of evaluation?
   a. Process
   b. Formative
   c. Cursory
   d. Outcome
   e. Longitudinal

Answer: d. Outcome is an assessment of the end point success of a program.

5. Which one of the following has the MOST influence on dental utilization rates?
   a. Socioeconomic status
   b. Ethnicity
   c. Race
   d. Gender
   e. Geographic location

Answer: a. Although all are factors, socioeconomic status is the MOST important influence on dental utilization rates.

Testlet #3

The city homeless shelter houses 559 adult men, 124 adult women, and 97 children younger than age 18. Fewer than 2% of sheltered adults hold full-time employment. City officials have recently implemented an employment training project for the homeless. Based on the results of a survey of prospective employers, the project will provide participants with assistance in reading and writing skills, resume and interview preparation, personal hygiene, appropriate attire, and working skills. Several dental hygienists and dentists have volunteered to assess the oral health needs of project participants using the OHI-S.[5]

1. The OHI-S is used to measure all of the following EXCEPT:

a. stain.
b. calculus.
c. material alba.
d. demineralization.
e. plaque.

Answer: d. The OHI-S is used to measure debris (plaque, material alba, stain, and food) and calculus on specific tooth surfaces, not tooth demineralization.

2. Every ninth adult listed on the alphabetized roster of shelter residents will be selected for assessment of oral hygiene needs. This sampling method is known as:
a. random.
b. convenience.
c. stratified.
d. systematic.

Answer: d. Systematic samplings are exemplified by selecting the nth person on a roster of individuals. A convenience sample, the least representative, entails selecting a sample that is not necessarily representative of the total population being studied. A stratified sample would allow proportional representation from each group but would not allow each member within a group an equal chance of selection. A random sample would allow each resident an equal opportunity to be selected but would not guarantee proportional representation from each age-group.

3. After watching a toothbrushing demonstration, the residents will be able to perform the Modified Stillman's toothbrushing technique. The "condition element" of this objective is:
a. after watching a toothbrushing demonstration.
b. the Modified Stillman's toothbrushing technique.
c. the residents.
d. will be able to perform.

Answer: a. The condition element of an instructional objective restricts or guides the participants as they attempt to meet the objective. In this ex-

ample, the audience element would be the residents, the behavior element would be "they will be able to perform," and the degree element of the objective is the Modified Stillman's toothbrushing technique.

4. Nearly 46% of project participants gained full-time employment within 3 months of project completion. Eighty-two percent of those remained employed for at least 2 years. This is an example of project:
a. supervision.
b. evaluation.
c. assessment.
d. implementation.
e. expectations.

Answer: b. Project evaluation is a judgment of the worth of a project. Assessment is the tool used to determine the needs of the population, implementation is putting the program into action, and supervision is the administration or overseeing of a project.

Testlet #4

You are the dental hygienist for a nursing home community of 150 residents. One of the administrator's goals is to improve the oral health status of the residents. She asks you to develop a program to achieve this goal.

1. You surveyed the nurses by written questionnaire concerning their understanding of dental health and oral hygiene procedures. Following compilation and evaluation of the answers, you planned the in-service program for the nurses. These activities parallel which of the following private practice activities?
a. History-taking and diagnosis
b. Diagnosis and treatment planning
c. History-taking, diagnosis, and treatment planning
d. History-taking, diagnosis, and treatment
e. History-taking, treatment planning, implementation, and evaluation

Answer: c. These activities most closely parallel history-taking, diagnosis, and treatment planning.

2. You must prioritize the oral health issues in the nursing home. Which of the following is NOT a criterion for determining whether a particular condition constitutes a public health problem?
   a. A condition that is widespread
   b. A condition that is a cause of morbidity
   c. A condition that is a cause of mortality
   d. The public believes it is a problem
   e. The disease is curable

Answer: e. Whether or not the disease is curable does not determine whether or not the disease is considered a public health problem.

3. Root Caries Index scores for a sample of this population were 2%, 3%, 3%, 4%, 4%, 5%, 5%, 5%, 6%, and 7%. Which of the following indicates the mode for this sample?
   a. 3%
   b. 4%
   c. 5%
   d. 6%
   e. 7%

Answer: c. The mode is the number that occurs most frequently in a population.

4. Which is the MOST effective way to provide oral hygiene instruction to the residents?
   a. Individualized instruction
   b. Lecture and demonstration
   c. Videotaped presentation
   d. Pamphlets
   e. General instructions posted in the bathrooms

Answer: a. Individualized instruction is the most effective educational approach, although not efficient for large groups. Lecture and demonstration is the most efficient way to provide oral hygiene instruction to large groups of people, but it is not as effective as individual instruction. Pamphlets are best as take-home tools after formal instruction.

5. The BEST measure of the effect of the program you develop for this group is:

a. total cost.
b. change in attitude.
c. health improvement.
d. resident happiness with the program.
e. staff happiness with the program.

Answer: c. Health improvement is the BEST measure of the effect of an oral health program. Cost measures, efficiency, attitude changes, and happiness may not result in oral health status change, which was the objective of the program.

Testlet #5

You have been contracted by a state health department to assess the oral health needs of the Medicaid population in the state. To assess the needs of this population, you provided oral screenings to all adult Medicaid applicants at the Medicaid office for 3 months. The children of the applicants were also screened. To aid in the effort, you hired two examiners. Prior to performing the screenings, the two examiners compared their techniques and diagnostic similarities using the chosen indices.

1. The type of sample used is a:
   a. random sample.
   b. stratified sample.
   c. judgment sample.
   d. convenience sample.
   e. quota sample.

Answer: d. A convenience sample is the simplest method, involving selecting a convenient group of participants.

2. The process of comparing techniques and diagnostic similarities among examiners is called:
   a. calibration.
   b. comparison.
   c. specificity.
   d. reliability.
   e. validity.

Answer: a. Calibration

3. The screenings revealed that 432 of 1000 people had moderate periodontitis. This is an example of:

a. incidence.
b. prevalence.
c. a percentage.
d. a range.
e. a mean.

Answer: b. Prevalence is the number of cases in a population at a given time.

4. The two examiners agreed in their diagnostic decisions 83% of the time. This is called:
   a. validation.
   b. interrater reliability.
   c. consistency.
   d. intrarater reliability.
   e. inconsistency.

Answer: b. Interrater reliability is the amount of agreement between two or more examiners.

5. If you found that 32% of the children had dental sealants, where would you look to determine whether that percentage was exceptional, at the national average, or low and needed to be a priority?
   a. Dental public health competency objectives
   b. American Clinical Guidelines Resource Guide
   c. Healthy People 2010 Objectives
   d. World Health Organization Survey Manual
   e. Local health department

Answer: c. The Healthy People 2010 Objectives list the national baseline and the objectives for the nation.

SUMMARY

Accredited dental hygiene programs provide a sound base of knowledge to prepare candidates for the NBDHE. Candidates preparing for the examination can enhance this foundation through a well-designed review process. Preparations should include knowledge of test-taking strategies, application of appropriate study techniques, and personal preparations. With a sound educational foundation, appropriate preparation, and a positive attitude, the dental hygiene candidate will achieve success in the National Board Dental Hygiene Examination.

RESOURCES

ADHA Center for Lifelong Learning (Review Course). Available at: http://www.adha.org.

Candidate's Guide for the NBDHE. Available at: http://www.ada.org/prof/ed/testing/natboardhyg/index.asp.

American Dental Association. National Board Dental Hygiene Examination. Available at: http://ada.org/prof/ed/testing/natboardhyg. Accessed January 2004.

Biron C. The Exam. RDH Student Focus. November: 2003;6–14,42.

Brian JN, Cooper MD. Complete Review of Dental Hygiene. Upper Saddle River, NJ: Prentice Hall, 2002.

Darby M. Mosby's Comprehensive Review of Dental Hygiene. 5th Ed. St. Louis, MO: C.V. Mosby, 2002.

DeBiase CB. Dental Hygiene in Review. Baltimore, MD: Lippincott Williams & Wilkins, 2001.

Felder R, Soloman B. Learning styles and strategies. Available at: http://www.ncsu.edu/felder-public/ILSdir/styles.htm.

Landsberger J. Study guides and strategies. Available at: http://www.iss.stthomas.edu/studyguides/tstprp. Accessed January 2004.

McKelvey ND. Saunders Review of Dental Hygiene. Philadelphia, PA: WB Saunders, 2000.

NBDHE reference texts. Available at: http://www.ada.org/prof/ed/testing/natboardgyg/reference.asp.

Search Terms: learning styles, study skills, ESL resources, ESL, examination skills, assessment and learning styles, and study guides.

REFERENCES

1. American Dental Education Association. Competencies for entry into the profession of dental hygiene, Exhibit 7.

J Dent Educ 2003;67(7):1–5. Available at: http://www.adea .org/cepr. Accessed February 2004.
2. Kolb D. Self-Scoring Inventory and Interpretive Booklet. Boston, MA: McBer, 1985.
3. Myers IB, McCaulley MH. Manual: A Guide to the Development and Use of the Myers-Briggs Type Indicator. Palo Alto, CA: Consulting Psychologists, 1985.

4. Felder R, Soloman B. Learning Styles and Strategies. Available at: http://www.ncsu.edu/felder-public/ILSdir/ styles.htm.
5. McKelvey ND. Saunders Review of Dental Hygiene. Philadelphia, PA: WB Saunders, 2000.

Appendix 1

ANSWERS TO REVIEW QUESTIONS

CHAPTER 1

1. e
2. d. The 1935 Social Security Act provided aid to states through Maternal Child Health (MCH) grants, which included oral health services.
3. c. The trials began in Michigan and New York in 1945.
4. b. The armed forces experience led to the development of the National Institute of Dental Research (NIDR), which addresses national dental problems.
5. e. The core functions of public health are a, b, and c.

CHAPTER 2

1. d. This person is most likely to have some type of dental insurance benefit and should be able to find an oral health care provider. The others have significant barriers (e.g., geographic, age).
2. d. More than 51 million school hours are lost to dental illness each year.
3. e. The fifth action seeks broad-based coalitions, not just collaborations among oral health professionals.
4. e. Although this may represent a collaborative effort, it is a city effort, not a national program.
5. c. Medicaid is already an entitlement program for children.
6. a. The other situations represent the opposite of current trends.
7. c. Several scientific groups are available (e.g., The Cochrane Group) that review studies and translate the research to practitioners.

CHAPTER 3

1. e
2. b
3. e

4. d
5. a
6. e

CHAPTER 4

1. e. The client is the community.
2. b. The American Dental Education Association
3. d

CHAPTER 5

1. b. All elements are required, other than crisis reaction. Careful planning should avoid the need to react to a crisis.
2. d. Although all elements are important, the most important consideration is to obtain community input.
3. c. A planner wants community input from the beginning of the needs assessment. Community involvement and input, however, are important throughout the planning process.
4. c. Determining the cost-effectiveness of a community program is part of program evaluation and the most similar to the evaluation of individual patient care.
5. e. All of these techniques can best use the available resources to plan effective programs.

CHAPTER 6

1. a. Although the need to publish a paper may be in the back of the planner's mind, it is not a reason for conducting a needs assessment. All other reasons given for conducting a needs assessment are valid considerations.
2. d. Repairing equipment is an indirect program activity. This activity is supportive in nature and not directly involved in planning or intervention delivery.
3. a. Goals and objectives are considered the heart of the program plan; they guide the intervention and are the basis for the evaluation.

4. b. False. This describes a program goal. It is more specific than a mission statement because it identifies what should change to work toward broad improvement in the mission of the program. A mission statement only describes the program's reason for existence.
5. a. True. It is important to do an extensive search for existing data to support the need for a program before going to the time and expense of collecting primary data.
6. a
7. c
8. b
9. d

Questions 6–9. The mission statement is a broad statement of directional change. The program goal identifies a desired change that should occur; the program objective guides program activities or interventions; and program intervention identifies a specific activity.

CHAPTER 7

1. c. It is important to raise awareness about the needs among interested parties before planning the program. This group should be involved throughout the planning, implementation, and evaluation process. It is important to have parent and school nurse participation, together with others in this group. It is too early in the process to determine whether children need to be rescreened. The adequacy of the state data will need to be determined.
2. e. All of the ways increase the capacity and effectiveness of programs. Coalitions or partnerships strengthen the effectiveness of programs. Grants supplement available funds. Combining resources with other health programs that have similar goals is a wise use of limited dollars.
3. d. Community water fluoridation would be the most cost-efficient, effective, safe way to reduce decay rates. Interventions that require daily compliance (e.g., tooth brushing education) would predictably only show short-term reductions in plaque levels and would not be as effective as interventions that do not. Treat-ment programs would reduce the unmet need but would not reduce caries rates.
4. b. Goals and objectives determine what a program intervention is designed to accomplish and form the basis for any evaluation.
5. e. All of these parties should be involved in the process.
6. c. It is important to determine the evaluation method during developmental stages.
7. b. A 1-year assessment of sound surfaces compared with decayed surfaces is a summative, or outcome, evaluation. It describes a desired health outcome. The other possible answers are all examples of formative, or process, evaluation.
8. b. It is best to target the areas with the highest need. Because teeth should be sealed shortly after eruption, many programs target children in first, second, fifth, and sixth grades. Sealants are indicated for teeth with deep pits and fissures.

CHAPTER 8

1. d
2. a
3. c
4. e
5. b. Other responses include topical applications.
6. e. Fluoride is beneficial to all age groups.
7. e. Primary prevention occurs before disease occurs. Remineralization is reversing early stages of the disease.
8. b. Oral disease is multifactorial.
9. a
10. c. Other responses are related to meso level or macro level social factors.

CHAPTER 9

1. d. To be considered successful, health education must result in behavioral change.
2. c. Age, gender, race, ethnicity, peer or reference group pressure, and prior knowledge about health problems are all factors that play a role in modifying beliefs and potential compliance with recommendations for health behaviors.

3. b. The major stages of the Stages of Change model are:
   - Precontemplation: unaware of the health problem, without any thought of need for change
   - Contemplation: aware of problem and thinking about the possibility of making a change
   - Decision/Determination: making a plan for change
   - Action: putting plan for change into action
   - Maintenance: continuing desired health action.
4. a. The factors that enhance acceptance and adoption of a new idea, behavior, product, or service innovation include relative advantage (superior to a past idea), compatibility (consistent with the adopters' experiences and values), complexity (ease of use), trialability (can be experimented with or tried on a limited basis), and observability (successful tangible results can be seen).
5. c. The Consumer Information Processing theory makes two key assumptions: (1) people are limited in how much information they can acquire, use, and remember; and (2) people combine bits of information into useable summaries and create decision rules to enable faster and easier choices. The application for health education (before people will use health information) is that it must be available, considered useful and new, and be user-friendly.
6. e. All of the phrases apply to focus groups.
7. d. Physiologic needs are basic survival requirements; ego/esteem needs are feelings of self-worth; social needs are needs for affectionate relationships and a place in one's culture, group, or family; self-fulfillment implies the ability to control one's needs rather than to be controlled by them and to achieve one's potential.
8. b. The learning ladder steps in sequence (from lowest to highest) are unawareness, awareness, self-interest, involvement, action, and habit.
9. b. Observational learning, or modeling, is a powerful learning tool that allows people to learn through observing others and seeing the results others derive from their actions.

10. a. Both statements refer to widely accepted learning principles.

CHAPTER 10

1. Lesson plans ensure that all information and material required to meet specific learning goals are presented in the most effective order and effectively supported by carefully chosen instructional materials. Additionally, instruction is stabilized if different individuals, using the same lesson plan, can present the same topic and accomplish the same learning goals.
2. b. An educational goal is a broad, general statement that describes the overall purpose of a block of instruction.
3. c. An instructional objective is a specific statement that clearly describes a behavior that can be observed and assessed to determine whether a learning experience has been successfully completed. *Demonstrate* is an action verb describing a behavior that can be assessed. *Know, appreciate,* and *understand* are vague terms; they do not specify when the knowing, appreciating, or understanding has been achieved.
4. a. *Instructional set* establishes the mood for the learning experience and makes learners aware of what they are to learn and why it has value for them. *Body* is the lesson information itself. *Closure* summarizes the presentation and reviews major points.
5. When incorporated into a carefully designed lesson, student-made posters can be educational for both those who make them and those who view them and can be used as learning activities to reinforce and review learning points. Using these projects as competing artwork in "poster contests" is not advised. There are legitimate concerns regarding placing students in competitive situations in which a prize is awarded. There are no assurances that the prizewinner develops a commitment to change and practices oral health behaviors.
6. These materials can be used for new information that may not yet be available in textbooks,

opportunities for extra or specialized reading for students who want and can manage more detailed information material for classroom teaching displays, bulletin boards, scrapbook collection topics, panel discussions of controversial issues, as well as materials for career guidance.

7. a and b. In Middle Eastern cultures, the importance of what is being said is conveyed by the loudness with which it is spoken. The louder one speaks, the more important he perceives his message to be. Anger, in contrast, is usually expressed by an intense, high-pitched voice. Importance is also conveyed through multiple repetition, as is characteristic in Muslim prayers.

8. d. Instructional planning is a purposeful, learner-centered activity, focusing on the target audience and their unique learning needs. Learning objectives, content, methods, materials, and activities are all chosen to accommodate need and ability.

9. Each strip is removed at the appropriate time, when the point is being discussed. The sequenced parts remain in view, showing how each part builds in relationship to the next.

10. b. Conversational distance space for Westerners is about 5 feet. For people from the Middle East, the appropriate distance is about 2 feet from the person with whom they are speaking. This closeness may make Westerners feel uncomfortable or "threatened" as others move in toward them during conversation.

CHAPTER 11

1. e
2. c
3. b
4. c
5. a
6. False. Incidence requires that you know the number of new cases during a specific *period*. Dental caries rates in the United States are based on the percentage of people who have disease at a certain *point in time*, therefore, they are prevalence rates.
7. d
8. b
9. d

CHAPTER 12

1. b. False. Both total caries experience and the amount of untreated decay has decreased.
2. c
3. a. True. For children aged 2–5 years, 27% of low-income children and 90% of higher income children have untreated decay. For children aged 15–18 years, 32% of low-income children and 17% of higher income children have untreated decay.
4. b
5. b. False. There has not been a substantial decline of caries experience in children aged 2–5 years and adults aged ≥46 years.
6. c
7. c
8. b. False. The prevalence of pocketing is relatively stable for those persons aged ≥25 years.
9. a, c, and d

CHAPTER 13

1. d
2. c
3. a. True
4. b. False. It means that 25% of their teeth with gingival recession have decay or fillings on the roots.
5. d
6. c
7. b. False. The Simplified Oral Hygiene Index (OHI-S) is becoming obsolete as periodontal research focuses more on subgingival, rather than supragingival, plaque and calculus as risk factors for periodontitis.
8. c
9. c
10. d

CHAPTER 14

1. Gender (a); because gender has two levels (male and female), it should be classified as a binary nominal categorical variable. Temperature (d); temperature is a continuous variable. Race (b); race can be categorized into many categories. However, because it has no natural order, it is a nominal categorical variable with >2 categories.

2. a. The median is the midpoint of the distribution of numbers. To facilitate finding this point, first put the observations in order: 0, 2, 3, 4, 5, 8, 10, 10, and 12. The median is the $[(n + 1)/2]^{th} = [(9 + 1)/2]^{th} = 5^{th}$ value, which, in this case, is 5.

3. c. Follow the steps in Box 14-6 to calculate the standard deviation:

   A. Compute the mean of the observations:

   The mean should be calculated using the formula

   $$\bar{x} = \frac{x_1 1 \, x_2 1 \, P \, x_n}{n}$$. In this case, the mean = [(12

   $+ 0 + 5 + 4 + 10 + 10 + 8 + 2 + 3)/9)] = 6.0$.

   B. Determine the squared difference between each observation x and the mean $\bar{x}$:

Observation x	Deviation x 2 $\bar{x}$	Squared Deviation (x 2 $\bar{x}$)²
0	0 − 6.0 = −6.0	(−6.0)² = 36.0
2	2 − 6.0 = −4.0	(−4.0)² = 16.0
3	3 − 6.0 = −3.0	(−3.0)² = 9.0
4	4 − 6.0 = −2.0	(−2.0)² = 4.0
5	5 − 6.0 = −1.0	(−1.0)² = 1.0
8	8 − 6.0 = 2.0	(2.0)² = 4.0
10	10 − 6.0 = 4.0	(4.0)² = 16.0
10	10 − 6.0 = 4.0	(4.0)² = 16.0
12	12 − 6.0 = 6.0	(6.0)² = 36.0
Total:	**0**	**138.0**

   C. Calculate the variance by determining the mean squared deviation:

   $$\text{Variance 5} \frac{\text{sum of squared deviations}}{\text{number of observations}} 5 \frac{138.0}{9} 5 \, 15.3$$

   D. Determine the standard deviation by taking the square root of the variance:

standard deviation = $1\overline{\text{ variance }}$ = $1\overline{15.3}$
= 3.91

4. a. Consult Table 14-3 to answer this question. There are three steps:

   A. Determine the probability that $Z \leq -1.0$:

   Although $Z \leq -1.0$ is not directly listed on the table, we can calculate it because we know that the probability that $Z \leq -1.0 = (1 - \text{Probability that } Z < 1.0)$. We can look up the probability that $Z < 1.0$ in the table; it is 0.8413. Hence, the probability $Z \leq -1.0 = 1 - 0.8413 = 0.1587$.

   B. Determine the probability that $Z \leq -2.0$:

   Following the same procedure as in Step A to determine that the probability that $Z \leq 2.0$ is 0.0227.

   C. Subtract (a) − (b) to determine probability that Z will lie between −2 and −1:

   Probability that Z will lie between −2 and −1 is $0.1587 - 0.0227 = 0.1360 = 13.6\%$.

5. d. We can answer this question in three steps, outlined in Box 14-7.

   A. Calculate the risk in the exposed:

   The risk in the exposed is $\frac{50}{100}$ 5 0.50.

   B. Calculate the risk in the unexposed:

   The risk in the unexposed is $\frac{50}{150}$ 5 0.33.

   C. Divide (a)/(b):

   The risk ratio is $\frac{0.50}{0.33}$ 5 1.52. Simply, this study found that smokers are 1.52 times as likely as nonsmokers to have gingivitis or periodontitis.

6. a. As dmft increases, DMFT also increases. Thus, the linear relationship between the two variables can be described as positive.

7. d. To test this null hypothesis, we would use ANOVA/F-test (see Boxes 14-9 and 14-12).

8. b. *Exposure* is the presence of periodontal disease, and *outcome* is the development of coronary heart disease; thus, a risk ratio of 1.5 is interpreted to mean that those with periodontal disease are 1.5 times more likely to develop coronary heart disease than those who did not have periodontal disease. As the name implies, the risk ratio is a ratio, not a difference; on this basis, you should have rejected answers *a* and *d*.

9. c. Because the authors rejected the null, we are concerned that an alpha error (α error) may have been committed. Alpha errors occur if you reject the null when the null is true. We are not concerned about beta errors (β errors) because beta errors are only a concern when you fail to reject the null. Sampling error may or may not be a concern in this study; however, a sampling error is not a type of statistical error.

10. b. No. Given a sufficiently large number of subjects, even small, clinically insignificant relationships may be statistically significant. As a clinician, it is your responsibility to judge whether a result is of clinical importance.

CHAPTER 15

1. d
2. e. Presenting findings at a professional meeting is a link in the diffusion of information, but not one of four components of evidenced-based dentistry (EBD).
3. a. Early adopters are the first to learn of innovations and to adopt them. As a result, they become opinion leaders for other later adopters and the public.
4. c. Presentations are usually made at professional meetings soon after a study is completed and, possibly, not yet published.
5. d. Clinical trials with control groups

CHAPTER 16

1. a
2. d
3. b
4. d
5. c
6. c
7. b
8. d
9. e
10. c

CHAPTER 17

1. c
2. c
3. c
4. e
5. e
6. d
7. b
8. e

Appendix 2

FEDERAL GOVERNMENT AGENCIES/ ACRONYMS (FIGURE 1-2)

Department of Health and Human Services (DHHS)
Program Support Center (PSC)
Administration on Aging (AoA)
United States Public Health Service (USPHS)
Centers for Medicare & Medicaid Services (CMS)
Office of Public Health and Science (OPHS)
Administration for Children and Families (ACF)

United States Public Health Service (USPHS)
Indian Health Service (IHS) (Ten area offices listed in Figure 1-2)
National Institutes of Health (NIH)
National Cancer Institute (NCI)
National Eye Institute (NEI)
National Heart, Lung, and Blood Institute (NHLBI)
National Human Genome Research Institute (NHGRI)
National Institute on Aging (NIA)
National Institute on Alcohol Abuse and Alcoholism (NIAAA)
National Institute of Allergy and Infectious Diseases (NIAID)
National Institute of Arthritis and Musculoskeletal and Skin Diseases (NIAMS)
National Institute of Biomedical Imaging and Bioengineering (NIBIB)
National Institute of Child Health and Human Development (NICHD)
National Institute on Deafness and Other Communication Disorders (NIDCD)
National Institute of Dental and Craniofacial Research (NIDCR)
National Institute of Diabetes and Digestive and Kidney Diseases (NIDDK)
National Institute on Drug Abuse (NIDA)

National Institute of Environmental Health Sciences (NIEHS)
National Institute of General Medical Sciences (NIGMS)
National Institute of Mental Health (NIMH)
National Institute of Neurological Disorders and Stroke (NINDS)
National Institute of Nursing Research (NINR)
National Library of Medicine (NLM)
Center for Information Technology (CIT)
Center for Scientific Review (CSR)
John E. Fogarty International Center (FIC)
National Center for Complementary and Alternative Medicine (NCCAM)
National Center on Minority Health and Health Disparities (NCMHD)
National Center for Research Resources (NCRR)
Warren Grant Magnuson Clinical Center (CC)

Centers for Disease Control and Prevention (CDC)
National Center on Birth Defects and Developmental Disabilities (NCBDDD)
National Center for Chronic Disease Prevention and Health Promotion (NCCDPHP)
National Center for Environmental Health (NCEH)
National Center for Health Statistics (NCHS)
National Center for HIV, STD, and TB Prevention (NCHSTP)
National Center for Infectious Diseases (NCID)
National Center for Injury Prevention and Control (NCIPC)
National Immunization Program (NIP)
National Institute for Occupational Safety and Health (NIOSH)
Epidemiology Program Office (EPO)

Public Health Practice Program Office (PHPPO)

Office of the Director (CDC/OD)

Health Resources and Services Administration (HRSA)

Bureau of Primary Health Care (BPHC)

Bureau of Health Professions (BHPr)

Maternal and Child Health Bureau (MCHB)

HIV/AIDS Bureau (HAB)

Office of Equal Opportunity & Civil Rights (OEOCR)

Office of Management and Program Support (OMPS)

Office of Legislation (OL)

Office of Planning and Evaluation (OPE)

Office of Information Technology (OIT)

Office of Performance Review (OPR)

Office of Minority Health (OMH)

Office of Rural Health Policy (ORHP)

Office of Special Programs (OSP)

Office of Financial Policy and Oversight (OFPO)

Office of International Health Affairs (OIHA)

Office of Communications (OC)

Food and Drug Administration (FDA)

Center for Biologics Evaluation and Research (CBER)

Center for Devices and Radiological Health (CDRH)

Center for Drug Evaluation and Research (CDER)

Center for Food Safety and Applied Nutrition (CFSAN)

Center for Veterinary Medicine (CVM)

National Center for Toxicological Research (NCTR)

Office of the Commissioner (OC)

Office of Regulatory Affairs (ORA)

Agency for Healthcare Research and Quality (AHRQ)

Center for Delivery, Organization, and Markets (CDOM)

Center for Financing, Access, and Cost Trends (CFACT)

Center for Outcomes and Evidence (COE)

Center for Primary Care, Prevention, and Clinical Partnerships (CP3)

Center for Quality Improvement and Patient Safety (CQuIPS)

Immediate Office of the Director (IOD)

Office of Communication and Knowledge Transfer (OCKT)

Office of Extramural Research, Education, and Priority Populations (OEREP)

Office of Performance Assessment, Resources and Technology (OPART)

Substance Abuse and Mental Health Services Administration (SAMHSA)

Center for Substance Abuse Treatment (CSAT)

Center for Substance Abuse Prevention (CSAP)

Center for Mental Health Services (CMHS)

Office of Policy, Planning and Budget (OPPB)

Office of the Administrator (OA)

Office of Program Services (OPS)

Office of Applied Studies (OAS)

Agency for Toxic Substances and Disease Registry (ATSDR)

Division of Health Assessment and Consultation (DHAC)

Division of Health Education and Promotion (DHEP)

Division of Health Studies (DHS)

Division of Toxicology (DT)

Division of Regional Operations (DRO)

Office of the Director (OD)

Office of Financial and Administrative Services (OFAS)

Office of Policy, Planning, and Evaluation (OPPE)

Office of Communication (OC)

Glossary

abandonment—withdrawing a patient's medical or dental care without providing sufficient notice to the patient

Aboriginal Health Worker—health care provider trained to provide basic health care services to remote aboriginal populations in Australia

abstract—a brief synopsis of a scientific report, study, or program, which allows the reader to determine if the information is relevant to their interests

access to care—an individual's ability to access needed health care services (e.g., if the nearest health care is more than 100 miles away, an individual has limited access to care)

activities—the component steps required to perform an intervention

administrative law—a branch of law that includes regulations developed by government agencies

Agency for Healthcare Research and Quality (AHRQ)—the health services research arm of the U.S. Department of Health and Human Services (DHHS), providing funding and technical assistance for health services research

Agency for Toxic Substances and Disease Registry (ATSDR)—a DHHS agency, providing health information to prevent harmful exposures and diseases related to toxic exposure

agent—a factor (e.g., a microorganism) by which the presence or absence (in deficiency diseases) is essential for disease occurrence

alternative hypothesis (H_a)—a statement that there is a relationship between an exposure and an outcome

American Association of Public Health Dentistry (AAPHD)—a professional organization of dental public health professionals and individuals concerned with improving the public's oral health

American Board of Dental Public Health (AB-DPH)—the national examining and certifying agency for the American Dental Association specialty of dental public health

American Dental Education Association (ADEA)—a professional organization representing dental educators and administrators

American Dental Hygienists' Association (ADHA)—the national professional organization representing dental hygienists in the United States

American Dental Hygienists' Association Types of Careers—a listing of different professional roles for dental hygienists

American Public Health Association (APHA)—the largest organization of public health professionals worldwide, representing members from more than 50 occupations

Analysis of Variance (ANOVA)—a statistical test that compares means across three or more categories; used when one variable is normally distributed (continuous) and one is multiple categorical

analytic study—examines associations or hypothesized causal relationships; generally concerned with identifying or measuring the effects of certain risk factors

anticipatory guidance—counseling a family about a child's current oral health status and what can be expected at upcoming developmental stages

APEX-PH (Assessment Protocol for Excellence in Public Health)—a planning tool within Healthy Communities 2000: Model Standards

assault—a willful attempt or threat to inflict injury; an intentional display of force to cause fear; can be committed without touching or striking

assignment—a classification of delegation or management by a dentist for a dental hygienist or dental assistant used in some jurisdictions; dentist need not be present

associated/association—a statistical dependence between two or more events or characteristics; an association may be positive or negative

Association of State and Territorial Dental Directors (ASTDD)—a national nonprofit organization representing the directors and staff of state public health agency programs for oral health

ASTDD Seven-Step model—a needs assessment tool; can be accessed through the Association of State and Territorial Dental Directors Web site

Atraumatic Restorative Technique (ART)—a non-traumatic procedure, which usually involves removal of necrotic tooth surface with a spoon instrument or slow-speed hand piece and placement of a temporary glass ionomer or composite restorative material

attitudes: intermediate variables that influence health

Autonomy: a principle of self-determination; respect

bar chart—a graphical representation of the frequency distribution of a categorical variable

barriers—the factors that hinder an individual from optimal health (e.g., social, psychological, physical)

Basic Screening Survey—a model for oral health surveillance developed by the Association of State and Territorial Dental Directors

battery—offensive touching of a person without the person's consent, which results in bodily harm

Behavioral Risk Factor Surveillance System—a state-based, ongoing data collection program designed to measure behavioral risk factors in adults in the United States

behaviors—intermediate variables that influence health

beneficence—principle of promoting what is good, kind, and charitable

beyond a reasonable doubt—highest level of proof required; necessary for a guilty verdict in a jury case

bias—the error in the estimation of a quantity not attributed to chance

bioethics—moral dilemmas and issues that result from advances in medicine and medical research

body—the component of a lesson plan that presents all major learning points; constitutes most lesson information

Canadian Association of Public Health Dentistry (CAPHD)—a Canadian national professional organization representing dental public health and related professionals

capitation—when managed care plans or clinics are paid a fixed amount per enrollee per month, regardless of whether that individual actually uses the services offered

career opportunities—the different pathways available for oral health professionals to take in the course of employment

case-control study—a study design in which persons with the disease of interest (cases) are compared with those without the disease (controls) in terms of exposure to some attribute or risk factor

case law—called common law; based on decisions made by judges

causative factors—factors associated with the development of disease

Centers for Disease Control and Prevention (CDC)—the leading federal agency involved with protecting the health and safety of the American people

chi-square test (χ^2)—a statistical test that compares proportions when both exposure and outcome are categorical variables

civil law—law concerned with civil or private matters, not criminal matters; includes torts and contract agreements

cleft lip—congenital defect of the lip; a fissure extending from the margin of the lip to the nostril; may be single or double

cleft palate—congenital failure of fusion between the right and left palatal processes

closure—the component of a lesson plan that summarizes the presented material; reviews the main points and gives a sense of unity to the entire lesson

cluster sampling—a nonprobability sampling in which the sample is divided into clusters, defined by geography or time, and a simple random sample is drawn from each cluster

coalitions—cooperative effort between partners to maximize efforts toward a common goal

code of ethics—a set of rules or guidelines that provides a framework for the behavior of a professional group

cohort—any designated group of persons followed or traced for a period

collaborative practice—model of oral health care delivery in which the dental hygienist provides educational, assessment, preventive, clinical, and therapeutic services without general supervision

Commissioned Corps—U.S. Public Health Service Commissioned Corp (USPHS); a uniformed service of the U.S. Government that does not bear arms; a career system for health professionals

common good—a focus on collaboration to benefit the larger good or that of the community

common risk factor approach—the integration of health improvement efforts that share disease risks

community—a group of people who live in a common geographic area or who have similar interests or needs

community coalitions—an alliance of community organizations or individuals gathered for a specific purpose (e.g., improve oral health of children)

community focus—a health education approach that addresses the impact of economy, politics, or other factors within the community; focuses on using community strengths to solve problems not effectively addressed by individuals or small groups

community needs assessment—an initial program planning step that determines to what extent certain needs exist and their salience compared with other problems and needs

Community Organization Theory—a behavioral theory that emphasizes development and active community participation to evaluate and solve health and social problems

Community Periodontal Index—measures periodontal health; developed and supported by the World Health Organization

community profile—a demographic description of a community, including total population, number of households, size, age distribution, household income, marital status, racial/ethnic composition, education geographic boundaries, political and economic atmosphere, and dental and medical resources

community water fluoridation—the process that optimizes fluoride levels in a community's water supply

compliance—acting in accordance with recommendations

confidence intervals—estimates a range of values likely to contain the true population parameter of interest

confidentiality—entrusted or held secret

confounding—a specific type of bias; occurs when a variable is related to the outcome of interest and is more likely to be present in one of the exposure groups

confounding variables—factors that can cause or prevent the outcome (disease) of interest

consideration—in contract law; something of value provided as part of an agreement

Consumer Information Processing Model—a marketing theory based on how consumers take in and use information when making decisions; it presumes that people can only acquire, use, and remember a limited amount of information and that, therefore, they summarize bits of information to enable faster and easier choices

contract law—the area of law that includes an enforceable agreement or obligation between two or more persons

convenience sample—a nonprobability sampling in which subject selection is based on researcher convenience, rather than any subject characteristic

core functions of public health—a set of core functions for public health agencies developed by the Institute of Medicine; centered on assessment, policy development, and assurance

correlation coefficient—a description of strength and direction of the linear relationship between two continuous or ordinal categorical variables

cost-benefit ratio—the difference between the expense of having a program versus the expense of not having the program

cost-effectiveness—the extent to which a program or intervention demonstrates enough benefit to justify the cost

Council on Linkages Between Academia and Public Health Practice—an organization comprised of leaders from various national organizations representing public health practice and academic communities

count—the number of occurrences of a disease

critical review—an assessment of the quality level of a scientific report

cross-sectional study—examines the relationship between disease and risk factors in a defined population at one particular time

cultural competence—possessing values and principles that allow one to interact effectively with individuals from different cultures

cultural knowledge—familiarity with the selected cultural characteristics of another ethnic group, including history, values, belief systems, and behaviors

cultural relevance—incorporating a specific group's health beliefs, dietary considerations, and communication styles in a health message to make it more meaningful

cultural sensitivity—an awareness and respect of cultural differences and similarities

damages—a monetary compensation awarded to a person who suffered loss or injury to their person, property, or rights; sum of money awarded to a person injured by tort

Dean's Fluorosis Index—measures the prevalence and severity of dental fluorosis

deceit—a deceptive misrepresentation to trick another; an untrue statement made with knowledge that it is false

defamation of character—published statement that injures a person's reputation

defendant—in civil cases, the person or organization that is sued; in criminal cases, the person being sued

degrees of freedom—the number of quantities free to vary

dental caries—demineralization of tooth enamel as a result of acid production by cariogenic bacteria

dental fluorosis—hypomineralization of the enamel as a result of excessive fluoride intake during tooth development

dental health professional shortage areas—geographic areas, special population groups, or facilities designated by the federal government as having a shortage of oral health personnel

dental home—a continuous, accessible source of comprehensive dental care

dental nurses/therapists—oral health care providers educated and trained to provide basic dental procedures

dental practice act—a single law, or compilation of laws, that regulates the practice of dentistry, dental hygiene, and dental assisting or other auxiliary individuals providing dental services

dental public health—one of nine dentistry specialties pertaining to the science and art of preventing and controlling dental diseases and promoting dental health through organized community efforts

Deontological Ethics—ethical theory that focuses on the morality, rather than the consequences of action

Department of Defense—the U.S. Government cabinet level department responsible for military security, flood control, oceanographic resources, and oil reserves management

Department of Education—the U.S. Government cabinet level department responsible for promoting educational excellence nationwide

Department of Health and Human Services (DHHS)—the U.S. Government cabinet level department primarily responsible for protecting the health of all Americans

Department of Justice—the U.S. Government cabinet level department responsible for law enforcement, public safety, immigration, and crime control

Department of Veterans Affairs—the U.S. Government cabinet level department responsible for patient care and benefit administration for U.S. veterans

dependent variables—the outcome(s) of interest in a study

descriptive statistics—numeric characteristics of a sample of a population of interest

descriptive study—describes the existing distribution of disease and other variables, without regard to causal or other hypotheses

df Index—measures dental caries in the primary dentition that include decayed and filled primary teeth or tooth surfaces

Diffusion of Innovations Theory—a behavioral theory that describes how new ideas, social practices, or products spread through a society or from one society to another

direct activities—the steps directly involved in the delivery of an intervention

direct supervision—a classification of delegation or management by a dentist for a dental hygienist or dental assistant; involves examination and diagnosis by a licensed dentist; dentist may be required to examine the patient before and after a procedure is completed

discussion—the section of a scientific report that presents study or program conclusions and discusses the relevance of the information presented

DMF Index—measures dental caries in the permanent dentition that include decayed, missing, and filled permanent teeth or tooth surfaces

duty—obligation or responsibility

educational goal—a nonspecific statement that serves as a foundation upon which to develop all subsequent plans

efficacious—produces a desired effect

efficiency—producing a desired result with minimum effort, expense, or waste

employment discrimination laws—state or federal laws that protect persons from being treated differently than others, based on uncontrollable factors, such as age, race, sex, national origin, or religion

enabling factors—health problem or behavioral factors that enable, or make it possible for, actions to occur; includes personal skills and available resources needed to perform a behavior

endemic—the constant presence of disease within a given population or geographic area

environmental factors—factors external to the individual human host that can influence disease

epidemic—the occurrence of disease in a given population or geographic area that clearly exceeds normal expectancy

epidemiology—the study of the distribution and determinants of disease and injuries in human populations

ethical dilemma—a situation that includes two or more important, opposing, ethical principles

ethical decision framework—a process to resolve an ethical dilemma, which considers ethical principles, codes of conducts, relevant facts, and results in an appropriate, ethically-based alternative

ethics—a branch of philosophy relating to morals or moral principles; rules or standards governing standards

evidence-based care—provides the most current, appropriate care for a patient population, based on the latest scientific evidence

evidence-based dentistry—oral health care that requires judicious integration of systematic assessments of clinically relevant scientific evidence relating to the patient's oral and medical condition and history with the provider's clinical expertise and the patient's treatment needs and preferences

evidence-based practice—integrating new evidence for effectiveness with expert opinion, clinical and community experience, and professional judgment

experimental study—a study in which the investigator directly controls the conditions

expressed contract—when both parties agree (written or oral) to the terms of an agreement

extrinsic motivation—the desire to change a behavior, based on external factors

false imprisonment—intentional, illegal detention or unjustified restraint of one's liberty or freedom of motion

Federal Poverty Level—an annual measurement of poverty in the United States issued by the DHHS; in 2003, the poverty guideline for a family of 4, in the 48 contiguous states, was $18,400

fidelity—principle of loyalty or faithfulness; keeping promises

financial barriers—limited access for patients because of their inability to pay for a service or because providers choose not to provide care for those with limited finances

flow charts—a diagram illustrating the flow of information through a system or program

fluoride varnish—a preventive procedure in which a highly concentrated varnish is painted directly on the teeth

focus group—a marketing technique to better understand consumer behavior; a guided discussion of a small group of people, used to collect information, including community needs, attitudes, and norms

Food and Drug Administration (FDA)—the DHHS agency responsible for protecting the public health, assuring the safety, efficacy, and security of human and veterinary drugs, biologic products, medical supplies, cosmetics, products that emit radiation, and the nation's food supply

formative evaluation—the measurement of program activities during implementation to determine problems and identify improvement opportunities

fraud—deception or misrepresentation, with intent to harm another or deprive them of their rights

frequency table—lists the number of observations in different value ranges

gatekeeper—the primary care provider (e.g., general dentist) who controls referrals to specialists

general supervision—a classification of delegation or management by a dentist for a dental hygienist or dental assistant that may require the dentist's examination and diagnosis for a procedure to be completed

Gingival Index—measures the prevalence and severity of gingival bleeding

gingivitis—reversible inflammation of gingival tissue

health—a state of complete physical, mental, and social well-being; not merely the absence of disease or infirmity

Health Belief Model—a theory that suggests that behaviors are directed by perceptions and beliefs of susceptibility, severity, beneficial behaviors, and the absence of barriers to action; suggests that whether a person engages in preventive health actions depends on these beliefs

health communication—the study and use of communication strategies to inform and influence individual and community decisions that enhance health

health disparities—the lack of available health care services generally affecting remote populations or people of low socioeconomic position

health education—educational interventions designed to help individuals or groups learn new health information and health behaviors; a process of communicating evidence-based methods of disease prevention and encouraging responsibility for self-care

health habits—repeated behaviors that influence health; either positive or negative (i.e., a regular exercise routine can be a positive health habit; however, smoking is considered a negative health habit)

health promotion—the science and art of helping change the lifestyle of individuals and society to attain optimal health, which places an emphasis on improving quantity and quality of life for all and enables people to improve their health, including the use of any preventive, educational, or administrative policy, program, or law

Health Resources and Services Administration (HRSA)—a DHHS agency, with the mission to improve and expand access to quality health care for all

Healthy Communities 2000: Model Standards—a guidebook and tool for planning public health efforts; used by local public health agencies to work toward Healthy People 2000 objectives

Healthy People 2010—a national health promotion and disease prevention initiative for the United States that includes identification of the most significant, preventable threats to health and elimination of health disparities among different population segments

Healthy People 2010 ToolKit—a planning guide, including technical tools and resources, to help states, territories, and tribes develop and promote successful, state-specific Healthy People 2010 plans

histogram—a graphical representation of a continuous variable frequency distribution

host factors—factors within the individual human host that can influence disease

hypothesis testing—a systematic, quantitative way to judge the evidence for a hypothesis

impact—the effect of a program on the community's health

implied contract—agreement inferred by the signs, inaction, or silence of a patient

implied duties—a responsibility of a provider to a patient, or patient to a provider, that is not specifically stated or written, but inferred by actions or status

incidence—the number of new disease cases within a specified period

independent variables—the exposure(s) of interest in a study

index—a graduated, numeric scale with upper and lower limits; scores on the scale correspond to specific criteria

Indian Health Service (IHS)—a DHHS agency that provides comprehensive, personal and public health services for American Indian and Alaska Native peoples

indirect activities—supportive activities required to carry out an intervention, such as equipment maintenance

indirect supervision—a classification of delegation or management by a dentist for a dental hygienist or dental assistant that may require examination and diagnosis by a dentist for a procedure to be completed; dentist must be on the premises

inferential statistics—analyses to determine whether results in a sample should be generalized to the entire population of interest

informed consent—an act (obtained orally and/or in writing) providing appropriate information to and obtaining the understanding of a patient regarding proposed treatments, risks, options, potential outcomes, and reasons for the recommended treatment, with an opportunity to answer the patient's questions

informed refusal—an act of providing appropriate information to and obtaining a decision to decline proposed treatment by a patient; if treatment is declined, information should include oral and general health risks and outcomes

initiative—a process in which an action is placed on the ballot by the request of a group of citizens

in-kind support—nonmonetary effort provided by an agency, or other entity, to illustrate a match for a portion of requested funds

Institute of Medicine—a nonprofit organization created to provide science-based advice on biomedical science, medicine, and health

instructional objectives—the lesson plan component that establishes the climate for an educational presentation, makes the learner aware of what they are to learn, and encourages the learning process

instructional planning—an organized approach to develop learner-appropriate educational plans that include analysis of the target audience; formulation of learning objectives; identification of relevant subject content; and selection of teaching methods, supporting materials, and learning experiences

instructional set—the component of a lesson plan that establishes the climate for an educational presentation and is intended to make learners aware of what it is they are to learn and to cause them to want to learn it

integration of oral and general health—the understanding that the mouth is an integral part of the whole body and that oral health is an important aspect of overall health

intentional tort—a civil wrong that occurs when an individual intended the results of an action or actions

interdisciplinary—when two or more professions are playing equal, often substitutionary or complementary, roles

interpersonal focus—a health education approach that focuses on a group, or groups, as the target of change; typically, uses small-group strategies to effect change

interval variables—a specific type of continuous variable

a. public health programs or efforts designed to improve or maintain health, alleviate needs, or decrease disease risks b. the activity or experience to which individuals in a target population will participate or be exposed to

intrapersonal focus—an health education approach that focuses on the individual as the target of change; typically uses behavior modification techniques to effect changes in knowledge, attitudes, or beliefs

intrinsic motivation—incentive to change behavior, based on internal factors

job description—a list of activities, roles, and duty divisions required in a staff position

juried—indicates that certain information or publications have been reviewed for scientific merit by experts in the field of study

justice—fairness; treatment without discrimination

knowledge—intermediate variables that influence health

law—a body of rules of action or conduct, prescribed by a governmental authority, that have a binding legal force

layout—the basic compositional form of an educational display; incorporates balance, emphasis, harmony, and contrast

leadership development—opportunity for developing a vision for the future, including the administration and advocacy skills that will translate that vision into action

Learning Ladder—a learning theory concept suggesting that people learn in a linear series of sequential steps, moving away from ignorance toward acquisition of information and adoption of a new behavior; decision-making continuum

learning styles—a characteristic processing of information and way of feeling and behaving in learning situations

lesson plan—a well-organized, written guide for presenting a specific block of instruction

leveraging resources—expanding program potential by combining resources with other programs, working in coalitions or with partners to accomplish mutual goals

libel—false or injurious written statements or materials, including photographs or videos, that are maliciously published

linear regression—a method to assess the relationship between a single, continuous outcome variable and one or more exposure variables, which may be continuous or categorical

literacy—the ability to read, write, and speak a language and to compute and solve problems at the levels of proficiency necessary to function on the job and in society

literature review—a comprehensive analysis and synopsis of the literature available on a particular topic

literature search—a search of medical, dental, or other scientific literature databases to gather information about a particular topic

loan forgiveness program—the payment of a dental professional's student loans after graduation by a facility, federal/state program, or other entity in exchange for the dental professional serving a specified period in an underserved area

logic model—a planning model that graphically illustrates the relationship between a program's ultimate aim and the strategies and activities used, with an outline of how progress is measured

logistic regression—a method that assesses the relationship between a single, binary outcome variable and one or more exposure variables, which may be continuous or categorical

macro level—social factors that influence society and cultural and political agencies

management information system—the organization of program data for program management and decision making

mapping—a tool that identifies trends, patterns, and opportunities in a population; uses geographical information systems to provide analysis and display of health-related data sets on maps

Maslow's Hierarchy of Needs—a human motivation theory that suggests inner forces (needs) drive a person into action and that some needs take precedence over others; suggests a hierarchical arrangement of needs as motivating factors

Maternal and Child Health—the HRSA bureau responsible for services and programs to assure the health of American mothers and children

mean—one measure of central tendency of a continuous variable; the sum of the values of the observations divided by the number of observations

media advocacy—strategic use of various media outlets and formats (e.g., TV and newspapers) to increase issue awareness and knowledge

median—one measure of central tendency of a continuous variable; the middle observation in a set of observations arranged in increasing order; 50th percentile

MEDLINE—see PubMed

meso level—social factors involving institutions, organizations, and social networks

methodology—the section of a scientific report that describes how the program, study, or evaluation was performed

micro level—social factors that influence an individual

midlevel provider—health care provider providing routine direct care; may or may not be required to work under the supervision of a physician or dentist (e.g., nurse practitioner, physician assistant, or dental nurse)

milk fluoridation—the addition of fluoride to milk to prevent dental caries

mission statement—a single statement that expresses a broad, overarching purpose for a program's existence

mobile and portable services—providing dental services from self-propelled mobile vans, mobile trailers that are parked at sites, or portable dental equipment that fits into an automobile or truck and can be set up in a home or other setting

Mobilizing for Action Through Planning and Partnership (MAPP)—a community-wide, strategic planning tool for improving community health

mode—one measure of central tendency of a continuous variable; the most frequent value in a set of observations

moral values—standards of conduct and thought influenced by family, religion, culture, and society

morbidity—sickness, illness

mortality—death

multifactorial—caused by more than one factor (e.g., dental caries is multifactorial because more than a single factor must be present to cause a lesion)

multiple causation—the concept that a given disease may have more than one cause

National Center for Health Statistics—the principal health statistics agency in the United States responsible for compiling statistical information to guide actions and policies to improve the health of U.S. citizens

National Health and Nutrition Examination Survey (NHANES)—an ongoing, national health survey conducted by the National Center for Health Statistics; part of the Centers for Disease Control and Prevention

National Institute of Dental and Craniofacial Research—the primary oral health research institute at the National Institutes of Health

National Institutes of Health (NIH)—a DHHS agency; the steward of medical and behavioral research for the U.S. Government

National Spit Tobacco Education Program (NSTEP)—an Oral Health America program aimed at preventing people, especially young people, from starting spit tobacco use and at helping all current users to quit

needs—services, conditions, and items required for health

needs analysis—a thoughtful prioritizing of problems

negligence—failure to perform professional duties to an accepted standard of care; carelessness

nominal variables—a categorical variable in which the categories cannot be put into any order (e.g., eye color)

nonmaleficience—principles of nonharm

nonprobability samples—a sample chosen in such a way that the probability of selecting a given subject from the population is unknown

normal distribution—bell-shaped distribution; mean = median = mode; 95% of all observations fall within two standard deviations of the mean

null hypothesis (H_0)—a statement that there is no relationship between an exposure and an outcome

observational study—a study design that does not involve intervention

oral/pharyngeal cancer—cancer of the lip, tongue, floor of the mouth, palate, gingiva and alveolar mucosa, buccal mucosa, or oropharynx

oral epidemiology—the study of the distribution and determinants of oral disease and injury in human populations

oral health disparities—certain population subgroups, defined by demographic factors, experience higher levels of oral disease

oral health education—a planned package of information, learning activities, or experiences that are intended to produce improved oral health

oral health infrastructure—programs and people who assure the public's oral health, (e.g., state and local government oral health programs)

oral presentation—a method of communicating scientific findings to an audience, usually at professional meetings

ordinal variables—a multiple categorical variable in which the categories can be sequentially arranged (e.g., never smoker, past smoker, current smoker)

Organizational Change Theory—a theory suggesting that organizations move through stages, or a series of steps, as they initiate and adopt changes to improve the problem-solving and renewal processes of large organizations or entire communities

organizational diagram—a graphic illustration of a group, department, or agency's chain of command and information flow

original source—the initial publication of an article by the original author

orofacial pain—pain associated with structures of the oral cavity or face

Ottawa Charter for Health Promotion—developed at the World Health Organization (WHO) First International Conference on Health Promotion (1986) in Ottawa, Canada

outcome evaluation—see summative evaluation

p-value—the probability of obtaining the observed data (or data that are more extreme) if the null hypothesis were true

Pan American Health Organization—an international public health agency that includes all 35 countries in the Americas

pandemic—a worldwide epidemic

parameter—a numeric characteristic of an entire population of interest

partners/partnerships—two or more people or groups joined in an activity

PATCH (Planned Approach to Community Health)—a planning tool within Healthy Communities 2000: Model Standards

peer-reviewed—indicates that certain information or publications have been reviewed for scientific merit by experts in the field of study

percentile—measures the spread of a continuous variable; a number that corresponds to a division of the range of a continuous variable, which is the value of the variable not exceeded by a specific percentage of all of the values in the sample (e.g., 75% of all values are below the value which defines the 75th percentile)

periodontitis—inflammation and infection of the ligaments and bones supporting the teeth

personal/cultural barriers—factors that inhibit patients from seeking care or following provider recommendations, based on personal or cultural beliefs

pilot test—a method of ensuring a program or survey is useable; determines if questions are interpreted as intended and that given answers include all possibilities

pit and fissure sealants—a plastic resin material applied to fissures in teeth to prevent dental caries

plain language movement—writing materials that enable people to quickly and easily find the needed information, understand what they read, and act on that understanding

plaintiff—person who initiates a lawsuit

planning models—structured guides or tools used when developing community programs

Plaque Index—measures the presence and amount of dental plaque

poster—a poster board display created to express an idea or results of a study to an audience

postprogram—evaluation outcomes assessed after a program is completed

power—probability of rejecting the null when the null is false; (1 – beta error)

Precede-Proceed—a planning model designed to explain health-related behaviors and to design and evaluate the interventions designed to influence both the behaviors and the living conditions that influence them and their sequelae

predictive value (positive)—for screening and diagnostic tests, the probability that a person with a positive test is a true positive (has the disease)

predisposing factors—factors related to health problems or behaviors that form the basis of, or motivation for, a behavior, including knowledge, beliefs, attitudes, values, cultural mores and folkways, and existing skills

preponderance of evidence—level of proof required to be successful in a civil action; jury must be at least 50% certain

preprogram and postprogram—measurements taken prior to a program or intervention are compared with measurements taken at the conclusion

preprogram and postprogrram, with a comparison group—measurements include the assessment of a group similar to the target group, but who did not receive the program; both target and comparison groups are assessed prior to the program, the program is delivered to the target group, and then both groups are assessed at the conclusion of the program

preprogram and postprogram, with a control group—an evaluation design method with random assignment from a target population to either a control or intervention group; both groups are assessed prior to the program/intervention and at the conclusion

prevalence—the number of disease cases in a population at a given time

Prevent Abuse and Neglect Through Dental Awareness (P.A.N.D.A.)—a public–private partnership committed to educating dental professionals on how to recognize and report suspected cases of child abuse

prevention—the act of preventing a disease or its sequelae

primary data—information collected on a target population for use in program development

primary prevention—the intervention in disease before it occurs (e.g., community water fluoridation, fluoride varnish, pit and fissure sealants, and preventive education)

probability sample—a sample chosen with a known probability of including a given subject from the population of interest

process evaluation—see formative evaluation

profession—a group of individuals with specialized knowledge, requiring advanced skill and knowledge that is self-regulating and guided by a code of ethics

professional responsibility—the obligation to fulfill specific requirements to maintain the expertise and knowledge associated with the profession

professionalism—representing qualities inherent in a professional, including technical skill, autonomy, self-monitoring, and adhering to a code of ethics

program evaluation—a measurement of intervention results against program objectives to determine whether a program successfully reduced or eliminated the identified need or problem

program goals—broad-based statement of desired long- or short-term changes to alleviate identified needs

program objectives—statements that define a desired change in the client or the environment

proportion—a ratio in which the numerator is included in the denominator

prospective study—a study design in which a group of individuals (cohort) are followed forward in time

public health—concerned with the aggregate health of a group, community, state, or nation

public health care financing programs—health/dental insurance programs for certain low-income or otherwise needy people (e.g., Medicaid)

public health practice—a career or setting that focuses on a community-based model for health care

PubMed—an English language bibliographic database that allows free Internet access through the National Library of Medicine

punitive damages—a monetary award to a victim, which is intended to punish the defendant and stop the conduct from being repeated

qualitative—descriptive, explanatory information

quality assurance—the accountability of a program as measured against best practices/standards

quality of life—the depth of meaning of a given life

quantitative—objective and measurable information

quantity of life—the actual number of years an individual has lived

quartile—measures the spread of a continuous variable; one of three values which divides the sample of values into four equal portions; i.e., the 25th (lower quartile), 50th (median), and 75th (upper quartile) percentiles

quota sample—a nonprobability sampling in which subjects in a block of predetermined size are selected

Ramfjord Index teeth—six index teeth often used when evaluating periodontal health; maxillary right first molar, left central incisor, left first premolar, mandibular left first molar, right central incisor, and right first premolar

ratio variable—a specific continuous variable

reading level—a measurement of written material readability; assesses the ease with which the material can be read and understood

refereed—indicates that information or publications have been reviewed for scientific merit by experts in the field of study

references—a list of sources used to prepare a presentation or written article

referendum—the process whereby an action by public officials is placed on the ballot for voter support

reinforcing factors—factors related to health problems or behaviors that provide incentive for repeating or persisting in existing health behaviors

reliable/reliability—different observers, looking at the same phenomenon, report similar levels; a particular technique applied repeatedly yields the same result each time

resources—available support (e.g., personnel, supplies, funds, buildings, and equipment)

results—the section of a scientific paper that states study or program outcomes

retrospective study—a study design in which inferences about exposure are based on past events or experiences

risk assessment—identifying protective factors or those that may place a person at risk for developing oral disease

risk factors—factors that place an individual at risk for a disease (e.g., tobacco use is considered a risk factor for oral cancer)

Root Caries Index—measures root caries; includes the number of exposed root surfaces as the denominator

round table—a method of presenting information in which participants discuss a topic in a group setting

safety net dental clinics—community-based clinics that serve uninsured or underinsured people or those who do not receive care in the private sector

salt fluoridation—the addition of fluoride to salt to prevent dental caries

sample—a selection of subjects from a population of interest

school-based programs—delivers oral health care at schools or in private practices to children unlikely to receive dental care

school water fluoridation—the process whereby a school system optimizes the school water supply, with fluoride levels much higher than recommended for community water supplies

secondary data—survey information that is available from other sources

secondary prevention—treating or controlling disease after it occurs (e.g., conservative amalgam restoration, remineralization of early caries, and conservative periodontal therapy)

secondary source—an article or study with quoted material from another source; not the initial author or source of information

sensitivity—the proportion of truly diseased persons in a screened population identified as having disease by the screening test

simple random sampling—a probability sample in which each subject has an equal and independent probability of being selected

Simplified Oral Hygiene Index—measures the presence of plaque and calculus; considered obsolete

slander—false oral statements or gestures

Social Cognitive Theory—the dominant version of Social Learning Theory; proposes that behaviors are learned socially, through direct or vicarious experiences and the observation of the actions of others and the results of those actions

social factors—factors caused by society that affect the health of an individual or a group (e.g., an individual's health may be affected by a policy)

social justice—fair distribution or allocation of resources

Social Learning Theory—suggests that people learn through their own experiences, as well as by the observation of the actions of others and the results of those actions

Social Marketing Theory—a technique used to increase public awareness of the relationship between behaviors and diseases and to influence people to take action to prevent or reduce disease

Social Security Act—passed by Congress in 1935, establishing benefits for the elderly and unemployed and providing state aid for health and welfare activities

socially equitable—the same or equal treatment for everyone, despite socioeconomic standing, race, or ethnicity

socioeconomic position—a person's status, based on both social and economic conditions

Special Olympics Special Smiles—an international organization dedicated to empowering individuals with intellectual disabilities to become physically fit, productive, respected members of society through sports training and competition

specificity—the proportion of truly nondiseased persons in a screened population who are identified by the screening test as not having disease

Stages of Change Model—suggests that whether a person engages in preventive health actions depends on a person's readiness to adopt a behavioral change; views behavioral change as a process, rather than an event, with people at varying levels of motivation or readiness

stakeholders—people, or groups, who have the potential to be affected or have a vested interest in a program

standard deviation—measures the spread of a normally distributed continuous variable; the average distance of each observation from the mean

standard error—an estimate of how well the sample statistic reflects the true population parameter of interest

standard of care—the ordinary skill and care expected of a reasonable, prudent practitioner

statistical inference—analytic methods to determine whether sample findings should be generalized to the entire study population of interest from which the sample was drawn or whether chance is a probable explanation for the findings

statistics—estimates of a population parameter from a sample of that population; the science of making statements about an entire population from a limited sample

statute of limitations—the period that a patient has to file a lawsuit

stratified random sample—a sample constructed by drawing simple random samples from two or more subgroups in a population; ensures sufficient numbers of subjects in each subgroup

structural barriers—barriers to care related to the number, type, concentration, location, or organizational configuration of health care providers

study skills—the techniques employed to enhance the seeking of knowledge

subject content—the main focus of the lesson plan; the information collected, researched, and selected for presentation about the topic

Substance Abuse and Mental Health Services Administration (SAMHSA)—government agency that works to improve the quality and availability of substance abuse prevention, addiction treatment and mental health services

summative evaluation—the judgment of the merit or worth of a program by a comparison of end results to goals

Surgeon General's Report on Oral Health (2000)—provides a comprehensive view of oral health in the United States and calls for public health professionals to address oral health issues

surveillance—the ongoing systematic collection, analysis, and interpretation of outcome-specific data for use in planning, implementing, and evaluating public health practices

t-test—compares means between two categories; used when one variable is normally distributed (continuous) and one is binary categorical

table clinic—a presentation method using a tabletop format; most appropriate for a hands-on demonstration

target audience—the intended learners for whom a specific educational plan is developed

target group/target population/targeting—the population segment identified to receive a public health intervention/program; limiting public health efforts to an identified group

technical battery—when a health care provider exceeds the provided patient consent

teledentistry—the use of electronic information and communications technology to provide and support health care delivered in distant locations

tertiary prevention—limiting disability from a disease or rehabilitation of an individual (e.g., a denture)

testlet—a short, descriptive scenario of a problem, situation, or event; differing from factual multiple choice questions in that the testlet format requires analysis and problem solving, rather than strict memorization

time line—a chart of events and procedures (e.g., target dates for completion of program activities)

title—a short description reflecting the content of an article; used as a guide by the reader and indexed for database reference

tooth loss—the loss of one or more permanent teeth

Tooth Surface Index of Fluorosis—measures prevalence and severity of dental fluorosis

tort law—the division of law that covers an act, or acts, that result in harm to another

total tooth loss—the loss of all natural permanent teeth (edentulous)

trends—consistent change over time

trespass—the act of going on another's property without expressed or implied consent

2×2 table—cross-tabulation of two binary variables

type I error—rejection of the null when the null is true; alpha error

type II error—failure to reject the null when the null is true; beta error

type font—lettering style (e.g., Times New Roman, Courier, Arial, Verdana, and Tahoma)

type size—the size of the lettering used for creating visual displays for educational programs

unintentional tort—a civil wrong that occurs when an individual does not intend the results of the action

United States Public Health Service (USPHS)—an agency of the US government responsible for monitoring and addressing health issues in the United States

unsupervised practice—treatment of a patient of record by a dental hygienist without a dentist on the premises; dental hygienist is practicing within an appropriate scope of practice

United States National Fluorosis Survey—a national survey of the prevalence of dental fluorosis conducted by the National Institute of Dental Research in 1986–1987

utilitarian ethics—ethical theory based on the principle of the greatest good for the greatest number; consequence-based ethical theory

valid/validity—objective measurement (i.e., does an instrument actually measure what was intended)

variable—anything that can be measured or manipulated in a study

variance—measures the spread of a normally distributed continuous variable; equal to standard deviation squared

veracity—truthfulness and honesty; refraining from deception or misrepresentation

virtue ethics—ethical theory that focuses on the character traits of an individual, not the individual's behavior

visuals—media materials for learning experiences (e.g., chalkboards, bulletin boards, flannel boards, posters, charts, audio and video recordings, models, and samples of authentic real-world objects)

volunteerism—providing services without receiving payment

Women, Infants, and Children (WIC) program—an agency of the US Department of Agriculture serving to safeguard the health of low-income women, infants, and children who are at nutritional risk

work statement—an action plan that explains what, where, and when a program's activities are accomplished

World Health Organization (WHO)—the directing and coordinating authority on international health work; proposes regulations and makes recommendations about global public health practices

xylitol—a non-cariogenic sugar alcohol used as a sugar substitute in food and snack items

Index

Page numbers in italics denote figures; those followed by a t denote tables; those followed by a b denote boxes.

A